STUDENT WORKBOOK FOR

CLINICAL PRACTICE OF THE

DENTAL HYGIENIST

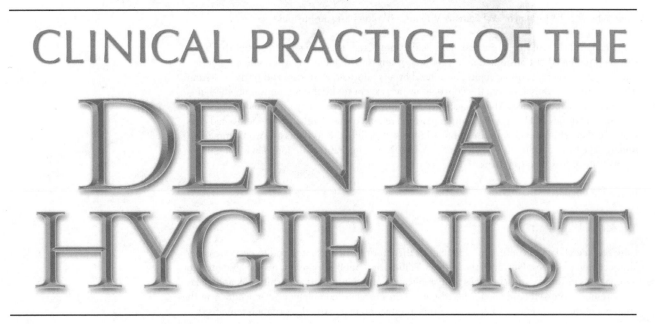

11th EDITION

Charlotte J. Wyche, RDH, MS
Department of Periodontics and Oral Medicine
University of Michigan School of Dentistry
Ann Arbor, Michigan

Esther M. Wilkins, BS, RDH, DMD
Department of Periodontology
School of Dental Medicine
Tufts University
Boston, Massachusetts

 Wolters Kluwer | Lippincott Williams & Wilkins
Health

Philadelphia · Baltimore · New York · London
Buenos Aires · Hong Kong · Sydney · Tokyo

Acquisitions Editor: Julie Stegman
Managing Editor: Meredith L. Brittain
Marketing Manager: Shauna Kelley
Designer: Doug Smock

Eleventh Edition

Printed in China

ISBN: 978-1-60831-72-95

Care has been taken to confirm the accuracy of the information presented and to describe generally accepted practices. However, the authors, editors, and publisher are not responsible for errors or omissions or for any consequences from application of the information in this book and make no warranty, expressed or implied, with respect to the currency, completeness, or accuracy of the contents of the publication. Application of this information in a particular situation remains the professional responsibility of the practitioner; the clinical treatments described and recommended may not be considered absolute and universal recommendations.

The authors, editors, and publisher have exerted every effort to ensure that drug selection and dosage set forth in this text are in accordance with the current recommendations and practice at the time of publication. However, in view of ongoing research, changes in government regulations, and the constant flow of information relating to drug therapy and drug reactions, the reader is urged to check the package insert for each drug for any change in indications and dosage and for added warnings and precautions. This is particularly important when the recommended agent is a new or infrequently employed drug.

Some drugs and medical devices presented in this publication have Food and Drug Administration (FDA) clearance for limited use in restricted research settings. It is the responsibility of the health care provider to ascertain the FDA status of each drug or device planned for use in his or her clinical practice.

LWW.com

*To **instructors** who ask open-ended questions and encourage reflection that helps students discover what they do not yet know. You understand that clinical dental hygiene practice is not a multiple-choice test.*

and

*To **students** who struggle to find answers for the open-ended questions their instructors ask them. You will soon discover that reflecting on what you don't know and working to find answers to real questions is what leads to real learning.*

There is no doubt that each student learns differently. Therefore, the aim of this workbook is to provide a variety of types of exercises so that you will be able to find something here to help you learn important concepts that are the foundation for dental hygiene practice. You are always encouraged, of course, to create additional learning experiences and activities that fit with your own learning style.

HOW TO USE THIS WORKBOOK

Some general guidelines for the exercises in the workbook are described below. Exercises in the **KNOWLEDGE** sections of the workbook provide lines for you to write your answers. Some chapters include crossword or word search puzzles to help learn terminology. For **COMPETENCY** and **DISCOVERY** type exercises, a separate word processing document, handwritten document, or a copy of the *Patient-Specific Dental Hygiene Care Plan* template from Appendix B may be required to provide a complete answer.

 KNOWLEDGE exercises in each chapter help you target important information and help you master the introductory material provided in the textbook. You will define terms, concepts, and principles in your own words; list the components of larger ideas; and reorganize information from the textbook in a variety of ways. Knowledge exercises comprise the largest, but by no means the most important, portion of this workbook.

COMPETENCY questions are found in each chapter and also in Section Summary areas of this workbook. Building competence in translating knowledge to practice is an essential component of becoming a dental hygiene professional. These exercises will ask you to use critical thinking skills to apply basic knowledge to clinical situations, analyze patient assessment data, create components of patient care plans, or document patient care activities. Some of the patient scenarios are written in paragraph form so you can learn to isolate important information, and some are formatted using the Assessment Findings section from the Care Plan template.

DISCOVERY activities are found in some of the chapters and also in each Section Summary. These exercises will help you learn to think beyond the basic knowledge. The Discovery activities will direct you to find and analyze current information about a topic introduced in the textbook by, for example, doing a scientific literature search, a Web-based Internet search, or a dental product analysis.

QUESTIONS PATIENTS ASK are also intended to encourage you to practice evidence-based decision-making skills. Reflecting on what additional or new knowledge is needed to address patient concerns is a key skill for lifelong learning and ultimately for providing evidence-based, comprehensive, and effective dental hygiene care.

EVERYDAY ETHICS activities challenge you to reflect on and apply ethical principles. An everyday Ethics scenario with "Questions for Consideration" is included in each textbook chapter. Many of these scenarios were created using real-life ethical situations faced by practicing dental hygienists. Each workbook chapter includes an Everyday Ethics box with **individual learning, cooperative learning,** or **discovery** activity prompts that will direct you to write about, discuss, or role play the ethics-related scenario and questions presented in the textbook.

FACTORS TO TEACH THE PATIENT cases ask you to outline or develop a patient/provider conversation using motivational interviewing techniques, patient-appropriate language, and knowledge gained from the textbook. Those brief conversations can then be compared with conversations written by your student colleagues, used for "role-play" exercises, or placed in your portfolio to illustrate your expertise in patient education.

 FOR YOUR PORTFOLIO suggestions are located in each Section Summary and in a few of the chapters. A learning portfolio is a collection of student work and reflection organized in such a way that it demonstrates an increase in student knowledge and professional competence over time. A student portfolio can be compiled simply and creatively using a three-ring binder with tabbed separators to organize the material into appropriate sections. An Internet search will help you locate online portfolio templates that can be used to develop a Web-based portfolio.

Development of a portfolio provides an opportunity for you to reflect on your growth as a dental hygiene professional. A portfolio that highlights your unique talents and provides evidence of special skills, competencies, or learning that goes beyond the requirements of your educational program can be useful during employment interviews or application to graduate education programs.

Answers for the workbook KNOWLEDGE questions along with rubrics and key considerations criteria that will help evaluate student responses to COMPETENCY exercises are located in the Faculty Resource Center at http://thepoint.lww.com/Wyche. Access to these answers is strictly limited to faculty only. If you have further questions concerning this workbook, please e-mail customerservice@lww.com.

COMPETENCIES FOR THE DENTAL HYGIENIST

The American Dental Education Association (ADEA) Competencies for Entry into the Allied Health Professions outline the areas in which a new graduate dental hygienist is expected to be able to apply knowledge to ensure that safe and effective patient care is provided. The title page for each section of this workbook lists specific ADEA competencies supported by learning the information from chapters included in that section of the textbook. A complete list of the competency statements found in Appendix A will provide a reference point to help you understand why learning specific concepts from each chapter is important for becoming a professional dental hygienist.

As you read the ADEA competency statements, you should note that your school may have adapted them somewhat for use in your dental hygiene program. Your school's competencies may be organized in a slightly different manner but will probably be very similar. You should make a point of receiving a copy of your school's competency statements for reference.

I encourage you to enjoy the process of learning and I hope that this workbook offers activities that will help you.

Sincerely,
Charlotte J. Wyche, RDH, MS
Dental Hygiene Educator

REVIEWERS

Barbara Adams, RDH, BS, MA
Dental Hygiene
Wallace State Community College
Hanceville, Alabama

Kimberlee Clark, RDH, BS, MEd
Dental Hygiene
Western Career College—San Jose
San Jose, California

Charles Crosby, DDS, JD
Dental Health Professions
York Technical College
Rock Hill, South Carolina

Sheila Gross, CDA, RDH, BA, MS
Health Sciences
Northeast Wisconsin Technical College
Green Bay, Wisconsin

Stephanie Harrison, BS, MA
Dental Hygiene
Community College of Denver
Denver, Colorado

Sherry Heaney, RDHAP, MEd
Dental Hygiene
Western Career College
San Jose, California

Suzette Jestin, CDA, PID, BEd
Dental
Vancouver Community College and University of British
  Columbia
Vancouver, British Columbia

Carolyn Ray, RDH, M.Ed.
Dental Hygiene
University of Oklahoma
Oklahoma City, Oklahoma

David Reff, BS, DDS
Dental Assisting and Dental Hygiene Programs
Apollo College
Boise, Idaho

Amanda Richardson, RDH, BS
Department of Dental Hygiene
University of Louisiana at Monroe
Caldwell Hall Monroe, Louisiana

Judy Romano, AS, BS, MA
Dental Hygiene/Dental Assisting
Hudson Valley Community College
Troy, New York

Natalie Vanoli, RDH, BS, RDHAP
Dental Hygiene
Western Career College
San Jose, California

ACKNOWLEDGMENTS

Ernestine R. Daniels, RDH, BS
(*Motivational Interviewing: A Patient-Centered Approach to Providing Oral Health Education*)

Marie Varley Gillis, RDH, MS
(*revision updates for workbook Chapters 29, 32, 40, 41, 44, 49, 51, and 64 in this editon*)

Joan McClintock, RDH, MEd
(*original author for workbook Chapters 6, 7, and 10 through 19 in the first edition*)

Marcia Williams, Medical and Scientific Illustrator
(*Figures for workbook and answer key and Care Plan templates*)

Textbook contributing authors who offered new ideas, feedback, suggestions for learning exercises, or case scenarios for "their chapters" in this edition of the workbook:

Pamela S. Kennard, BSN, RDH, MA (Chapter 45)

Ernestine R. Daniels, RDH, BS (Chapter 64)

Jan B. Selwitz-Segal, RDH, CDA, MS (Chapter 65)

Barbara Dawidjan, RDH, MEd (Chapter 67)

Donna Homenko, RDH, MEd, PhD (Everyday Ethics boxes)

Thank you for your help in making this workbook possible.

CONTENTS

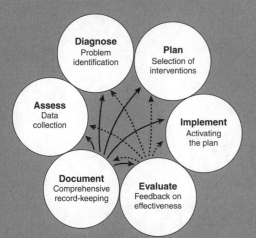

Diagnose
Problem identification

Plan
Selection of interventions

Assess
Data collection

Implement
Activating the plan

Document
Comprehensive record-keeping

Evaluate
Feedback on effectiveness

Orientation to Clinical Dental Hygiene Practice

Chapters 1–3

■ LEARNING OBJECTIVES

Completing the exercises in this section of the workbook will prepare you to:

1. Identify the characteristics of a dental hygiene professional.
2. Apply ethical, legal, cultural, and personal professional standards to the practice of dental hygiene.
3. Use an evidence-based decision making process to locate and evaluate current scientific evidence related to dental hygiene interventions.
4. Apply the principles of effective health communication.

■ COMPETENCIES FOR THE DENTAL HYGIENIST (APPENDIX A)

Competencies supported by the learning in Section I:

Core Competencies: C1, C2, C3, C4, C5, C6, C7, C8, C9, C10, C11, C12.

Health Promotion and Disease Prevention: HP2, HP4, HP5.

Professional Growth and Development: PGD1, PGD3.

The Professional Dental Hygienist

Learning Objectives

Upon successful completion of these exercises, you will be able to:

1. Identify and define key terms and concepts related to the professional dental hygienist.
2. Define the scope of dental hygiene practice.
3. Identify and define the components of the Dental Hygiene Process of Care.

4. Identify and apply components of the Dental Hygiene Code of Ethics.
5. Explain legal, ethical, and personal factors affecting dental hygiene practice.
6. Apply concepts in ethical decision making.

 KNOWLEDGE EXERCISES

Write your answers for each question in the space provided.

1. Identify and (in your own words) briefly define the healthcare-related roles your dental hygiene education will prepare you to fulfill.

_____

_____

_____

_____

_____

2. How is the role of public health related to the other roles?

_____

3. Describe a dental hygienist using the terminology associated with integrated practice roles, healthcare focus, and services provided by dental hygienists.

_____

_____

_____

4. Identify three personal factors that affect the way an individual dental hygienist is perceived as a representative of the entire profession of dental hygiene.

_____

_____

_____

5. Define dental hygiene care.

_____

_____

_____

1-13
30
31

6. Identify three types of services provided by the dental hygienist.

   _____

   _____

   _____

7. Define health promotion.

   _____

8. What dental hygienist role was emphasized by Dr. A.C. Fones, who is considered the father of dental hygiene?

   _____

9. What is the primary goal of each dental hygienist with respect to patient care?

   _____

10. List at least three personal goals the professional dental hygienist will strive for in clinical practice.

    _____

    _____

    _____

    _____

    _____

11. In what way is the dental hygienist a cotherapist?

    _____

12. In your own words, explain the three types of prevention.

    _____

    _____

    _____

13. List three ways in which a dental hygienist can specialize.

    _____

    _____

    _____

14. The Dental Hygiene Process of Care provides the framework for offering individualized dental hygiene services based on identified patient needs. In your own words, briefly define each of the six phases of the Dental Hygiene Process of Care.

■ Assessment

   _____

   _____

■ Diagnosis

   _____

   _____

■ Planning

   _____

   _____

■ Implementation

   _____

   _____

■ Evaluation

   _____

   _____

■ Documentation

   _____

   _____

15. Both _____ (observed) and _____ (perceived) data are collected in the assessment phase of the Dental Hygiene Process of Care.

16. Identify three factors involved in analyzing assessment data before formulating the dental hygiene diagnosis.

    _____

    _____

    _____

17. In your own words, describe the purpose of dental hygiene diagnosis statements.

    _____

    _____

    _____

18. What is a dental hygiene care plan?

    _____

    _____

    _____

19. Identify the steps that are important to include when you are planning dental hygiene care.

_____

_____

_____

_____

_____

_____

20. Define oral hygiene.

_____

_____

21. Define dental hygiene intervention.

_____

_____

22. Define dental hygiene prognosis.

_____

_____

23. Dental hygienists usually provide dental hygiene care under the supervision of a dentist. Identify and briefly define four levels of supervision.

_____

_____

_____

_____

24. At what point in the Dental Hygiene Process of Care is a patient's continuing care interval determined?

_____

25. In what ways are the assessment and the evaluation phases of the dental hygiene process of care similar?

_____

26. What six special factors apply to members of a group defined as having professional status?

_____

_____

_____

_____

_____

27. What is a code of ethics?

_____

_____

28. Name at least two professional organizations that have developed codes of ethics for the practice of dental hygiene.

_____

_____

_____

29. Briefly define each of the following seven core values in dental hygiene in your own words:

Autonomy and respect: _____

_____

Confidentiality: _____

_____

Societal trust: _____

_____

Non-malfeasance: _____

_____

Beneficence: _____

_____

Justice and fairness: _____

_____

Veracity: _____

_____

30. What is the difference between an ethical issue and an ethical dilemma?

_____

_____

31. Describe the four steps that can help direct your decision making when resolving an ethical situation.

_____

_____

_____

_____

COMPETENCY EXERCISES

Use paper and pen or create an electronic document to answer these questions.

1. Provide examples from dental hygiene practice, education, and licensure to explain why a dental hygienist can be considered a primary healthcare professional. In your discussion, refer to the definition of *primary healthcare* and to the definition of a *profession* (Box 1-1 in the textbook).

2. Explain why the notion of lifelong learning is considered an ethical component of dental hygiene practice.

3. Dental hygiene interventions play a major role in all levels of prevention of oral disease. Give examples (different from those included in the textbook) of a dental hygienist's role in each level of prevention.

4. David Martin is a 13-year-old who chews bubble gum and sips a sugar-sweetened carbonated beverage all day long, especially when he is studying. An oral examination indicates that he has extensive dental decay. Write a dental hygiene diagnosis statement for David.

 ## QUESTIONS PATIENTS ASK

What sources of information can you identify that will help you answer your patient's questions in this scenario?

Your patient, Jessica Miles, who is a junior in high school, comments, "My mom and I were talking about where I will be going to college after next year. She said to ask you where you went. She thinks what you do would be real cool. Did you have to take a lot of sciences? Do they have dental chairs and all the equipment right in the school and do people come in for you to learn from? I know you clean our teeth—why do you like working in people's mouths?"

Everyday Ethics

Before completing the learning exercises below, reread and reflect on the *Everyday Ethics* scenario and *Questions for Consideration* in this chapter of the textbook. It may also be useful to review the *Dental Hygiene Ethics* discussion in Chapter 1, the *Ethical Applications* in the introduction pages for each section in the textbook, as well as the *Codes of Ethics* in Appendices I, II, and III.

Individual Learning Activity
Imagine that you are the dental hygienist in this scenario. Answer each of the questions for consideration at the end of the scenario.

Collaborative Learning Activity
Work as a group to develop a 2- to 5-minute role-play that introduces the Everyday Ethics scenario described in the chapter (a great idea is to video record your role-play activity). Then develop separate 2-minute role-play scenarios that provide at least two alternative approaches/solutions to resolving the situation. Ask classmates to view the solutions, ask questions, and discuss the ethical approach used in each. Ask for a vote on which solution classmates determine to be the "best."

 ## Factors To Teach The Patient

This scenario is related to the following factors listed in this chapter of the textbook:

■ *The role of the dental hygienist as cotherapist with each patient and with members of the dental profession.*
■ *The moral and ethical nature of becoming a dental hygiene professional person.*
■ *The patient's potential state of oral health, and how it can be improved and maintained.*

Sarah, your really good friend, has agreed to be a patient for your first clinical experience as a dental hygiene student. When you call her to remind her of her appointment tomorrow, she asks you a bit about what you will do during the appointment. You excitedly begin to explain the procedures.

Sarah interrupts saying that it all sounds quite boring to her. She asks you to tell her why you are studying so hard to become a dental hygienist. Write a statement explaining your knowledge and interest in dental hygiene practice to Sarah.

Evidence-Based Dental Hygiene Practice

Upon successful completion of these exercises, you will be able to:

1. Explain evidence-based dental hygiene practice and identify the skills needed to practice evidence-based dental hygiene care.
2. Discuss research approaches and connect research types to the strength of evidence each provides.
3. Describe a systematic approach to finding science-based information in the healthcare literature.
4. Describe skills needed for analyzing Internet-based health information.

 KNOWLEDGE EXERCISES

Write your answers for each question in the space provided.

1. List four factors that interact to direct the selection of patient care interventions in an evidence-based dental hygiene practice.

   _____

   _____

   _____

   _____

2. Place the steps for a systematic approach to evidence-based dental hygiene practice in the correct order by placing the numbers 1 through 6 in the space beside each step.

ORDER	DESCRIPTION OF STEP
	Develop a researchable question
	Evaluate the results
	Search for the evidence
	Analyze the evidence
	Determine the clinical issue
	Apply the evidence

3. What is a refereed publication?

_____

_____

4. List four types of research studies.

_____

_____

_____

_____

5. What is the difference between qualitative and quantitative research approaches?

_____

_____

6. What type of research looks at the strength and types of relationships between variables?

_____

7. What is the difference between experimental and quasi-experimental research?

_____

_____

8. What is *in vitro* research?

_____

_____

9. What is the difference between a case report and a case study?

_____

_____

10. What is a case-control study?

_____

_____

What does retrospective mean?

_____

11. Randomized controlled double-blind studies help eliminate _____ by placing study participants randomly in either the experimental or control group and by "blinding" the researchers to which participant is in which group.

12. Place the levels of evidence in order from most valuable to support evidence-based practice (1) to less valuable (6) for making decisions related to clinical dental hygiene care.

ORDER	TYPE OF EVIDENCE
	Analysis of all studies that investigate a specific question
	Opinions of journal editors or other "expert" practitioners
	Prospective studies that follow groups or retrospective studies that compare groups of research subjects
	Research that does not include human subjects
	RCT studies
	Studies that describe or analyze one or more cases of an unusual condition

13. What six actions can help the dental hygiene practitioner analyze the content of health information found on the Internet for validity and reliability?

_____

_____

_____

_____

_____

_____

14. List two ways to help determine the accuracy of health information found on the Internet?

_____

_____

15. List ways to help determine whether or not a health-related website is providing biased information (checking for objectivity).

_____

_____

CHAPTER 2 Evidence-Based Dental Hygiene Practice

8

16. Informed consent forms and Institutional Review Board approval help protect the rights of _____ _____ (2 words) in research studies.

17. What is a PICO question?

_____

_____

18. List the components of a PICO question.

_____

_____

_____

_____

COMPETENCY EXERCISES

Use paper and pen or create an electronic document to answer these questions.

1. Your patient is a 1-year-old child who has evidence of early childhood caries (ECC). You know that to help decrease risk for further caries activity and help remineralize white spot lesions, this child needs to be provided with topical fluoride application even at this young age. However, you are unsure whether the topical gel application or the fluoride varnish would be the best choice. Write a PICO question that will help direct your search for information to support the intervention you select for this very young child.

2. Explain why a peer-reviewed journal is more likely than a commercial-based health magazine to contain the type of evidence that is appropriate to support clinical recommendations that a dental hygienist includes in a patient's care plan?

? QUESTIONS PATIENTS ASK

What sources of information can you identify that will help you answer your patient's questions?

"I just heard about this cool new dental product from my friend!! Do you think it is any good?" "Will it clean my teeth as well as what I am doing now?" "I know my situation is different than some other people, so will it work for me?"

Everyday Ethics

Before completing the learning exercises below, reread and reflect on the Everyday Ethics scenario and Questions for Consideration in this chapter of the textbook. It may also be useful to review the Dental Hygiene Ethics discussion in Chapter 1, the Ethical Applications in the introduction pages for each section in the textbook, as well as the Codes of Ethics in Appendices I, II, and III.

Individual Learning Activity
Identify a situation you have experienced that presents a similar ethical dilemma. What did you learn from how the situation was (or was not) resolved at the time it occurred?

Discovery Activity
Ask a friend or relative who is not involved in healthcare to read the scenario and discuss it with you from the perspective of a "patient" who receives services within the healthcare system. Discuss what you learned from the concerns, insights, or difference in perspective that person expressed.

Factors To Teach The Patient

This scenario is related to the following factors listed in this chapter of the textbook:

■ *A result from one study doesn't necessarily provide the best answer.*

Your patient, Marcus, tells you that he just read a newspaper article citing new research study that contradicts a recommendation you have made for his self-care. How will you respond to his assertion that the research proves that this new technique is probably better than the one that you have recommended?

WORD SEARCH

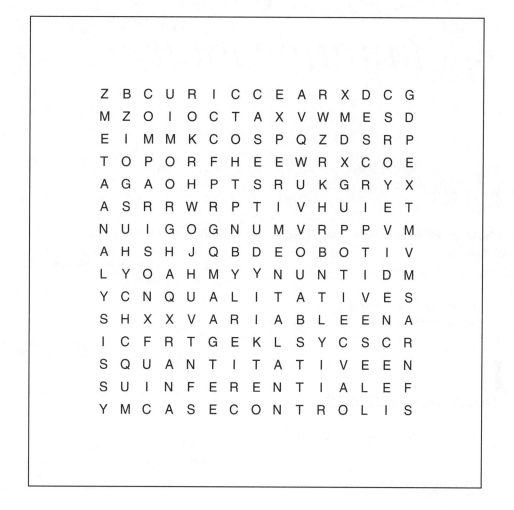

```
Z  B  C  U  R  I  C  C  E  A  R  X  D  C  G
M  Z  O  I  O  C  T  A  X  V  W  M  E  S  D
E  I  M  M  K  C  O  S  P  Q  Z  D  S  R  P
T  O  P  O  R  F  H  E  E  W  R  X  C  O  E
A  G  A  O  H  P  T  S  R  U  K  G  R  Y  X
A  S  R  R  W  R  P  T  I  V  H  U  I  E  T
N  U  I  G  O  G  N  U  M  V  R  P  P  V  M
A  H  S  H  J  Q  B  D  E  O  B  O  T  I  V
L  Y  O  A  H  M  Y  Y  N  U  N  T  I  D  M
Y  C  N  Q  U  A  L  I  T  A  T  I  V  E  S
S  H  X  X  V  A  R  I  A  B  L  E  E  N  A
I  C  F  R  T  G  E  K  L  S  Y  C  S  C  R
S  Q  U  A  N  T  I  T  A  T  I  V  E  E  N
S  U  I  N  F  E  R  E  N  T  I  A  L  E  F
Y  M  C  A  S  E  C  O  N  T  R  O  L  I  S
```

WORD SEARCH CLUES

1. A type of study in which the same subjects are followed over time
2. A retrospective study that compares individuals who have a certain condition with others who do not have that condition
3. In-depth description of several cases of individuals who have an unusual or complex condition
4. A type of study in which results are reported in numbers
5. The group in a research study that does not receive the intervention
6. A factor that is manipulated and measured during a research study
7. The highest level of evidence to support best practices
8. Type of statistical analysis that can help determine the frequency with which something exists
9. Type of numerical statistic that allows generalization from a sample to a population
10. Supports efforts to determine or demonstrate the truth
11. Type of study in which intervention variables are manipulated to find the effect of one on another
12. Acronym sometimes used to indicate a randomized controlled double-blind study
13. A subjective research approach in which study results are reported using a narrative

Effective Health Communication

Upon successful completion of these exercises, you will be able to:

1. Discuss the skills and attributes of effective health communication.
2. Explain how the patient's age, culture, and health literacy level affect health communication strategies.

3. Identify barriers to effective communication.
4. Identify communication theories relevant to effective health communication and motivational interviewing.

 KNOWLEDGE EXERCISES

Write your answers for each question in the space provided.

1. Define health communication in your own words.

   _____

   _____

2. To establish the kind of rapport that enhances communication with a patient of any age, gender, or culture, the dental hygienist will _____ more than _____, especially at the beginning of the appointment.

3. List as many as you can of the abilities/attributes of a dental professional who is able to establish rapport with each patient in order to provide effective health communication.

   _____

   _____

   _____

   _____

   _____

   _____

4. What factors contribute to the efficacy of the health information provided for patient education?

   _____

   _____

   _____

   _____

   _____

5. List and briefly define in your own words the three types of communication.

   _____

   _____

   _____

6. List as many factors as you can remember that can affect the way that health messages are understood during patient education sessions.

   _____

   _____

_____

_____

_____

_____

7. The level of a patient's health literacy does NOT only depend on the individual's _____ level but rather on the interaction of a complex set of _____ and _____ skills as well as personal health-related knowledge.

8. List some ways that the dental hygienist can address health literacy issues in the dental hygiene practice.

_____

_____

_____

_____

_____

9. Match each communication theory in column 1 with the appropriate brief description in column 2.

COMMUNICATION THEORY	DESCRIPTION
Health Belief Model _____	A Based on the concepts of individual beliefs and normative beliefs.
Theory of Reasoned Action _____	B Based on belief that actions will affect outcomes.
Self-Efficacy _____	C Based on perception of susceptibility, seriousness of threat, ability to prevent, and personal capability making changes.
Locus of Control _____	D States that individuals decide to change health behaviors by moving along a continuum of predictable steps.
Transtheoretical Model and Stages of Change _____	E Based on perception of whether internal or external factors determine disease and health.

10. Which theory does a motivational interviewing approach to oral health education build from?

_____

11. Identify the key components of motivational interviewing as an approach for providing health education interventions during patient care.

_____

_____

_____

_____

_____

12. In the space provided below, list as many factors as you can to complete the following statement. A dental hygienist who can effectively use a motivational interviewing technique to inspire and support health behavior changes has the ability to:

_____

_____

_____

_____

_____

_____

13. Match the age group in column 1 with the correct description of a key point related to communicating with that age group in column 2.

AGE GROUP	COMMUNICATION-RELATED DESCRIPTION
Infants _____	A Marked desire to have their viewpoint and needs considered with respect.
Toddlers and Preschoolers _____	B Like to assert independence and maintain control over situations.
School-Aged Children _____	C Physical and cognitive changes may impact ability to communicate.
Adolescents _____	D Communicate primarily through senses.
Older Adults _____	E Developing ability to relate the impact of external events to themselves.

14. True or False (circle one). Using "terms of endearment" to address a frail elderly patient is a communication approach that will put the patient at ease as well as demonstrate the care provider's empathy.

15. True or False (circle one). When communicating with a caregiver who is in the treatment room while you are providing oral hygiene instructions for the patient, maintain eye contact with the caregiver as the primary focus of the conversation so that he or she does not feel left out.

16. In your own words, describe the effect that ethnic or cultural background can have on your patients' health status or the way they respond to your dental hygiene interventions.

_____

_____

_____

_____

17. _____ _____ (two words) delivery of dental hygiene care, including respect for and responsiveness to the unique culture-related characteristics, values, and needs of each patient can make a positive difference in oral health outcomes.

18. _____ _____ (two words) is a skill that can be developed by exploring and learning to appreciate the wide variety of differences among the individuals who are your patients.

19. List attributes of a dental hygienist who strives to deliver effective healthcare for patients of all cultures.

_____

_____

_____

_____

_____

_____

20. List ways to enhance awareness of culture-related needs during patient care.

_____

_____

_____

_____

_____

_____

21. List ways to enhance language-related communication with all patients.

_____

_____

_____

_____

22. When communicating with a patient while using an interpreter, whom do you speak directly to when asking questions?

_____

23. What factors related to communication and culture are appropriate to document in a patient's permanent record?

_____

_____

_____

_____

COMPETENCY EXERCISES

Apply information from the chapter and use critical thinking skills to complete the competency exercises. Write responses on paper or create electronic documents to submit your answers.

1. Numerous factors can interfere with effective communication. Table 3-1 in the textbook describes or defines what each factor means. Provide a brief example from your own life experience (not necessarily related to dental hygiene) that illustrates each of the types of barriers. For example, an **interpersonal barrier** to effective communication could be illustrated by describing a time when you could only seem to argue, rather than discuss, with a friend who had taken a political stand opposite yours. After you describe the situation, jot down any thoughts you have about how you might have overcome that barrier and been more effective in communicating.

2. Use the information in Table 3-5 in the textbook to create a brief statement that describes the difference between a traditional approach to dental hygiene education and the use of motivational interviewing to encourage a patient to embrace healthy behaviors.

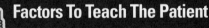

Everyday Ethics

Before completing the learning exercises below, reread and reflect on the Everyday Ethics scenario and Questions for Consideration in this chapter of the textbook. It may also be useful to review the Dental Hygiene Ethics discussion in Chapter 1, the Ethical Applications in the introduction pages for each section in the textbook, as well as the Codes of Ethics in Appendices I, II, and III.

Individual Learning Activity

Imagine the scenario from the patient's perspective. How might the patient's response to the questions following the scenario be different from those of the dental hygienist involved?

Collaborative Learning Activity

Work with a small group to develop a 2- to 5-minute role-play that introduces the Everyday Ethics scenario described in the chapter (a great idea is to video record your role-play activity). Then develop separate 2-minute role-play scenarios that provide at least two alternative approaches/solutions to resolving the situation. Ask classmates to view the solutions, ask questions, and discuss the ethical approach used in each. Ask for a vote on which solution classmates determine to be the "best."

Factors To Teach The Patient

This scenario is related to the following factors listed in this chapter of the textbook:

■ *The dental hygienist's ability to provide good dental hygiene care is enhanced by the willingness and ability of the patient to communicate accurate and complete information about health status, needs, and concerns.*

Mr. Romine has been a patient in the clinic for many, many years. You are a new dental hygienist in the practice who is scheduled to provide his regular maintenance care today. You discover that his health history form, which notes some significant health history issues including history of an infectious disease, arthritis, hypertension, and an undefined "heart problem," has not been updated in several years. When you politely ask him to fill out a new one, he angrily states, "Information about my health is my private business."

What are some ways that you might approach Mr. Romaine to help build rapport and establish enough trust to help him share the information you need to provide safe and effective dental hygiene care for him? Share your ideas with student colleagues. Was their approach similar to yours or very different? What did you learn from the discussion?

CROSSWORD PUZZLE

ACROSS

1. Nonword cues that help provide meaning during verbal communication
4. Type of communication that sends wordless messages (two words)
7. An approach to communication with elderly patients that may include baby and using terms of endearment that can be perceived as patronizing or demeaning
10. Easy-to-read written health information (two words)
11. Translation of a thought using words, gestures, or signs
15. Refers to communication with patients from other cultures than one's own (two words)
16. The process of sharing messages related to health and wellness (two words)
17. An individual's belief that actions will affect outcome (two words)
18. A set of cognitive and psychosocial skills that determines ability to obtain, understand, and respond to health messages (two words)

DOWN

1. A form of communication based on words
2. A common set of learned beliefs, attitudes, values, and behaviors

3. Cultural _____ that can affect communication or delivery of dental hygiene care are documented in a patient's record
5. What a dental hygienist should do more often than talking during a health education conversation with a patient
6. The ability to provide health messages for persons with limited English (or other language) proficiency is referred to as _____ competence
8. Communication through touching
9. Making an effort to understand behaviors of diverse groups is referred to as being culturally _____
12. If a dental hygienist possesses a set of skills that enables effective cross-cultural health-related communication with individuals of another culture, that dental hygienist is considered to be culturally _____
13. The study of how people use language and the impact of language
14. An attitude or judgment about others that is usually not based on personal experience but rather learned from other sources

Orientation to Clinical Dental Hygiene Practice

■ Chapters 1–3

 COMPETENCY EXERCISES

Apply information from the chapter and use critical thinking skills to complete the Competency exercises. Write responses on paper or create electronic documents to submit your answers.

Read the Section I Patient Assessment Summary to help you answer questions 1 and 2.

SECTION I—PATIENT ASSESSMENT SUMMARY

Patient Name: *Christopher Michaels*	Age: 10	Gender: ☒ M ☐ F	☑ Initial Therapy
			☐ Maintenance
Student (Clinician) Name: D.H. Student	Date: Today		☐ Re-evaluation

Chief Complaint:

Toothache and swollen area in lower left jaw. Ulcerated lesion on left upper lip.

ASSESSMENT FINDINGS

Medical History
- No current findings
- ASA II and ADL level 0

Social and Dental History
- No dental exam in 5 years
- Ulcerated, crusted lesion on left upper lip, spreading to nose.
- High sucrose intake (juice, candy)
- Poor dental biofilm control

Dental Examination
- Enlarged left submandibular lymph node
- Large lesion on mandibular left primary second molar
- Numerous small carious lesions
- Generalized gingivitis

At Risk For:
- N/A

At Risk For:
- Low health literacy (of parents)
- Pain and secondary infection due to active herpetic lesion
- Increased incidence of dental caries
- Increased risk of periodontal infection

At Risk For:
- Secondary infection
- Possible endodontic infection and pain from dental caries
- Further incidence of dental caries
- Gingival infection/periodontal disease

Periodontal Diagnosis/Case Type and Status:

Gingivitis

Caries Management Risk Assessment (CAMBRA) Level:

☐ Low ☐ Moderate ☐ High ☑ Extreme

1. The clinical issue: It is likely that the ulcerated lesion you observe on Christopher's upper lip is caused by an infectious condition and you are worried that providing treatment for him while the lesion is active can cause the infection to spread or that you could be infected. Write a PICO question that you can use to help guide your search for evidence to help make a decision about providing dental hygiene treatment today.

2. You decide to use a motivational interviewing technique to help educate both Christopher and his mother that drinking juice all day long is a health-related behavior that needs to change in order to reduce the risk for additional dental caries. However, Mrs. Michaels insists that he really enjoys drinking the juice and that she gives him at least five containers each day because she believes that juice is a healthy way for him to drink lots of liquids when he is active. Describe Mrs. Michael's readiness to change her behavior related to reducing Michael's consumption of the sugary beverage. Outline a Motivational Interviewing approach you can use at this appointment in an effort to help her move toward the next stage of willingness to change both her and Christopher's behavior.

3. Core values in dental hygiene practice include **autonomy and respect.** An example of this value is that you, as the dental hygienist, must respect your patient's right to refuse dental hygiene recommendations or treatment, even when your professional opinion is that doing so may cause deterioration of their oral health status.

   Select another one of the core values in dental hygiene practice and give an example to illustrate it. Discuss your example with student colleagues.

4. Identify an expression, gesture, or movement that you commonly make (see Box 1-4 for some ideas). Explain how your action can have unintended meaning or be the cause of a misunderstanding that will have a negative effect on the relationship you are developing with a patient of cultural background that is different than your own.

5. Explain why systematic reviews and meta-analysis articles are considered to constitute the highest level of evidence to support the selection of dental hygiene interventions for patient care.

DISCOVERY EXERCISES

1. Box 1-4 in the textbook lists questions for self-assessing personal values. Write brief answers for each of the five questions. Identify how your personal values relate to your future as a dental hygiene professional.

2. Obtain a copy of the rules or laws that govern the practice of dental hygiene in your state or country. Answer the following questions.

   - What type of supervision must dental hygienists have when they provide care for the patients?
   - Does your state have any provisions that allow dental hygienists to provide care in a collaborative practice or under reduced supervision for underserved populations or in any specific kinds of public health settings?
   - What specific services are the dental hygienists in your state or area licensed to provide?
   - What are continuing education requirements for dental hygienists who practice in your state or country?

3. Find a contact person for the dental hygiene professional association nearest to you and ask questions about membership, continuing education, and leadership opportunities.

4. Explore *The Provider's Guide to Quality and Culture: Health Disparities* Web site (available from the Managers Electronic Resource Center at: http://www.erc.msh.org). Click on the link to the Provider's Guide on the left hand side of the page. Take the quiz to identify misconceptions you have about characteristics common to individuals of other cultures. Return to this Web site to review more specific information when you are planning care for a patient whose cultural background is different from your own.

5. Explore the Health on the Net Foundation/HONcode Web site by typing http://www.hon.ch into your browser and then clicking on the Medical Professional link at the top of the page. Click on the "Trustworthy Medical Information" link and then type in the word "dental" in the search engine to get a list of HONcode certified Web sites that provide dental information. Try typing other words related to dental hygiene care into the search engine to see what "hits" you receive.

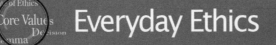

Everyday Ethics

*Surf health-related Web sites, government Web sites, online health literature databases, or any other online resource to find information related to ethics in health care, research, or public health. In particular, topics such as informed consent, HIPAA, public health access, licensure, and so on provide good topics to investigate on the internet. Identify a URL that others can use to locate the Web site or resource you discover, and then **annotate*** the*

citation by writing a brief description, providing an overview of the contents, and explaining how the resource might be helpful for the study of professional ethics.

Combine what you discover with ethics-related materials identified by other student colleagues to develop an annotated bibliography of online resources everyone can use to help further explore the Everyday Ethics scenarios throughout the textbook.

*****annotate***: to provide a critical or explanatory description.*

FOR YOUR PORTFOLIO

Use the basic information from the three chapters in Section I of the textbook to write a personal philosophy of dental hygiene practice statement. Describe how you believe yourself to be as a dental hygiene professional. Identify characteristics that describe the way you will provide dental hygiene care. Do this at the beginning of your training just after you complete these chapter and section exercises, and then do it again just before you graduate (don't peek at what you wrote the first time, please). Finally, write a summary of how these two documents reveal your personal growth during your training as a professional.

CROSSWORD PUZZLE

ACROSS

1. Refers to the components of a researchable question
4. Self-_____ is an essential element of attaining both personal and professional goals and objectives.
5. A type of communication that can be particularly important to consider if effective health communication is desired with a patient whose culture differs from that of the care provider
7. The skill set related to this health literacy domain includes skills and knowledge developed during previous health-related experiences.
9. Dental hygiene role that is interrelated with all the other roles (two words)
13. _____ signs for yes and no vary between cultures. (two words)
16. One of the databases commonly used by dental hygienists for locating biomedical information related to patient care
17. The ability to build relationships, assess readiness to change behaviors, and pay attention to patient's attitudes and beliefs are important _____ of effective health communication.
18. A _____ approach to finding applicable and current scientific information is an important component of evidence-based dental hygiene practice.
19. An individual who is blind and cannot hear well has a _____ barrier to communicating.

DOWN

2. This barrier to effective health communication can happen when too much information is provided on too many topics at one time and no written reinforcement is provided.
3. An acronym that refers to a group of individuals within an institution who review research proposals in order to protect the rights and welfare of volunteer research subjects.
4. When the patient perceives a lack of respect on the part of the care provider, an _____ barrier to communication may exist.
6. A collaborative organization that produces and disseminates systematic reviews of healthcare interventions.
8. A type of dental hygiene practice relationship in which a consulting dentist provides oversight but not necessarily direct or general supervision.
10. When the patient is in this stage of readiness, the focus for dental hygiene education is on assisting the patient to examine pros and cons of the proposed health-related behavior change.
11. In evidence-based dental hygiene practice, patient _____ or values are a factor in determining patient care interventions.
12. Effective health communication is enhanced if the practitioner is _____ regarding a patient's culturally related health practices and beliefs.
14. The general standards of right and wrong that guide the behavior of members of a profession.
15. Dental hygiene role related to influencing change in agencies and organizations to resolve problems and improves access to care.

SECTION II

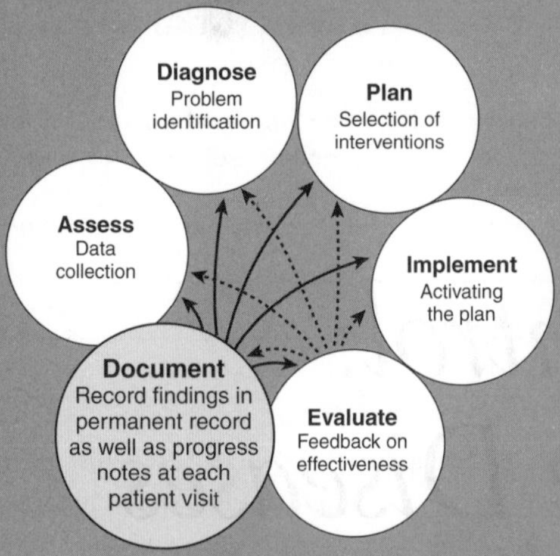
Diagnose
Problem identification
Plan
Selection of interventions
Assess
Data collection
Implement
Activating the plan
Document
Record findings in permanent record as well as progress notes at each patient visit
Evaluate
Feedback on effectiveness

Preparation for Dental Hygiene Practice

Chapters 4–8

■ LEARNING OBJECTIVES

Completing the exercises in this section of the workbook will prepare you to:

1. Apply concepts of infection/exposure control to protect the safety of self and patient during the dental hygiene appointment.
2. Position self, patient, and equipment to promote comfort, safety, and efficiency during the dental hygiene appointment.
3. Document all aspects of patient care.

■ COMPETENCIES FOR THE DENTAL HYGIENIST (APPENDIX A)

Competencies supported by the learning in Section II:

Core Competencies: C2, C3, C4, C5, C6, C9, C11, C12.

Health Promotion and Disease Prevention: HP2, HP3, HP4, HP6.

Patient/Client Care: PC1, PC2, PC3, PC4, PC5.

Exposure Control: Barriers for Patient and Clinician

Learning Objectives

Upon successful completion of these exercises, you will be able to:

1. Identify and define key terms and concepts related to exposure control, clinical barriers, and latex allergies.
2. Apply and remove clinical barrier materials without cross-contamination.

3. Identify and explain the rationale for hand washing and other exposure-control techniques used during patient care.
4. Identify criteria for selecting appropriate protective barrier materials.

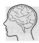 **KNOWLEDGE EXERCISES**

Write your answers for each question in the space provided.

Also refer to Sections III, IV and V in the CDC Guidelines for Infection Control in Dental Health-Care Settings *(Appendix IV in the textbook) as you complete the exercises for this chapter.*

1. An organized system for exposure control that treats body fluids of all patients as though they were infectious is a description of _____.

2. Identify the term or concept related to each of the following statements:

   ■ Physically blocks exposure to bodily fluids to prevent disease transmission.

   _____

   ■ A specific, potentially health-threatening bodily contact with infectious material while you are providing dental hygiene care.

   _____

   ■ Contact with infectious material that is reasonable to expect as a component of providing dental hygiene care.

   _____

3. List three purposes for having a written exposure control plan.

   _____

   _____

   _____

4. Define the following terms in your own words:
   ■ Immunization

   _____

   _____

   ■ Inoculation

   _____

   _____

■ Toxoid

_____

_____

■ Vaccine

_____

_____

■ Vaccination

_____

_____

■ HCP

_____

_____

■ DHCP

_____

_____

5. Unscramble the following words; definitions are included to help you.

■ hiiinrts (_inflammation of the mucous membrane of the nose_)

_____

■ toxmanu (_a test for the presence of active or inactive tuberculosis_)

_____

■ bcMytaercoiumr cykitbreysos (_droplet nuclei, ranging from 0.5 to 1 μm, that are a risk in health care settings_)

_____

_____

6. Updating immunizations against a number of diseases is an important protective factor for DHCP. What is a booster immunization?

_____

7. List the basic immunizations recommended for DHCP.

_____

_____

_____

8. List the factors that describe an appropriate clinic gown or uniform.

_____

_____

_____

_____

_____

_____

9. During patient care, long hair should be fastened back, and facial hair should be covered by _____.

10. List the essential characteristics of an ideal face mask.

_____

_____

_____

_____

11. Particles in aerosols smaller than _____ can remain suspended up to 24 hours.

12. What size particle can penetrate to the alveoli of lungs when inhaled?

_____

13. What size are the tuberculosis-causing bacterium particles?

_____

14. When should a clinician wear a face shield over a regular mask?

_____

15. How is a contaminated mask removed from your face?

_____

16. Who wears protective eyewear during dental hygiene care?

_____

17. List types of eyewear appropriate for wear during patient care.

_____

_____

_____

_____

INFOMAP 5-1

METHOD	PREPARATION	LATHERING METHOD	SITUATION IN WHICH THE TECHNIQUE IS RECOMMENDED
Routine Handwash			
Antiseptic Handwash			
Surgical Antisepsis			
Antiseptic Hand Rub			

 ## COMPETENCY EXERCISES

Apply information from the chapter and use critical thinking skills to complete the competency exercises. Write responses on paper or create electronic documents to submit your answers.

1. Fill out Infomap 5-1 to compare the methods of handwashing. Then use the information in the Infomap to describe verbally the differences between the methods to a fellow student or a patient.

2. Use the information in Chapter 3 to develop a step-by-step checklist, in proper sequence, for getting ready to provide patient care. Consider the sequence for handwashing as well as applying all of the personal protective barriers that you use in your clinic. Pay careful attention to creating a detailed system that minimizes the possibility of cross-contamination.

3. Compare your checklist to the lists that other student colleagues have created or to one provided by your instructor. Refine your list and use it as part of your own personal written exposure control plan.

4. Describe at least three ways you can prevent cross-contamination during handwashing in the clinic at your school.

5. Practice removing gloves using the system illustrated in Figure 3-4 in the textbook. Explain how this procedure will prevent cross-contamination.

6. Explain why it is necessary to document a latex allergy on the patient's permanent record. Identify how that information is recorded in the patient records at your school.

Everyday Ethics

Before completing the learning exercises below, reread and reflect on the Everyday Ethics scenario and Questions for Consideration in this chapter of the textbook. It may also be useful to review the Dental Hygiene Ethics discussion in Chapter 1, the Ethical Applications in the introduction pages for each section in the textbook, as well as the Codes of Ethics in Appendices I, II, and III.

Individual Learning Activity

Imagine that you are the dental hygienist in this scenario. Answer each of the questions for consideration at the end of the scenario.

Collaborative Learning Activity

Work with a small group to develop a 2- to 5-minute role-play that introduces the Everyday Ethics scenario described in the chapter (a great idea is to video record your role-play activity). Then develop separate 2-minute role-play scenarios that provide at least two alternative approaches/solutions to resolving the situation. Ask classmates to view the solutions, ask questions, and discuss the ethical approach used in each. Ask for a vote on which solution classmates determine to be the "best."

? QUESTIONS PATIENTS ASK

What sources of information can you identify that will help you answer your patient's questions in this scenario?

How do I know this room was cleaned after the last patient was in here? Did you wash your hands? Is everything you use brand new for each patient? How do I know that I won't be exposed to an infectious disease during my dental hygiene treatment?

Factors To Teach The Patient

- *Purposes for use of barriers (face mask, protective eyewear, and gloves) by the clinician for the benefit of the patient.*
- *Importance of eye protection.*

Mrs. Johnson is bringing her 3-year-old son, Jimmy, in for his first dental hygiene appointment. She states that he is frightened by the mask and asks you not to wear it during the appointment. She is also concerned because she has never been asked to wear glasses during previous dental hygiene appointments at another dental office. She states that Jimmy will probably protest at having to wear the child-size glasses you have ready.

Write a paragraph you will use to explain to Mrs. Johnson the importance of, and the rationale for, using these barriers. Include some comments that will help explain their use to Jimmy.

25. Briefly describe a system for remembering to monitor regularly sterilization effectiveness.

    _____

    _____

26. How are instruments stored following sterilization so that they remain contamination free?

    _____

    _____

27. List three uses for chemical disinfectants.

    _____

    _____

    _____

28. Describe the three levels of chemical disinfectants.

    _____

    _____

    _____

29. List the factors you will consider when selecting a chemical disinfectant for use in your dental hygiene treatment room.

    _____

    _____

    _____

    _____

    _____

    _____

30. What information on a product label tells you about the effectiveness of the chemical agent you use for disinfection?

    _____

    _____

31. List the product label items to look for when you prepare and use a chemical disinfectant.

    _____

    _____

    _____

    _____

    _____

    _____

32. Define each of the following types of waste:

    ■ Infectious waste _____

    _____

    ■ Contaminated waste _____

    _____

    ■ Hazardous waste _____

    _____

    ■ Toxic waste _____

    _____

    ■ Regulated waste _____

    _____

33. Items such as needles are disposed of in a _____

    _____

34. Correctly number the sequence of steps for disinfecting environmental surfaces in the treatment room by placing the numbers 1 through 4 in the space provided.

STEP #	DESCRIPTION OF STEP
4	Spray surfaces and allow to air-dry
1	Put on PPE, including heavy-duty household gloves
3	Scrub surfaces with gauze sponges or paper towels
2	Spray all surfaces liberally and completely

35. According to CDC recommendations, water lines should be flushed for _____ at the beginning of the day and, according to the CDC 2003 guidelines, for _____ between patients to reduce microbial counts.

36. Identify two oral procedures that can reduce microbial counts before dental hygiene treatment.

    _____

    _____

37. What additional patient-related factors can be included as standard procedures that will help manage infection control during treatment?

_____

_____

_____

_____

38. Describe a permucosal exposure to blood or other body fluids.

_____

39. What basic procedures are followed when a clinician experiences a percutaneous exposure to blood or contaminated body fluids?

_____

_____

_____

_____

40. Why is it important to clean the exposed parts of your face regularly during your clinical day?

_____

41. What three components regarding infection control are included in an office policy manual?

_____

_____

_____

42. Refer to Appendix IV in the textbook (*CDC 2003 Guidelines for Infection Control in Dental Health-Care Settings*) as you answer the following questions:

CDC 1. Section VI A of the CDC guidelines recommend that you use only FDA-cleared medical devices and that you follow manufacturers' instructions for sterilization. The category for this recommendation is 1B. What does a category 1B recommendation mean?

_____

_____

CDC 2. What procedure does Section VI F of the CDC guidelines recommend in case of a positive spoor-monitoring test?

_____

_____

_____

CDC 3. The CDC 2003 guidelines, Section VII, recommends the use of _____-level chemical disinfectants on clinical contact surfaces that are visibly contaminated with blood.

COMPETENCY EXERCISES

Apply information from the chapter and use critical thinking skills to complete the competency exercises. Write responses on paper or create electronic documents to submit your answers.

1. **Putting it all together:** Review both Chapters 5 and 6 to answer this question. Write brief statements or lists to summarize all of the procedures you can follow every day to maintain the chain of asepsis and prevent disease transmission in each of the following categories:
   - You and your colleagues
   - Your patient
   - The clinic
   - During treatment
   - Post-treatment

2. Explain the difference between decontamination, disinfection, and sterilization.

3. Identify specific ways that planning ahead before seating a patient in the dental chair can ensure that you will maintain asepsis and eliminate cross-contamination during patient treatment.

4. The textbook describes features of dental treatment room equipment that facilitate optimum infection control. Describe the features in your school clinic that meet these criteria.

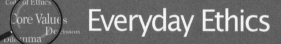

Everyday Ethics

Before completing the learning exercises below, reread and reflect on the Everyday Ethics scenario and Questions for Consideration in this chapter of the textbook. It may also be useful to review the Dental Hygiene Ethics discussion in Chapter 1, the Ethical Applications in the introduction pages for each Section in the textbook, as well as the Codes of Ethics in Appendices I, II, and III.

Individual Learning Activity
Imagine that you are the dental hygienist in this scenario. Answer each of the questions for consideration at the end of the scenario.

Collaborative Learning Activity
Ask a dental hygienist who has been practicing for a year or more to read the scenario. Share the responses you have made to answer each question and ask that person to discuss the situation with you. What insights did you have or what did you learn during this discussion?

Factors To Teach The Patient

- *The meaning of* standard precautions *and what is included under the term; how these precautions protect the patient and the dental team members.*
- *Methods for sterilization of instruments, including hand pieces, and how the autoclave or other sterilizer is tested daily or weekly.*

Mrs. Norton is on the telephone again. She recently made a first dental appointment for Daniella, her 3-year-old daughter, and she is clearly nervous about it. This is the second time she has called in with questions. This time, she wants to be assured that her daughter will not be exposed to any infectious diseases during dental hygiene treatment.

Using the information you learned in Chapters 5 and 6 of the textbook, write a statement explaining infection control procedures and reassuring Mrs. Norton.

WORD SEARCH

```
S  W  A  N  T  I  M  I  C  R  O  B  I  A  L  C  T
P  C  O  N  T  A  M  I  N  A  T  I  O  N  L  A  A
O  D  V  B  S  A  Q  J  A  O  W  I  O  A  E  S  G
R  I  X  E  R  T  S  K  J  U  C  T  C  S  E  L  C
E  S  V  X  N  R  E  Q  R  M  T  I  X  N  H  I  J
T  I  B  B  P  V  P  R  L  E  T  O  I  R  T  A  T
E  N  I  O  C  X  I  I  I  G  L  C  P  A  N  N
S  F  O  D  J  R  F  R  R  L  R  U  E  L  O  C  K
T  E  B  C  I  O  I  C  O  E  I  S  L  I  A  G  F
I  C  U  H  I  S  I  T  T  N  I  Z  T  A  S  V  R
N  T  R  B  Z  M  P  A  I  T  M  A  A  I  T  G  E
G  A  D  E  E  T  W  O  N  C  T  E  S  T  O  E  T
C  N  E  S  Y  T  D  A  S  I  A  P  N  T  I  H  D
X  T  N  H  I  P  R  R  N  A  E  L  M  T  W  O  H
O  Y  W  N  J  T  P  A  R  S  B  H  D  A  A  G  N
T  B  U  B  W  I  S  B  A  H  S  L  M  W  I  L  X
J  O  K  A  S  P  O  R  I  C  I  D  E  H  X  K  H
```

WORD SEARCH CLUES

1. Agent that kills or suppresses microorganisms
2. Applied to living tissue to prevent growth or action of microorganisms
3. The number of contaminating organisms contained within a biomaterial
4. Surface film that contains microorganisms
5. Introduction of infectious material into a tissue or onto a surface
6. Agent that destroys microorganisms but may not kill bacterial spores
7. Term used by OSHA that refers to infectious waste
8. A cleaning process that reduces the level of, but does not completely eliminate, biocontamination.
9. Substance that kills microbiologic spores
10. Process that kills all forms of life
11. Disinfection/sterilization category that refers to surfaces such as counter tops in the treatment room
12. Disinfection/sterilization category that refers to objects that penetrate soft tissue or bone
13. Disinfection/sterilization category that refers objects that touch but do not penetrate oral tissues and are sterilized or treated with high-level disinfection after use
14. Regularly required to verify proper use and functioning of the sterilizer (two words)
15. A place in which biofilm can form and contaminate water used during patient care (three words)
16. This level of disinfectant inactivates spores and all forms of bacteria, fungi, and viruses
17. Steam under pressure describes the method of sterilization provided by an _____
18. Refers to one-use instruments or other materials used during patient care.
19. U.S. government organization that provides regulations and guidelines for disposal of infectious waste
20. Obtained by exclusion, removing, or killing all contaminating organisms

Introduction to Documentation

Upon successful completion of these exercises, you will be able to:

1. Identify and define key terms and concepts related to written and computerized dental records and charting.
2. Describe concepts related to ensuring confidentiality and privacy of patient information.
3. Compare three tooth-numbering systems.
4. Discuss the various components of the patient's permanent, comprehensive dental record.
5. Recognize and explain a systematic method for documenting patient visits.

 KNOWLEDGE EXERCISES

Write your answers for each question in the space provided.

1. Why do dental professionals document patient care activities and maintain a permanent, comprehensive patient record?

   _____
   _____
   _____
   _____
   _____
   _____

2. What actions regarding a patient record are essential to ensure accurate documentation of patient care in case the record is needed during a legal action?

   _____
   _____

   _____
   _____

3. Identify the important components of the patient record.

   _____
   _____
   _____
   _____
   _____
   _____

4. Handwritten records are recorded legibly and written in _____.

5. What is HIPAA?

   _____
   _____

6. What are the three components of HIPAA?

_____

_____

_____

7. List patient rights that are protected by HIPAA.

_____

_____

_____

_____

_____

8. List HIPAA-designated responsibilities of health-care providers and employers.

_____

_____

_____

_____

_____

_____

9. In your own words, define the term *sign*.

_____

_____

10. Define the term "symptom."

_____

_____

11. Identify the purposes of complete and accurate periodontal and dental charting.

_____

_____

_____

_____

_____

12. Identify the types of chart forms that can be used to record your patient's dental charting.

_____

_____

_____

13. Define "systematic procedure" as it relates to dental charting.

_____

_____

14. In your own words, briefly describe the clinical observations that are included in your patient's periodontal charting.

■ *Gingival changes* _____

_____

_____

■ *Items charted* _____

_____

_____

■ *Deposits* _____

_____

_____

■ *Factors related to occlusion* _____

_____

_____

■ *Radiographic findings* _____

_____

_____

15. What items are documented in a dental charting record?

_____

_____

_____

_____

_____

_____

_____

16. List all 5 types of documentation discussed in this chapter that comprise a permanent, comprehensive patient record.

_____

_____

_____

_____

_____

17. List 4 types of information that are NEVER included in a patient record.

_____

_____

_____

_____

18. What factors are included in a patient progress note?

_____

_____

_____

19. Describe each of the components in the SOAP note method for documenting patient visits.

_____

_____

_____

_____

_____

20. Because different tooth numbering systems are used in dental offices and clinics, it is necessary for you to be familiar with all of them. Refer to Figures 8-1, 8-2, and 8-3 in the textbook to provide guidance as you complete Infomap 8-1. Completing this exercise will help you compare the three types of tooth numbering systems.

INFOMAP 8-1					
TOOTH NUMBERING SYSTEM	**ORGANIZATION (ARCHES OR QUADRANTS)**	**PERMANENT DENTITION**	**PRIMARY DENTITION**	**ADDITIONAL FEATURES**	**EXAMPLE: MAXILLARY RIGHT CENTRAL INCISOR**
Palmer System Tooth Numbering					
International Tooth Numbering (Fédération Dentaire Internationale)					
Universal Tooth Numbering (American Dental Association)					

COMPETENCY EXERCISES

Apply information from the chapter and use critical thinking skills to complete the Competency exercises. Write responses on paper or create electronic documents to submit your answers.

1. Caroline Lacy arrives for your 10:00 appointment. She is 3 years old and has never had her teeth charted. Identify the correct tooth number for the two teeth listed below using each of the tooth numbering systems.

	MANDIBULAR LEFT PRIMARY FIRST MOLAR	MAXILLARY LEFT PRIMARY FIRST MOLAR
Palmer		
FDI		
Universal		

2. The dental practice where you work has decided to change from a chart that uses anatomic drawings of the complete teeth to a chart that contains only geometric diagrams. The plan is to chart both restorative and periodontal findings on the new form. You are asked for your opinion at the staff meeting. What would you say?

3. Flip through the various chapters in Section VIII of the textbook and randomly select three or four of the "Example Progress Notes" located in each chapter. Analyze each example you select to determine which information in the example is related to each of the SOAP note components. Boxes 8-2 and 8-3 in the chapter should provide some guidance for this exercise. Is information missing from any of those example progress notes?

4. Examine the previous progress notes from a patient chart in your school clinic. Analyze each to determine whether the SOAP components have been included in each entry.

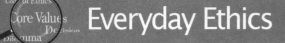

Everyday Ethics

*Before completing the learning exercises below, reread and reflect on the **Everyday Ethics Scenario and Questions for Consideration in this chapter of the textbook**. It may also be useful to review the Dental Hygiene Ethics discussion in Chapter 1, the Ethical Applications in the introduction pages for each Section in the textbook, as well as the Codes of Ethics in Appendices I, II, and III.*

Discovery Activities
- Ask a dental hygienist who has been practicing for a year or more to read the scenario. Provide them with a

copy of the Code of Ethics as well. Share the responses you have made to answer each question and ask that person to discuss the situation with you. What insights did you have or what did you learn during this discussion?
- Ask a friend or relative who is not involved in healthcare to read the scenario and discuss it with you from the perspective of a "patient" who receives services within the healthcare system. Discuss what you learned from the concerns, insights, or difference in perspective that person expressed.

Factors To Teach The Patient

- Interpretation of all recordings; meaning of all numbers used, such as for probing depths

You have just completed the periodontal and dental charting during a patient's initial appointment. The patient asks you to explain all those numbers and letters you were

calling out to the dental assistant who was writing everything down for you.

List the main points you would want to cover in a conversation that explains all kinds of numbers and letters that are used to document periodontal and dental conditions.

Read the Section II Patient Assessment Summary to help you answer questions 1 and 2.

1. Prior to seating the patient, you are handed the information in the Assessment Summary on the previous page, received during a pre-appointment telephone call. This is a first-ever dental appointment for young Jean Luc Aristide who has recently arrived in this country from Haiti to live with a foster family while he receives medical treatment. He speaks very little English, but his bright smile and curious gaze capture your attention and make you smile back at him. Marge Black, a social worker who is arranging access to healthcare services, accompanies him to the dental appointment. What questions will you need to ask his guardian in order to determine Jean Luc's health status before providing dental hygiene care?

2. What steps will you take to protect both Jean Luc and yourself while you are collecting the rest of your assessment data and providing oral hygiene instructions during this first appointment?

3. Compile a personal immunization log. Identify any missing immunizations and make arrangements to receive them.

4. Examine the personal protective barrier equipment (protective eyewear, masks, gloves, etc.) that you have selected for your own use in the clinic and describe how they meet the characteristics of acceptable exposure-control barriers.

5. Locate the eyewash station in your clinic that is nearest to your treatment area. Practice using the eyewash.

 DISCOVERY EXERCISES

1. Search online or in the library to discover the purpose and function of each of the following federal, state, and local government organizations and discuss how they relate to the practice of dental hygiene.

   ▪ *CDC*
   ▪ *EPA*
   ▪ *FDA*
   ▪ *OSAP*
   ▪ *OSHA*
   ▪ *Department of Community Health*

2. The CDC 2003 Guidelines for Infection Control in Dental Health-Care Settings that you will find in Appendix IV in the textbook contains only the outlined recommendations, not the full text of the report. You can access the complete report in your library by looking for the Centers for Disease Control and Prevention's *Guidelines for Infection Control in Dental Health Settings—2003* (MMWR 2003;52, no. RR-17) or online at http://www.cdc.gov/mmwr/preview/mmwrhtml/rr5217a1.htm. Scroll down to explore the full report to find and read the section titled "Contact Dermatitis and Latex Hypersensitivity." Write a brief summary of what you learned. When you have time, explore the information in other sections of the report.

3. Investigate the sterilization methods and procedures that are used at your school clinic.

4. If the guidelines for your school clinic require a different approach than the SOAP notes approach for documenting information in patient care progress notes, compare the two approaches and identify similarities and differences between the two approaches regarding the factors that are documented.

5. Investigate to determine your school clinic's protocol for procedures to follow if you experience a percutaneous or permucosal exposure to blood or other bodily fluids in the clinic.

6. Imagine that you have been asked to select a new handwashing soap that will be used in your clinic. Search for scientific evidence of effectiveness of antibacterial agents commonly used in handwashing soaps that are available for use by dental hygienists. Select the best alternative, and explain why you made your selection. (*Hint*: Check the soap that is currently in use in your clinic as well as some dental supplier catalogs to find the most commonly used antibacterial agents, and then develop a PICO question that will help you review the scientific literature for research evidence of effectiveness.)

7. Investigate dental supply catalogs to determine the types of gloves available for use in dental clinics and the cost of each type. What scientific evidence is available to help you determine which type of glove provides the most effective barrier to microorganisms you are likely to encounter during patient care?

CROSSWORD PUZZLE

ACROSS

1. Carpal Tunnel Syndrome is a _____ disorder that commonly affects dental hygienists.
3. To apply substances that destroy most (but not all) infective organisms onto an inanimate object
5. Refers to the period of time when an infectious agent can be transferred from an infected person to another person
7. To kill all forms of life, as with an autoclave
9. Refers to the exposure to disease that may result from the performance of one's usual duties
12. A virus, microorganism, or other substance that causes disease or infection
13. Process of introducing a substance into the body to produce immunity to a specific disease
14. Particles suspended in air
15. Repetitive movements, use of a forceful grasp, and vibration are commonly recognized ergonomic _____ (two words).
17. A state that can occur if a patient is suddenly brought upright after being in a supine position for a long period of time
18. Refers to the transmission of potentially infectious agents between one place or person and another person or place (two words).

DOWN

1. Useful for protecting face and respiratory system from aerosols when providing dental hygiene treatment
2. Eye, mouth, mucous membrane, nonintact skin, or parenteral contact with blood or other potentially infectious material (two words)
4. A chemical _____ is used to change the color of a marker on autoclave tape to indicate that the package has been brought to a specific temperature.
6. A type of dental hygiene practice that includes attention to equipment, work layout and work processes that decreases strain and fatigue and protects the functional health and well-being of both the clinician and the patient (two words)
8. A preventive, functional-movement strategy that, performed daily, can help reduce the dental hygienist's risk for musculoskeletal injury and prevent pain
10. Refers to the people, equipment and other materials identified as a link in the Chain of Disease Transmission.
11. Agent that can be used to reduce surface pathogens on mucosa or skin
16. Wiping, scrubbing or other process that reduces bioburden, but does not completely eliminate contamination on clinical instruments or surfaces

FOR YOUR PORTFOLIO

1. Develop a personal, written exposure-control plan. Do not forget to include an appropriate reference list to indicate that you have based your personal plan on scientific evidence. Consider making the plan in a format that could be easily updated and adapted to any setting later on when you are a practicing dental hygienist.

2. List your personal selections/recommendations for handwashing soap, gloves, and any other infection-control supplies used in dental hygiene care. Support each recommendation with a brief written summary of product characteristics and how the product meets the criteria for acceptability.

3. Develop a personal, written, long-term plan to avoid cumulative trauma injuries related to dental hygiene practice. Update this plan yearly as you learn more about working conditions that compromise your comfort and effectiveness when you are providing dental hygiene care.

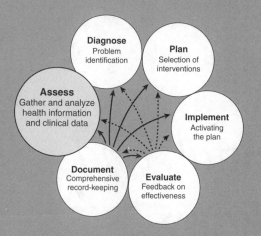

Assessment

Chapters 9–22

■ LEARNING OBJECTIVES

Completing the exercises in this section of the workbook will prepare you to:

1. Identify components of a complete patient assessment.
2. Apply a variety of assessment methods to gather data and document the patient's health status.
3. Determine individual and community oral health status using a variety of dental indices.
4. Document assessment findings.

■ COMPETENCIES FOR THE DENTAL HYGIENIST (APPENDIX A)

Competencies supported by the learning in Section III

Core Competencies: C5, C8, C10, C11, C12, C13, C14

Health Promotion and Disease Prevention: HP2, HP3, HP4, HP5, HP6

Community Involvement: CM1, CM2, CM6

Patient/Client Care: PC1, PC2, PC3, PC4

Personal, Dental, and Medical Histories

Upon successful completion of these exercises, you will be able to:

1. Identify and define key terms and concepts related to preparing patient histories.
2. Discuss the purposes of the personal, medical, and dental histories.
3. List and discuss the types, systems, forms used, question types, and styles used to collect patient history data.
4. Recognize considerations for patient care that are identified by various items recorded on the patient history.

KNOWLEDGE EXERCISES

Write your answers for each question in the space provided.

1. In your own words, explain why taking a complete and accurate patient history is necessary before providing dental hygiene care.

_____

_____

2. List the purposes of taking personal, medical, and dental histories during patient assessment.

_____

_____

_____

_____

_____

_____

_____

3. In your own words, describe each of the following systems for obtaining the patient's history.

■ *Pre-appointment information:* _____

_____

_____

■ *Self-history:* _____

_____

_____

■ *Brief history:* _____

_____

_____

■ *Complete history:* _____

_____

_____

4. List the characteristics of an adequate patient history form.

_____

_____

_____

_____

_____

5. What factors can affect the accuracy of a patient history?

_____

_____

_____

_____

_____

6. Describe each type of patient-history questionnaires in your own words.

■ *System oriented:* _____

_____

_____

■ *Disease oriented:* _____

_____

_____

■ *Symptom oriented:* _____

_____

_____

■ *Culture oriented:* _____

_____

_____

7. Why is it important for the dental hygienist to record contact information for the patient's physician in the personal history? _____

_____

_____

8. Identify the advantages associated with each method of collecting patient data. Each answer may be used more than one time.

METHODS OF DATA COLLECTION	ADVANTAGE
A. Questionnaire	____ Legal written record with patient's signature
B. Interview	____ Consistent
	____ Development of rapport
	____ Time-saving
	____ Flexibility for individual needs

9. List factors that can contribute to success in gaining patient cooperation during the history interview.

_____

_____

_____

_____

_____

_____

10. List three types of medical consultation related to the development of patient history.

_____

_____

_____

11. List the health conditions that require antibiotic premedication prior to dental and dental hygiene treatment.

_____

_____

_____

_____

12. Which dental hygiene procedures require antibiotic premedication for patients at risk for endocarditis?

_____

_____

13. State the standard antibiotic premedication regimen prescribed for at-risk adult patients prior to dental procedures.

_____

_____

COMPETENCY EXERCISES

Apply information from the chapter and use critical thinking skills to complete the Competency exercises. Write responses on paper or create electronic documents to submit your answers.

1. Review the patient history questionnaire forms used in your practice setting (either your dental hygiene program clinic or the dental practice where you receive care). Use the information in the "Considerations for Appointment Procedures" located in the right-hand column of Tables 9-1, 9-2, and 9-3 in the textbook to identify the reason for including each of the items on the form.

2. Compare the patient history form used in your practice with the ADA form included in the textbook chapter. What are the similarities and differences between the forms?

3. Using the format required in your dental hygiene program clinic, document an imaginary patient appointment during which personal, dental, and medical histories are obtained.

DISCOVERY EXERCISE

Search online to find patient health history questionnaires in languages other than English.

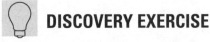

Everyday Ethics

*Before completing the learning exercises below, reread and reflect on the **Everyday Ethics Scenario and Questions for Consideration in this chapter of the textbook.** It may also be useful to review the Dental Hygiene Ethics discussion in Chapter 1, the Ethical Applications in the introduction pages for each Section in the textbook, as well as the Codes of Ethics in Appendices I, II, and III.*

Individual Learning Activity
Imagine that you are the dental hygienist in this scenario. Answer each of the questions for consideration at the end of the scenario.

Discovery Activity
Ask a dental hygienist who has been practicing for a year or more to read the scenario. Provide them with a copy of the Code of Ethics as well. Share the responses you have made to answer each question and ask that person to discuss the situation with you. What insights did you have or what did you learn during this discussion?

Factors To Teach The Patient

This scenario is related to the following factors listed in this chapter of the textbook:

- The need for obtaining the personal, medical, and dental history before performing dental and dental hygiene procedures and the need for keeping the histories up to date
- The assurance that recorded histories are kept in strict professional confidence
- The relationship between oral health and general physical health
- The interrelationship of medical and dental care

You are just starting to treat Jon Wojeckick, who is 37 years old. You begin to ask questions about his medical history. You notice he has stopped making eye contact

and is hesitating over some of the answers. You have a feeling that he is not giving you accurate information, and you want to be sure you are obtaining all the data you need to provide optimum safe care. You know from studying Tables 9-1, 9-2, and 9-3 in the textbook that items from the patient history have a connection to how you provide dental hygiene care for your patient.

Use the examples of patient conversations in Appendix D of this workbook as a guide to write a statement explaining the relationship between oral health and physical health and the need for accurate information to facilitate treatment planning. Include at least three examples of appointment considerations that are linked to items in the patient history. Be sure to assure Mr. Wojeckick that recorded histories are kept in strict professional confidence.

CHAPTER 10

Vital Signs

Upon successful completion of these exercises, you will be able to:

1. Identify and define key terms and concepts related to recording vital signs.
2. Identify four vital signs and describe the range of expected values.
3. Describe procedures for determining and recording a patient's temperature, pulse, respiration, and blood pressure.
4. Discuss the importance of regular determination of vital signs for a patient receiving dental hygiene care.

 KNOWLEDGE EXERCISES

Write your answers for each question in the space provided.

1. The vital signs patient record stamp that is illustrated in Figure 10-1 in the textbook suggests recording a fifth vital sign. What is it?

   _____

2. Describe how you will position your patient to explain and record vital signs.

   _____
   _____

3. If your patient's vital signs are not within normal range, what should you do?

   _____
   _____

4. What are the normal adult ranges for each of the vital signs?

   _____
   _____

   _____
   _____

5. What factors should you consider when you are deciding whether to take your patient's temperature?

   _____
   _____
   _____
   _____

6. Normal average temperature varies among individuals, but in general, the average temperature of an adult over 70 years old is slightly _____ than the adult average, and the temperature of a child under 5 years old may be slightly _____.

7. List the factors that can increase body temperature.

   _____
   _____
   _____
   _____

8. The most common location for taking temperature is the mouth. What contraindications would lead you to select another location?

_____

_____

9. What emergency situations may cause your patient to exhibit an increased pulse rate? (*Hint*: See Tables 69-4 and 69-5 in Chapter 69, Emergency Care, of the textbook)

_____

_____

_____

_____

10. In your own words, describe how to obtain and record your patient's pulse.

_____

_____

_____

11. Define a respiration.

_____

12. Describe the factors to observe while you are counting your patient's respiration rate.

_____

_____

_____

_____

13. Describe the procedure for counting respirations.

_____

_____

14. What emergency situations can cause a change in your patient's respiration?

_____

_____

15. What physical factors determine the maintenance of blood pressure?

_____

_____

_____

16. Emergencies such as fainting, blood loss, and shock will cause blood pressure to _____.

17. What action should you take if your patient's blood pressure is at a prehypertension level or above?

_____

_____

18. How frequently should your patient's blood pressure be taken and recorded during dental hygiene treatment?

_____

_____

COMPETENCY EXERCISES

Apply information from the chapter and use critical thinking skills to complete the Competency exercises. Write responses on paper or create electronic documents to submit your answers.

1. You have just seated Maura Kennedy in the dental chair for her dental hygiene maintenance appointment. You read in her patient record that she is 33 years old, has no remarkable health problems, and is taking no medications. She reports that the only change in her health history today is that she has had a sinus infection for the last 2 weeks. She reports that she started taking antibiotics the day before yesterday and is feeling a bit better, but her nasal passages are still all stuffed up. Write a brief statement that you will use to inform Maura that you are going to determine and record her vital signs.

2. When you take Maura's temperature, you find that it is normal. Her pulse rate is 70 beats/min; while you still have your fingers on her wrist, you count her respirations. Her respiration is slightly fast, 20/min, and you note that she takes several shallow breaths followed by one or two gulps of air and that she wheezes a bit when she exhales. However, you note that her color is good, so she must not be having any real problem with air exchange, and her breathing problems may just be the result of her stuffy nose. You wrap the blood pressure cuff around her right arm, pump it up, and place the stethoscope. You hear the sounds begin at the 122 mark on the manometer, and the last sound you hear is at 83. After a discussion with Maura and with Dr. Ichero, you all decide to reschedule Maura for her maintenance visit in a couple of weeks when her sinus infection is gone.

Using your institution's guidelines for writing in patient records, document that you assessed Maura's vital signs at this appointment and rescheduled her appointment for a future date.

3. Create a brief step-by-step guide for determining and recording all of the vital signs on a 3-by-5-inch card (this is sometimes called a "job aid"). If you can laminate your job aid, you will be able to disinfect it to use during patient care. Practice using your step-by-step guide to determine and record vital signs for family members, friends, or student colleagues. If you practice with a dental hygiene instructor as your patient, you can receive valuable feedback on your techniques!

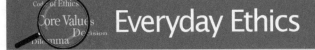

Everyday Ethics

*Before completing the learning exercises below, reread and reflect on the **Everyday Ethics Scenario and Questions for Consideration in this chapter of the textbook**. It may also be useful to review the Dental Hygiene Ethics discussion in Chapter 1, the Ethical Applications in the introduction pages for each Section in the textbook, as well as the Codes of Ethics in Appendices I, II, and III.*

Individual Learning Activity
Identify a situation you have experienced that presents a similar ethical dilemma. What did you learn from how the situation was (or was not) resolved at the time it happened?

Collaborative Learning Activity
Answer each of the questions for consideration at the end of the scenario in the textbook. Compare what you wrote with answers developed by another classmate and discuss differences/similarities.

Factors To Teach The Patient

This scenario is related to the following factors listed in this chapter of the textbook:

- How vital signs can influence dental and dental hygiene appointments
- The importance of having a blood pressure determination at regular intervals

Mr. Borman Gorbachov, the CEO of a large manufacturing firm, is always in a hurry. He simply cannot seem to sit still for his whole appointment and is always chiding you that you should work faster so that he can be done and get back to work. Today he sighs heavily and then protests loudly when you tell him that you are going to take and record his vital signs. He states that he just had his blood pressure taken a month or so ago at his doctor's office and there is nothing wrong with him. You look in his patient record to discover that the previous blood pressure, taken almost 2 years ago, was normal.

Use the examples of patient conversations in Appendix D as a guide to prepare a conversation you can use to educate Mr. Gorbachov about the reasons for determining a patient's vital signs at each appointment. Use the conversation you create to educate a patient or friend, and then modify it based on what you learned from the interaction.

WORD SEARCH

```
E F O O A N O X I A A P N E A D R G M Y
G F M R D I S T O L E P O M L H H I I C
F K L I X M P T K U V X Q Y Z F Y Z S H
E Y K A U S C U L T A T I O N V T L S K
O L B Z Y S Q B L I L W G K B Y H M A I
P U N C P P P R X G J K Z E N P M I H Y
S E O W C H U A G X E V A I Y Y M K F P
K L R R N Y L D P J X M X V K R K C H S
M X M D K G S Y C D R F E X E E O T N T
B Y O I M M E C X T S M K H L X R K D A
R R T L E O H A C A R O T I D I O O G C
A O E C R M H R I T H O E B E A T V W H
C F N H C A J D B W P L I Z D E K X U Y
H D S F U N V I W Y P S N N Z K O I N C
I W I Q R O R A H Q W Q Z Y T I F O J A
A C V H Y M V I T A L S I G N S F R T R
L O E Y W E T Y M P A N I C A B B Q Q D
C U F F L T H Y P E R T E N S I O N K I
L V R S T E X S Y S T O L E U G C L V A
X L A E L R R A D I A L Y T I U M O O T
```

WORD SEARCH CLUES

1. All four: body temperature, pulse, respiratory rate, and blood pressure (two words)
2. Artery in the neck that is the site for taking a pulse during cardiopulmonary resuscitation
3. Device for determining blood pressure
4. A contraction of the heart ventricles during which blood is forced into the aorta and the pulmonary artery
5. A count of heartbeats; can also refer to the pressure that is the difference between systolic and diastolic blood pressure (40 mm Hg)
6. Element used in a device that records body temperature and also in a device that records blood pressure
7. Fever; temperature values greater than 37.0°C or 98.6°F
8. Heartbeat at a rate greater than 100 beats per minute
9. Inflatable component of a sphygmomanometer that wraps around the patient's arm during recording of blood pressure
10. Listening for sounds produced within the body
11. The lower number in a recorded blood pressure fraction; marks the pressure at the last distinct tap heard on the sphygmomanometer
12. Lower-than-normal body temperature; values below 96.0°F
13. Normal tension or tone; pertaining to having normal blood pressure
14. Noted along with volume and strength when counting the pulse rate
15. Oxygen deficiency
16. Pulse taken using fingertips placed at the wrist
17. The site used to find the pulse for an infant
18. The sound of blood passing through blood vessels that is produced by vibratory motion of the arterial wall
19. A systolic blood pressure of 140 mm Hg or greater and diastolic blood pressure of 90 mm Hg or greater
20. Temporary cessation of spontaneous respirations
21. A type of thermometer that is gently inserted into the ear canal
22. Unusually slow heartbeat and pulse; below 50 beats per minute

CHAPTER 11

Extraoral and Intraoral Examination

Upon successful completion of these exercises, you will be able to:

1. Identify and define key terms and concepts related to providing an intraoral and extraoral patient examination.
2. List and describe the objectives of the examination of the oral cavity and adjacent structures by the dental hygienist.
3. List and describe the steps for a thorough examination.
4. Accurately describe conditions and lesions found during an oral examination.
5. List the warning signs of oral cancer and discuss the follow-up procedure for a suspicious lesion.

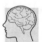 **KNOWLEDGE EXERCISES**

Write your answers for each question in the space provided.

1. Briefly list a dental hygienist's objectives for performing extraoral and intraoral examinations.

   _____
   _____
   _____
   _____
   _____
   _____
   _____
   _____
   _____

2. As you get ready to perform an examination for your patient, you should

   ■ *Review:* _____
   _____

   ■ *Examine:* _____
   _____

   ■ *Explain:* _____
   _____

3. In your own words, explain the advantages of using a systematic sequence for patient examination.

   _____
   _____

4. Match the types of palpation with the appropriate definition and description. There are two answers for each type of palpation.

TYPES OF PALPATION	DEFINITION/DESCRIPTION
Digital: _____ and _____ **Bimanual:** _____ and _____ **Bilateral:** _____ and _____ **Bidigital:** _____ and _____	A. Use of finger or fingers and thumb from each hand applied simultaneously in coordination B. Use of a finger C. Two hands used at the same time to examine corresponding structures on opposite sides of the body D. Use of finger and thumb of the same hand E. Palpation of the lips F. Index finger applied to the inner border of the mandible beneath the canine-premolar area to determine the presence of a torus mandibularis G. Index finger of one hand palpates the floor of the mouth inside, while a finger or fingers from the other hand press on the same area from under the chin externally H. Fingers placed beneath the chin to palpate the submandibular lymph nodes

5. In your own words, define the following types of documentation recorded for each oral lesion.

■ *History:* _____

_____

_____

■ *Location and extent:* _____

_____

_____

■ *Size and shape:* _____

_____

_____

■ *Color:* _____

_____

_____

■ *Surface texture:* _____

_____

_____

6. Identify the characteristics you would expect to observe for each of the following types of oral lesions.

a. *Indurated:* _____

b. *Blisterform:* _____

c. *Pustule:* _____

d. *Plaque:* _____

e. *Ulcer:* _____

f. *Erythema:* _____

g. *Torus:* _____

h. *Papillary:* _____

7. Early oral cancer takes many forms. Write a brief description of the characteristics you might observe for each of the five basic forms listed below.

White Areas: _____

_____

_____

Red Areas: _____

_____

_____

Ulcers: _____

_____

_____

Masses: _____

_____

_____

Pigmentation: _____

_____

_____

8. What characteristics indicate that a lesion should be biopsied?

_____

_____

_____

_____

9. When is a cytologic smear technique used to evaluate an oral lesion?

_____

_____

10. Briefly describe exfoliative cytology in your own words.

_____

_____

11. If the slide is found to be inadequate for diagnosis, explain in your own words why this happened.

_____

_____

12. Match each laboratory report category with its description.

LABORATORY REPORT CATEGORY	DESCRIPTION
_____ Class I	A. Normal
_____ Unsatisfactory	B. Uncertain (possible for cancer)
_____ Class V	C. Slide is inadequate for diagnosis
_____ Class II	D. Probable for cancer
_____ Class IV	E. Atypical, but not suggestive of malignant cells
_____ Class III	F. Positive for cancer

13. Using the information in Box 11-1, Table 11-1, and Figure 11-9 in the textbook, imagine that your patient presents with the conditions listed in Infomap 11-1. Complete the Infomap by identifying the indications and influences on the appointment associated with each observation.

INFOMAP 11-1

ORDER OF EXAMINATION	OBSERVATION	INDICATION AND INFLUENCES ON THE APPOINTMENT
Overall appraisal of patient	Labored breathing	
Face	Evidence of fear or apprehension	
Skin	Multiple light brown macules	
Eyes	Eyeglasses (corrective)	
Nodes Submental; submandibular	Lymphadenopathy	

ORDER OF EXAMINATION	OBSERVATION	INDICATION AND INFLUENCES ON THE APPOINTMENT
Temporomandibular joint	Tenderness; sensitivity; noises (clicking, popping, grating)	
Lips	Blisters, ulcers	
Breath odor	Cigarette odor	
Labial and buccal mucosa	Multiple red nodules on left buccal mucosa	
Tongue	Coating	
Floor of mouth	Limitation or freedom of movement of tongue	
Saliva	Evidences of dry mouth; lip wetting	
Hard palate	Tori	
Soft palate, uvula	Large uvula	
Tonsillar region, throat	Large tonsils	

✓ COMPETENCY EXERCISES

Apply information from the chapter and use critical thinking skills to complete the Competency exercises. Write responses on paper or create electronic documents to submit your answers.

1. List the steps (in the correct order) that you will follow to prepare for an EXTRAORAL examination of your patient.

2. List the steps (in the correct order) that you will follow to prepare for an INTRAORAL examination of your patient.

3. Your patient, Kurt Bachleim, age 23 years, presents with localized, coalescing multiple lesions on the right buccal mucosa. Mr. Bachleim also has an exostosis extending from tooth 12 to tooth 15 and trismus. Describe what you would expect to see and any possible adaptations you will need to make for the appointment.

4. Your patient, Yoon Chang, presents with a tiny (about 1 mm) bluish-black lesion on the top right half of her tongue. She said that it was not bothering her at all. You palpate the lesion, but do not feel anything unusual. Ms. Chang reports that the same thing had come up on her palate a few weeks ago. As you continue to question her, she mentions that she has had a broken blood vessel or two on her fingers in the past. She had actually forgotten about it until you started asking questions. Dr. Pine is not in the office today, so you document the lesion in the patient record in order to discuss it with him tomorrow and decide appropriate follow-up procedures. Use your institution's guidelines for writing in the patient record and the information in Chapter 11 to describe the lesion on Ms. Chang's tongue.

Everyday Ethics

*Before completing the learning exercises below, reread and reflect on the **Everyday Ethics Scenario and Questions for Consideration in this chapter of the textbook**. It may also be useful to review the Dental Hygiene Ethics discussion in Chapter 1, the Ethical Applications in the introduction pages for each Section in the textbook, as well as the Codes of Ethics in Appendices I, II, and III.*

Collaborative Learning Activity
NOTE: The Everyday Ethics Scenario in this chapter contains two different ethical components for the dental hygienist: providing information for her patient and approaching her coworkers to change office policies. Work with a group of students to provide alternate approaches for each of the two ethical concerns in the scenario.

■ Work with a small group to develop a 2- to 5-minute role play that introduces the Everyday Ethics scenario described in the chapter (a great idea is to video record your role play activity). Then develop separate 2-minute role play scenarios that provide at least two alternative approaches/solutions to resolve the situation. Ask classmates to view the solutions, ask questions, and discuss the ethical approach used in each. Ask classmates to vote for the "best solution."

Factors To Teach The Patient

This scenario is related to the following factors listed in this chapter of the textbook:

■ The reasons for a careful extraoral and intraoral examination at each maintenance appointment
■ A method for self-examination (The examination should include the face, neck, lips, gingiva, cheeks, tongue, palate, and throat. Any changes should be reported to the dentist and the dental hygienist.)
■ The warning signs of oral cancer

Aishia Williams presents for a new patient examination. During your assessment, you discover that she has previously been treated for oral cancer and is at risk for recurrence. She has not been evaluated for 18 months.

Use the examples of patient conversations in Appendix D of this workbook as a guide to write a statement explaining the need for careful follow-up and frequent evaluation by a dental professional as well as the need for Ms. Williams to perform a regular oral self-examination and to be aware of the warning signs of oral cancer.

Use the conversation you create to role play this situation with a fellow student. If you are the patient in the role play, be sure to ask questions. If you are the dental hygienist, try to anticipate questions and answer them in your explanation.

Dental Radiographic Imaging

Learning Objectives

Upon successful completion of these exercises, you will be able to:

1. Identify and define key terms, abbreviations, and concepts related to exposing and processing dental radiographs.
2. Describe procedures for producing and processing x-rays and digital x-ray images.
3. Identify measures to protect yourself and your patient from ionizing radiations.
4. Select film size and type, film-holding devices, and clinical radiographic techniques for patient surveys.
5. Describe the positioning of individual intraoral film packets based on the area of the mouth and clinical technique.
6. Use guidelines to determine the indication for exposure of dental radiographs.
7. Identify probable causes of common radiographic inadequacies.

KNOWLEDGE EXERCISES

Write your answers for each question in the space provided.

EXPOSING AND PROCESSING RADIOGRAPHS

1. In your own words, state two important objectives of dental radiology.

   _____

   _____

2. Using the diagrams and descriptions in the textbook as a reference, describe in your own words how x-rays are produced after the power switch on the x-ray machine is activated.

   _____

   _____

   _____

3. Collimation refers to:

   _____

   _____

   _____

4. How does a change in mA affect the final radiographic image?

   _____

5. Identify how increasing the kilovoltage affects the image density.

   _____

6. How is image contrast affected by increasing the kilovoltage?

   _____

   _____

7. List two advantages of high kVp.

_____

_____

8. List three advantages of lengthening the target-to-film distance during exposure of patient radiographs.

_____

_____

_____

9. How can the target-to-film distance lengthened when using an individual x-ray unit?

_____

10. Identify three components to consider when selecting dental radiograph film.

_____

_____

_____

11. What are the advantages of using digital radiography?

_____

_____

_____

_____

_____

_____

12. Correctly sequence the following steps in producing an INDIRECT digital radiograph, numbering them from 1 to 5 (1 = first step; 5 = final step).

_____ Electronic charge activates the sensor

_____ Image is scanned using a laser scanner

_____ Image stored on the PSP plate

_____ Sensor placed in patient's mouth

_____ Image displayed on computer

13. What type of digital imaging uses a sensor with a cord attached?

_____

14. The digital radiograph captures an image using _____ shades of gray.

RADIATION SAFETY

1. Identify three factors that influence the biologic effects of radiation on cells.

_____

_____

_____

2. List human tissues and organs that are highly radiosensitive.

_____

_____

_____

_____

3. List three ways to protect yourself from primary and leakage radiation while making patient radiographs.

_____

_____

_____

4. Relative to your patient's head, where can you best stand to protect yourself from secondary radiation?

_____

_____

5. List the ways you can protect your patient during exposure of dental radiographs.

_____

_____

_____

CLINICAL TECHNIQUES

1. Describe a complete dental radiographic survey.

_____

_____

2. When a rectangular position-indicating device (PID) is used for beam collimation when you expose dental radiographs, how do you adjust the x-ray machine to accommodate both horizontal and vertical film positioning?

_____

_____

3. Match the area of the mouth or teeth listed below with the radiographic film or sensor size most frequently used. Each film/sensor size may be used more than once.

INTRAORAL AREA	FILM/SENSOR SIZE
_____ Overlapping anterior teeth	A. Size No. 0
_____ Permanent dentition bitewings	B. Size No. 1
_____ Primary teeth	C. Size No. 2
_____ Adult posterior (periapical view)	
_____ Child maxillary (occlusal view)	

4. Select one correct answer to complete the following statement. When exposing a periapical film of tooth 12, directing the central ray with too much vertical angle will produce an image of the tooth that has roots that appear to be very _____.

5. Identify three reasons why the paralleling technique usually produces better images with increased patient safety than the bisecting-angle technique.

_____

_____

_____

6. When positioning the film inside the patient's mouth, the stippled or colored side of the film packet is placed:

_____

7. To maintain a visually open contact on a bitewing x-ray, the horizontal angle of the central beam is directed:

_____

_____

8. How do you position the patient's head when you are making an occlusal survey image of the mandibular teeth?

_____

9. If the patient's head is tilted to the side or the occlusal plane is not parallel with the floor, the angle of the PID must be altered to adapt the central ray to the patient's position. List two conditions that must be met when you are using the paralleling technique to expose periapical radiographs.

_____

_____

10. List the reasons why images of oral structures on a panoramic x-ray may have poor detail or be distorted even if you are very careful to use proper techniques when exposing the radiograph.

_____

_____

_____

_____

11. Identify one reason that a panoramic image may be ordered instead of or in addition to periapical films for an individual patient.

_____

_____

IN AND OUT OF THE DARKROOM

1. Exposure to radiation changes the silver halide crystals coating x-ray film to _____ and _____ ions.

2. After developing the film, only the amount of _____ _____ corresponding to radiolucency and radiopacity remains.

3. The fixer solution removes the _____ _____ crystals that were not exposed to radiation.

4. Correct processing temperature and time for optimal manual processing are _____ °F and _____ minutes.

5. If the temperature of the solutions is higher than the optimal, the amount of time that the film remains in the developer should be _____.

6. What kind of safelight filter is used in a darkroom when processing both intraoral and extraoral films?

_____

_____

7. Match the image inadequacy commonly found on dental x-rays (first column) with the most probable cause of the problem (second column).

IMAGE INADEQUACY	PROBABLE CAUSE
____ Dark lines across film	A. Extreme increase in vertical angle
____ Double image	B. Film exposed twice
____ Foreshortening	C. Bent film
____ Large dark stain on one end of the film safelight	D. Unsafe safelight
____ Light image with a pattern overlaying the image	E. Sudden temperature change in processing solutions
____ Puckered surface	F. Static electricity
____ Stretched appearance of images	G. Film placed backwards in mouth
____ Whole film too dark	H. Overlap of film in developer

8. List anatomic landmarks (besides the teeth) that you might locate on an x-ray of your patient's mandibular incisor area.

_____

_____

_____

9. Name a mandibular structure that could appear on a maxillary third molar x-ray.

_____

10. Identify the factors that will enhance interpretation of images on patient radiographs.

_____

_____

_____

_____

_____

_____

✓ COMPETENCY EXERCISES

Apply information from the chapter and use critical thinking skills to complete the competency exercises. Write responses on paper or create electronic documents to submit your answers.

1. In your own words, explain the relationship between the tooth, the film, and the central beam of radiation when using the paralleling technique. (*Hint:* Use your hands as a three-dimensional way to "draw" the images so you can visualize them as you try to explain.)

2. Mrs. Honey Davis, age 42, presents in your clinic for her initial appointment. She states that she has come because she needs her teeth cleaned and because a tooth on the upper left side of her mouth has been bothering her. She has not been to visit a dentist for 2 years. She states that she had a lot of x-rays taken when she was last examined by her previous dentist just before she moved to your town but that she did not bring them with her today.

   When collecting your initial assessment data, you identify no positive clinical signs/symptoms of periodontal disease and no clinical evidence of active dental caries. She has six small amalgam restorations in her posterior teeth; only tooth 19 has a restoration on a proximal surface. However, Mrs. Davis reports intermittent use of mint candy to combat a feeling of dry mouth caused by a medication she takes. You also note an accumulation of biofilm on proximal tooth surfaces.

   You are planning to ask Dr. Gray, your employer, to examine Mrs. Davis. You know that he will probably order some x-rays. Using Tables 12-4, 12-5 and 12-6 in the textbook, determine which x-rays would be recommended for Mrs. Davis and why.

3. You plan to expose a periapical radiograph of Mrs. Davis's tooth 15 using the paralleling technique. Explain the following:
   a. Where the front edge of the film should be positioned.
   b. How the film is placed relative to the long axis of tooth 15 and the mesial/distal line of that tooth.
   c. How the central beam of radiation is directed relative to the long axis of tooth 15.
   d. Where the lingual cusp of tooth 15 should rest in a disposable styrofoam film holder.

4. After you take all of the films prescribed for Mrs. Davis and place them in a paper cup, you will go into the darkroom to process the films. Create a step-by step procedure for infection control and processing the films.

5. In spite of your attempts to reassure him of the appropriateness and safety of the bitewing x-rays prescribed by the dentist, your patient, Jeff Darlington, has refused to have any x-rays taken

at his recall appointment. Using your institution's guidelines for writing in patient records, document that he has refused the recommended exposures.

6. Gather a variety of dental radiographs taken in your clinic that are currently not being used for patient care. Place them in x-ray mounts for easy viewing. Evaluate the radiographs using Table 12-10, Analysis of Radiographs, in the textbook.

   Identify any errors in the technique or processing and describe possible causes and corrections you can make to eliminate the problem. Compare your evaluation of the films with those made by one or two of your student colleagues. Discuss any differences in the way you each evaluated the same x-ray or the corrective measures you described for an error.

DISCOVERY EXERCISE

Gather a variety of dental radiographs taken in your clinic that are currently not being used for patient care. Place them in x-ray mounts for easy viewing. What additional resources will help you to identify the anatomic landmarks visible on each film?

Everyday Ethics

*Before completing the learning exercises below, reread and reflect on the **Everyday Ethics Scenario and Questions for Consideration in this chapter of the textbook.** It may also be useful to review the Dental Hygiene Ethics discussion in Chapter 1, the Ethical Applications in the introduction pages for each Section in the textbook, as well as the Codes of Ethics in Appendices I, II, and III.*

Individual Learning Activity
Imagine that you are the dental hygienist in this scenario. Answer each of the questions for consideration at the end of the scenario.

Discovery Activity
Ask a friend or relative who is not involved in healthcare to read the scenario and discuss it with you from the perspective of a "patient" who receives services within the healthcare system. Discuss what you learned from the concerns, insights, or difference in perspective that person expressed.

Factors To Teach The Patient

This scenario is related to the following factors listed in this chapter of the textbook:

■ When the patient asks about the safety of radiation

As you talk with Mr. Glazier, you realize that not only is he concerned about why additional x-rays are necessary, but he is extremely concerned about the safety and negative effects of the additional dose of radiation he will receive. Using the examples of patient conversations from Appendix D as a guide, write a statement explaining all of the safety factors in place in your clinic to protect him from excessive exposure to radiation.

Use the conversation you create to role play this situation with a fellow student. If you are the patient in the role play, be sure to ask questions. If you are the dental hygienist, try to anticipate questions and answer them in your explanation.

CROSSWORD PUZZLE

ACROSS

1. Acronym that refers to the collimator cone of the x-ray machine
3. The secondary shadow that surrounds the periphery of the primary shadow; a blurred margin
5. The appearance of dark images on a radiograph as a result of the greater amount of radiation that penetrates low-density objects
7. As low as reasonably achievable
9. Refers to the dose that results from repeated exposure to radiation
11. Filmless radiography system that stores images on a computer
12. Refers to the minimum dose that produces any detectable effect on body tissues
14. Refers to the maximum dose of radiation a person can receive and not expect significantly harmful results
17. The appearance of light (white) images on a radiograph as a result of the amount of radiation that is absorbed by dense objects
18. Beam of radiation directed at right angles to the film or sensor when using the paralleling technique (two words)
19. Refers to body cells, with the exclusion of germ cells
21. The technique used for controlling the size and shape of the primary radiation beam that exits the position indicating devise
22. The art and science of making radiographs
23. Radiation that has been deviated from its primary direction during passage through a substance; a form of secondary radiation

DOWN

1. Refers to the beam of x-ray photons that bounces in all directions from the anode of an x-ray machine
2. Refers to the dose of radiation absorbed when the central beam passes through body tissue
4. Refers to the beam of primary radiation that comes off the anode to exit the x-ray machine directly through the position indicating device
6. The dose of radiation that is, or could be, sufficient to cause death
8. Refers to the dose of radiation imparted at a specific exposure point
9. Tungsten filament, which is a coiled wire heated to generate a cloud of electrons; has a negative charge
10. Small intraoral detector that captures a digital radiographic image
13. That branch of science that deals with the use of radiation in the diagnosis and treatment of disease
15. Refers to the dose of radiation that produces the appearance of redness on human skin
16. An error of technique that results when the beam of radiation does not completely cover the film being exposed (two words)
20. A tungsten target embedded in a copper stem, positioned at an angle to the electron beam; has a positive charge

Study Casts

Learning Objectives

Upon successful completion of these exercises, you will be able to:

1. Identify and define key terms and concepts related to making oral study casts.
2. List and discuss the purposes and uses of study casts.
3. Identify the supplies, steps, and procedures involved in taking an impression.
4. List the supplies, steps, and procedures involved in making a study cast.

 KNOWLEDGE EXERCISES

Write your answers for each question in the space provided.

1. Your patient wants to know why you are recommending taking an impression for a study cast and how can study casts be used for different kinds of patients, not just her. In your own words, describe the uses and purposes of study casts.

_____

_____

_____

_____

_____

_____

_____

_____

_____

2. You are asked to order all the supplies you will need for taking patient impressions and pouring study casts. List the supplies you will order.

_____

_____

_____

_____

_____

_____

_____

_____

_____

3. You have tried in the impression tray for your patient.

   a. In checking the width of the tray, you allowed for an adequate thickness of impression material on the facial and lingual surfaces of each tooth to provide _____ and _____ to the impression.

b. Your patient has a tooth in prominent linguoversion, so you allowed for a minimum thickness of _____ in.

c. When you checked the length of the tray, you made sure to allow coverage of the _____ area of the mandible and the _____ of the maxilla.

4. The steps involved in taking a maxillary impression are listed below. You have already tried in and prepared the tray. Number the list in the correct order (1 = first step; 6 = last step).

_____ Seat the tray from posterior to anterior.

_____ Maintain equal pressure on each side of the tray.

_____ Rinse under cool running water and proceed with disinfection for maxillary cast.

_____ Insert the tray with a rotary motion.

_____ Elevate the cheek over the edge of the impression to break the seal, and remove the impression with a sudden jerk.

_____ Ask the patient to form a tight O with the lips to mold the impression material.

5. Mark each of the following statements **true or false** by circling the correct answer. If the statement is false, correct it, and write the true statement in the space provided.

a. **True or False** The material used for the interocclusal record is placed over the occlusal surfaces, and the patient is directed to close in habitual occlusion.

_____

_____

b. **True or False** When the leftover material on the spatula has lost its surface stickiness, the impression should be held in position in the patient's mouth for two more minutes.

_____

_____

c. **True or False** You stand behind the patient to take a mandibular impression.

_____

_____

d. **True or False** A removable oral prosthesis is left in the patient's mouth while the impression is taken.

_____

_____

e. **True or False** Spatulating the impression material for 2 minutes will allow the chemical reactions to proceed uniformly.

_____

_____

f. **True or False** Plaster produces a cast fairly susceptible to breakage.

_____

_____

g. **True or False** Ideal gelation time for impression material is between 7 and 9 minutes when the room temperature is 20 to 21°C (68 to 70°F).

_____

_____

h. **True or False** The patient is positioned in a supine position when you take an impression.

_____

_____

i. **True or False** To lower the surface tension, the patient should take a deep breath.

_____

_____

j. **True or False** The teeth are wet with the air/water syringe before the impression is taken.

_____

_____

k. **True or False** The most frequent error in the use of the alginates for impressions is delay in pouring the cast.

_____

_____

l. **True or False** You stand at the side and toward the back of the patient to take a maxillary impression.

_____

_____

m. **True or False** If you have delayed trimming after separating the impression from the cast, the cast must be thoroughly soaked in water before trimming.

_____

_____

n. **True or False** You can wait until you have a break in your schedule before you pour the alginate impression.

_____

_____

o. **True or False** The impression tray is seated with a rotary motion.

_____

_____

p. **True or False** Dust particles from the alginate impression material can cause serious irritation to the eyes.

_____

_____

q. **True or False** Seat the posterior portion of the tray before the anterior portion.

_____

_____

r. **True or False** A wax rim around the borders of the tray prevents discomfort.

_____

_____

s. **True or False** The maxillary cast is trimmed to a point, and the mandibular cast is rounded.

_____

_____

t. **True or False** Rock the impression back and forth to release it.

_____

_____

u. **True or False** Vestibular areas, occlusal surfaces, and undercut areas should be precoated with wax.

_____

_____

v. **True or False** Wax is the only material available for obtaining a bite registration.

_____

_____

6. The steps involved in mixing dental stone are given below. First complete the sentences, and then number the list in the correct order (1 = first step; 6 = last step).

____ Sift in the powder gradually to _____ _____ _____ and to allow each particle to become _____.

____ Measure the water and powder according to the manufacturer's specifications. (The ratio of water to powder is _____ ml of water for _____ grams of stone.)

____ Stir briefly until all powder is wet, then vibrate the mix to release _____ _____.

____ Place measured water (which is at _____ temperature) in a clean, dry mixing bowl.

____ The result is a _____ _____ _____ mix.

____ Use a vacuum mixer.

7. Dental stone is sensitive to changes in the relative humidity of the atmosphere. List some strategies that protect the stone.

_____

_____

_____

8. Water controls the strength, rigidity, and hardness of the cast.

■ Increasing the water to dental stone ratio _____ the strength of the cast.

■ Temperature affects the setting time of the dental stone: _____ water increases it, and _____ water decreases it.

9. Complete the following sentences to describe the process of pouring the anatomic portion of the cast.

a. Shake any _____ out of the impression.

b. Start at the most posterior tooth and allow the mix to flow through the impression. Use _____ amounts and vibrate continually. _____ the impression so that the material passes into the tooth indentions and flows slowly down the side, across the _____ surface or the _____ edge.

c. Air is trapped when the process is hurried or ____ _____.

d. When all tooth indentations are covered, add larger amounts of mix to slightly _____ the impressions. Vibrate.

10. The base of the cast can be made using a variety of techniques. List the steps for each of the following techniques.

■ Rubber model base former

_____

_____

_____

■ Two-step or double pour

_____

_____

_____

_____

■ Boxing technique

_____

_____

_____

_____

11. The exact proportions of the study casts and the steps required to accomplish the trimming and finishing depend on several factors. List these factors.

_____

_____

_____

12. In your own words, describe the features of an acceptable study cast. Use the figures in Chapter 11 of the textbook to help you visualize your descriptions.

_____

_____

_____

_____

13. Complete the following sentences related to finishing and polishing of the completed cast.

a. Allow casts to dry thoroughly for _____.

b. Smooth the art portion with _____ _____.

c. Soak in heated soap solution for _____.

d. Rub with a _____.

e. _____ may be used to help polish the cast.

COMPETENCY EXERCISES

Apply information from the chapter and use critical thinking skills to complete the competency exercises. Write responses on paper or create electronic documents to submit your answers.

Privesh Doshi is a dental assistant at the dental clinic in which you are practicing. Dr. Pecharo has asked you to teach Privesh how to take an impression (assume that you are in a state or province where it is legal for dental assistants to make impressions). You decide the best way to teach is to make a checklist so Privesh can follow it every time he is taking an impression.

1. Create the checklist.

2. Privesh is concerned about making the patient gag. Give him some suggestions on how to prevent this.

3. Privesh is concerned about taking the impressions. He needs more information on how to mix the alginate material and wants to know how much time he has to insert the material into the patient's mouth. Explain these procedures.

4. The alginate impression that Privesh took this morning has been sitting on the counter in the laboratory for 4 hours. What are your concerns?

Everyday Ethics

*Before completing the learning exercises below, reread and reflect on the **Everyday Ethics Scenario and Questions for Consideration in this chapter of the textbook.** It may also be useful to review the Dental Hygiene Ethics discussion in Chapter 1, the Ethical Applications in the introduction pages for each Section in the textbook, as well as the Codes of Ethics in Appendices I, II, and III.*

Discovery Activities

■ Ask a dental hygienist who has been practicing for a year or more to read the scenario. Provide them

with a copy of the Code of Ethics as well. Share the responses you have made to answer each question and ask that person to discuss the situation with you. What insights did you have or what did you learn during this discussion?

■ Ask a friend or relative who is not involved in healthcare to read the scenario and discuss it with you from the perspective of a "patient" who receives services within the healthcare system. Discuss what you learned from the concerns, insights, or difference in perspective that person expressed.

Factors To Teach The Patient

This scenario is related to the following factors listed in this chapter of the textbook:

■ Importance and purposes of study casts; reasons for comparative casts after treatment or at a later date
■ Use of the casts of other patients to show effects of treatment or what can happen if the prescribed treatment is not carried out

You have just seated your patient, Mrs. Lorna Patel. Refer the Section III Summary exercises if you would like to review her

care plan. Before this appointment, Mrs. Patel was unaware of the generalized moderate attrition in her mouth.

Using the example of patient conversations in Appendix D as a guide, write a statement explaining to Mrs. Patel the need to take the alginate impression to make study casts so you can document her condition. Be sure to discuss the need to fabricate a night guard and why study casts will help you do that. Compare your conversation with one developed by a student colleague to identify any missing information.

CHAPTER 14

The Periodontium

Learning Objectives

Upon successful completion of these exercises, you will be able to:

1. Identify and define key terms and concepts related to the gingiva.
2. Identify the clinical features of the periodontal tissues that must be examined for a complete assessment.
3. List the markers for periodontal infection and classify them by type, degree of severity, and causative factors.
4. Identify gingival landmarks and discuss their significance.

 KNOWLEDGE EXERCISES

Write your answers for each question in the space provided.

1. Match each term with the appropriate definition.

TERMS RELATED TO THE GINGIVA	DEFINITION
Generalized _____ Marginal _____ Clinical crown _____ Papillary _____ Anatomic root _____ Diffuse _____ Anatomic crown _____ Localized _____ Clinical root _____	A. A change that is confined to the free or marginal gingiva. B. The gingiva is involved about all or nearly all of the teeth throughout the mouth. C. A change that involves a papilla but not the rest of the free gingiva around a tooth. D. Spread out, dispersed; affects the gingival margin, attached gingiva, and interdental papillae; may extend into alveolar mucosa. E. Indicates the gingiva around a single tooth or a specific group of teeth. F. The part of the tooth above the attached periodontal tissues; can be considered the part of the tooth where clinical treatment procedures are applied. G. The part of the tooth below the base of the gingival sulcus or periodontal pocket; the part of the root to which periodontal fibers are attached. H. The part of the tooth covered by enamel. I. The part of the tooth covered by cementum.

2. Define the following terms in your own words. (*Hint:* You may want to think about location as you define each term.)

   ■ Masticatory mucosa

   _____

   _____

   ■ Lining mucosa

   _____

   _____

   ■ Cementum

   _____

   _____

   ■ Alveolar bone

   _____

   _____

   ■ Free gingival groove

   _____

   _____

   ■ Gingival sulcus (crevice)

   _____

   _____

   ■ Interdental gingiva

   _____

   _____

   ■ Col

   _____

   _____

3. Draw and label the periodontal ligament in the correct position on Figure 14-1.

4. Use the following terms to label Figure 14-1 with each of the components of the gingiva and periodontium.

   ■ Alveolar bone

   ■ Alveolar mucosa

   ■ Attached gingiva

   ■ Cementoenamel junction

   ■ Enamel

   ■ Free gingiva

   ■ Free gingival groove

   ■ Gingival margin

   ■ Gingival sulcus

   ■ Junctional epithelium

   ■ Mucogingival junction

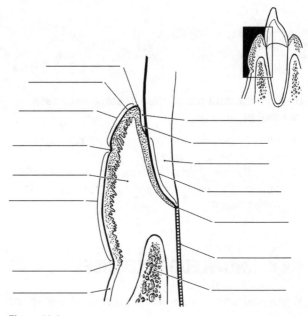

Figure 14-1

5. Draw the following gingival fibers in their correct position on the Figure 14-1 diagram. Use colored pencils to help differentiate.

   ■ Alveologingival fibers

   ■ Circumferential fibers

   ■ Dentogingival fibers

   ■ Dentoperiosteal fibers

6. Use the following terms to label the diagram of teeth and gingiva in Figure 14-2.

   ■ Alveolar mucosa

   ■ Attached gingiva

- Free gingiva

- Interdental papilla

- Mandibular labial frenum

- Maxillary labial frenum

- Mucogingival junction

7. Match the gingival fiber group with the correct location and purpose.

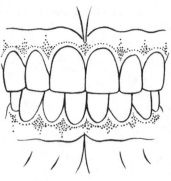

Figure 14-2

GINGIVAL FIBER GROUP	LOCATION AND PURPOSE
Dentogingival fibers_____ Transseptal fibers_____ Dentoperiosteal fibers_____ Apical fibers_____ Inter-radicular fibers_____ Circumferential fibers_____ Oblique fibers_____ Alveolar crest fibers_____ Alveologingival fibers_____ Horizontal fibers_____	A. From the cervical area of one tooth across to an adjacent tooth (on the mesial or distal side only) to provide resistance to separation of teeth. B. From the cementum in the cervical region into the free gingiva to give support to the gingiva. C. From the root apex to adjacent surrounding bone to resist vertical forces. D. From the root above the apical fibers obliquely toward the occlusal to resist vertical and unexpected strong forces. E. From the alveolar crest into the free and attached gingiva to provide support. F. From the cervical cementum over the alveolar crest to blend with fibers of the periosteum of the bone. G. From the cementum in the middle of each root to the adjacent alveolar bone to resist tipping of the tooth. H. From the alveolar crest to the cementum just below the cementoenamel junction to resist intrusive forces. I. Continuous around the neck of the tooth to help maintain the tooth in position. J. From the cementum between the roots of multirooted teeth to the adjacent bone to resist vertical and lateral forces.

8. To complete this exercise using Figure 14-2 you will need red, blue, and green pencils.

- On the left side of the diagram, color the interdental papilla in both the maxillary and mandibular arch in red.

- On the right side of the drawing, color the free gingiva in blue.

- On the right side of the drawing, color the attached gingiva in green.

9. You are getting ready to do an examination of Patrice Davis, who is a professional ice skater and is curious about everything. She wants to know exactly how you are going to check her "gum tissues," and she does not want you to "skate over anything." She really wants to have a nice smile for the competitions! Explain the purpose of the examination to Patrice and list the markers you will use to describe the appearance of her oral tissues.

_____

_____

_____

_____

_____

_____

_____

_____

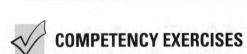 **COMPETENCY EXERCISES**

Apply information from the chapter and use critical thinking skills to complete the competency exercises. Write responses on paper or create electronic documents to submit your answers.

1. Your patient, Tucker McLeimgreen, presents with clinically normal-appearing gingiva. Describe in your own words what you expect to observe as you examine Tucker's gingival tissues both visually and with a probe.

2. Your patient, Xin Singer, is very concerned about the areas of localized, wide, shallow recession she has

on teeth 6 and 7 and the narrow, deep (with missing attached gingiva) recession she has on teeth 24 and 25. Using Figures 12-1 and 12-2 as a guide, draw a sketch of the recession that is described here. Then identify the points you will discuss with Xin.

3. Your patient, Frank Catty, presents with gingiva that looks like the tissue pictured in Figure 14-10B in the textbook. On the basis of your understanding of this condition, describe Frank's gingival tissue using the following markers: color, size, shape, consistency, surface texture, position of the gingival margin, and bleeding.

4. You are providing care for Kathleen Gallagher. She is a research scientist particularly interested in inflammation. You have just completed the gingival examination and are planning to discuss the information you have gathered and the causes for the oral changes you have documented. Kathleen has not received dental care for 5 years, and she is worried about her "bleeding gums" and wants to know exactly why these changes are occurring. Refer to Table 14-1 in the textbook to help you collect your thoughts and then explain the *reasons* for each change listed in the next column.

- Color: bright red

- Size: enlarged

- Shape: bulbous papillae

- Consistency: soft, spongy (dents readily when pressed with probe)

- Surface texture: smooth, shiny gingival

- Position of gingival margin: enlarged; higher on the tooth, above normal; pocket deepened

- Position of junctional epithelium: probing is within normal limits

- Bleeding: spontaneous

- Exudate: none on pressure

5. For some kinds of patient records, you will need to describe a patient's condition in sentence form. Document a brief gingival description that you will include in Kathleen Gallagher's record.

Everyday Ethics

Before completing the learning exercises below, reread and reflect on the Everyday Ethics scenario and Questions for Consideration in this chapter of the textbook. It may also be useful to review the Dental Hygiene Ethics discussion in Chapter 1, the Ethical Applications in the introduction pages for each section in the textbook, as well as the Codes of Ethics in Appendices I, II, and III.

Individual Learning Activities
Identify a situation you have experienced that presents a similar ethical dilemma. Write about you would do differ-

ently now than you did at the time the incident happened— support your discussion with concepts from the dental hygiene codes of ethics.

Discovery Activity
Summarize this scenario for faculty member at your school and ask them to consider the questions that are included. Is their perspective different than yours or similar? Explain.

Factors To Teach The Patient

This scenario is related to the following factors:

- Characteristics of normal healthy gingiva
- The significance of bleeding; healthy tissue does not bleed
- Relationship of findings during a gingival examination to the personal daily care procedures for infection control

You have just seen Kathleen Gallagher, the patient described in Competency Exercise 4. She is very anxious now that you have told her about all the implications of your findings from the gingival examination.

Working with the data you have collected and the causative factors you have identified, and using the examples of patient conversations in Appendix D as a guide, write a statement explaining what type of tissue changes you would like to see at Kathleen's next appointment.

Use the conversation you create to role-play this situation with a fellow student. If you are the patient in the role-play, be sure to ask questions. If you are the dental hygienist, try to anticipate questions and answer them in your explanation.

CROSSWORD PUZZLE

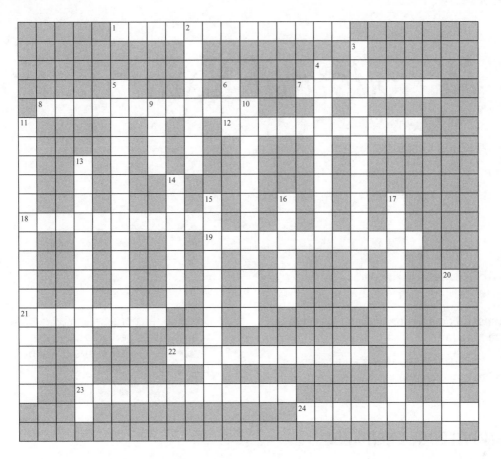

ACROSS

1. One of two structures that together create a cell junction and form an attachment between junctional epithelial cells and the tooth surface.
7. A fibrous change of the mucous membrane as a result of chronic inflammation.
8. Tissue that surround and support the teeth.
12. Formation of pus.
18. Increase in size of tissue or organ caused by an increase in size of its constituent cells.
19. Variation in gingival color related to complexion or race.
21. Fibrous connective tissue that surrounds and attaches the roots of teeth to the alveolar bone.
22. The act of chewing.
23. Characterized by increased blood flow, increased permeability of capillaries and increased collection of defense cells and tissue fluid/usually produces alterations in color, size, shape, and consistency of tissue.
24. Base of the sulcus; formed by cementum, periodontal ligament, and the alveolar bone.

DOWN

2. A space between two natural teeth.
3. The development of a horny layer of flattened epithelial cells.
4. Fiber-producing cell of the connective tissue.
5. The type of mucosal lining in which the stratified squamous epithelial cells retain their nuclei and cytoplasm.
6. Contains leukocytes, degenerated tissue elements, tissue fluids, and microorganisms.
9. The type of epithelial tissue that serves as a liner for the intraoral mucosal surfaces.
10. Junction between the attached gingiva and the alveolar mucosa.
11. Measured from the CEJ to the base of the sulcus or pocket (two words).
13. Abnormal thickening of the keratin layer (stratum corneum) of the epithelium.
14. Fills the interproximal area between two teeth.
15. Abnormal increase in volume of a tissue or organ caused by formation and growth of new normal cells.
16. Narrow fold of mucous membrane that passes from a more fixed to a more movable area of the oral mucosa.
17. The distance from the gingival margin to periodontal attachment at the base of the pocket (two words).
20. The pitted, orange-peel appearance frequently seen on the surface of the attached gingiva.

Periodontal Examination

Learning Objectives

Upon successful completion of these exercises, you will be able to:

1. Identify and define key terms and concepts related to oral examination procedures.

2. Describe the purpose and procedure for the use of each instrument in a basic examination setup.

3. Discuss the implications of various oral findings identified during the examination.

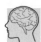

KNOWLEDGE EXERCISES

Write your answers for each question in the space provided.

1. Match each term with the correct definition.

EXAMINATION PROCEDURES TERM	DEFINITION
Horizontal bone loss_____	A. A slender instrument, usually round in diameter with a rounded tip, designed for examination of the teeth and soft tissues
Clinical attachment level_____	B. Probing depth as measured from the cementoenamel junction (or other fixed point) to the location of the probe tip at the coronal level of attached periodontal tissues
Explorer_____	
Bifurcation_____	
Fremitus_____	C. Determination of the accuracy of an instrument by measurement of its variation from a standard
Tactile_____	D. The distance from the gingival margin to the location of the periodontal probe tip at the coronal border of attached periodontal tissues
Explorer tip_____	
Calibration_____	
Probe_____	E. A slender stainless-steel instrument with a fine, flexible, sharp point used for examination of the surfaces of the teeth to detect irregularities
Probing depth_____	
Tactile discrimination_____	F. A vibration perceptible by palpation
	G. Pertaining to touch
	H. The ability to distinguish relative degrees of roughness and smoothness
	I. Two roots
	J. Slender, wirelike, circular in cross section, and tapering to a fine, sharp point
	K. When the crest of the bone is parallel with a line between the cementoenamel junctions of two adjacent teeth

2. The mouth mirror is made up of three parts: the _____, the _____, and the _____ _____.

3. Describe the types of mirror surfaces in your own words.

_____

_____

_____

_____

4. Identify the purposes and uses of mouth mirrors.

_____

_____

_____

_____

5. How does the application of air improve assessment procedures?

_____

_____

_____

6. The probe is a slender instrument with a _____ _____ tip designed for the examination of the _____ and the topography of an area. It can be made of steel or plastic. Refer to Table 15-1 and Figure 15-1 in the textbook and identify the type of probe used at your school. Notice the markings and be sure you know how to read the probe you are using.

7. Fill in the blanks as you read these facts about pocket characteristics.

   a. A pocket is measured from the _____ of the pocket to the _____ margin.

   b. The pocket (or sulcus) is _____ around the entire tooth, and the entire sulcus is measured.

   c. The _____ of the pocket varies around an individual tooth; rarely measuring the same all around a tooth or even around one side of a tooth.

   d. The _____ of attached tissue assumes a varying position around the tooth.

   e. The _____ margin varies in its position on the tooth.

   f. Proximal surfaces must be approached by entering from both the _____ and the _____ aspects of the tooth.

   g. Gingival and periodontal infections begin in the _____ area more frequently than in other areas around the tooth.

   h. Probing depth may be _____ directly under the contact area because of crater formation in the alveolar bone.

   i. Anatomic features of the _____ wall of the pocket influence the direction of probing. Examples are concave surfaces, anomalies, shape of the cervical one-third, and position of _____.

8. The probe reading in part A of Figure 15-1 is _____. The probe reading in part B of the figure is _____. Given these readings, identify which figure part in Figure 15-1 demonstrates tissue that is within normal limits and which demonstrates periodontal

_____

_____

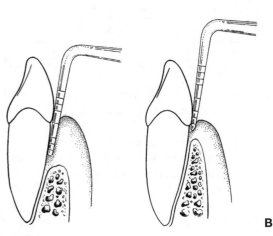

A   B

Figure 15-1

9. Match the health status of the periodontium with the appropriate location of the probe tip.

PERIODONTAL STATUS	LOCATION OF PROBE TIP
Gingivitis and early periodontitis _____ Normal healthy tissue _____ Advanced periodontitis _____	A. At the base of the sulcus or crevice, at the coronal end of the junctional epithelium B. Penetrates through the junctional epithelium to reach attached connective tissue fibers C. Within the junctional epithelium

10. The probe is adapted to individual teeth and surfaces. In your own words, describe how to adapt the probe for each of the following structures.

■ Molars and premolars _____

_____

_____

_____

■ Anterior teeth _____

_____

_____

_____

■ Proximal surfaces _____

_____

_____

_____

11. Mark each of the following statements true or false. If the statement is false, correct it.

a. True or False (circle one). When the crest of the bone is parallel with a line between the cementoenamel junctions of two adjacent teeth, the term vertical bone loss is used.

_____

_____

b. True or False (circle one). Attachment level refers to the point at which periodontal tissues are attached at the base of a sulcus or pocket.

_____

_____

c. True or False (circle one). Radiographs show pockets; soft tissue is seen in a radiograph.

_____

_____

d. True or False (circle one). Clinical attachment level is measured from a changeable point (usually the free gingiva) to the attachment, whereas the probing depth is measured from a fixed point (the crest of the cementoenamel junction) to the point of attachment.

_____

_____

e. True or False (circle one). Stability of attachment level is characteristic in health.

_____

_____

f. True or False (circle one). When there is visible recession, the probing depth is greater than the clinical attachment loss.

_____

_____

g. True or False (circle one). To calculate attachment level, if the gingival margin is above the cementoenamel junction, subtract the distance (in millimeters) from the cementoenamel junction to the gingival crest from the total probing depth.

_____

_____

h. True or False (circle one). A tooth with fremitus has excess contact, possibly related to a premature contact.

_____

_____

i. True or False (circle one). Probing depth is greater than the clinical attachment level when the cementoenamel junction is covered by free gingiva.

_____

_____

j. True or False (circle one). Inflammation in the periodontal ligament leads to degeneration or destruction of the fibers.

k. True or False (circle one). Anatomic variations that complicate furcation examination are fused roots; anomalies, such as extra roots; and low or high furcations.

l. True or False (circle one). To examine a furcation you may use the probe in a diagonal or a horizontal position to examine between roots when there is gingival recession or a flexible, short, soft pocket wall that permits access or you can use a furcation probe, such as a Nabers 1N or 2N, to examine advanced furcation.

m. True or False (circle one). To examine the mucogingival junction, look for blanching at the mucogingival junction while doing the tension test.

n. True or False (circle one). Mucogingival involvement is not present when the probe passes through the pocket directly into the alveolar mucosa.

o. True or False (circle one). When periodontal disease is active, pocket formation and migration of the attachment along the cemental surface continue.

p. True or False (circle one). Subtract the probing depth from the total gingival measurement to get the width of the attached gingiva.

q. True or False (circle one). The use and adaptation for which the explorer was designed determines whether the shank is straight, curved, or angulated.

r. True or False (circle one). The slender, wirelike working end of the explorer has a degree of flexibility that decreases tactile sensitivity.

s. True or False (circle one). For increased acute tactile sensitivity, a lightweight handle is more effective.

t. True or False (circle one). A wide-diameter instrument handle with serrations for friction while grasping can prevent finger cramping from too tight a grasp.

u. True or False (circle one). With a lighter grasp, tactile sensitivity is decreased.

v. True or False (circle one). When an explorer tip is sharp and tapered, more pressure is required to increase tactile sensitivity.

w. True or False (circle one). The function of each type of explorer is related to its adaptability to specific surfaces of teeth at particular angulations.

x. True or False (circle one). Because fremitus depends on tooth-to-tooth contact, determination is made only on the mandibular teeth.

y. True or False (circle one). When inflammation is present and a pocket extends to or through the mucogingival junction, a streak of color (red, bluish red) that shows the inflammatory changes from the gingival margin to the mucogingival junction may be apparent.

_____

_____

z. True or False (circle one). The periodontal ligament is connective tissue and hence appears in a radiograph as a radiolucent (dark) line next to the root surface.

_____

_____

12. Mark each of the following statements true or false. If the statement is false, correct it.

a. True or False (circle one). The development of the ability to use an explorer and a probe is achieved first by learning the anatomic features of each tooth surface and the types of irregularities that may be encountered on the surfaces.

_____

_____

b. True or False (circle one). Probes vary in diameter; the thicker types may provide greater tactile sensitivity.

_____

_____

c. True or False (circle one). As an explorer or probe moves over the surface of enamel, cementum, a metallic restoration, a plastic restoration, or any irregularity of tooth structure or restoration, a particular surface texture is apparent. With each contact, sound may be created.

_____

_____

d. True or False (circle one). The probing depth equals the clinical attachment level when the free gingival margin is level with the cementoenamel junction.

_____

_____

e. True or False (circle one). When the probe is used, it is quiet over clean, smooth enamel but is scratchy or noisy on rough cementum or calculus. Sometimes a metallic restoration may cause a squeak or metallic ring. With experience, the clinician can differentiate among surfaces.

_____

_____

f. True or False (circle one). A mobility rating of "I" means the tooth shows severe movement and may move in all directions, vertically as well as horizontally.

_____

_____

g. True or False (circle one). With adequate light, a source of air, proper retraction, and the use of mouth mirror, dried supragingival calculus can generally be seen as either chalky white or brownish yellow, in contrast to the tooth color. A minimum of exploration can confirm the finding.

_____

_____

h. True or False (circle one). An intact surface where remineralization may be occurring must be explored vigorously. An aggressive examination can be made by using the side of the explorer's tip.

_____

_____

i. True or False (circle one). Calculus deposits may obstruct direct passage of the probe to the base of the pocket. Lift the tip slightly away from the tooth surface and follow over the deposit to proceed to the base of the pocket.

_____

_____

j. True or False (circle one). Tactile sensations pass through the instrument to the fingers and hand and to the brain for registration and action.

_____

_____

k. True or False (circle one). When probing, you can use a walking stroke, in a vertical or diagonal (oblique) direction.

_____

_____

l. True or False (circle one). The maximum depth of each stroke during exploring should be 3 mm.

_____

_____

m. True or False (circle one). In a shallow pocket, the exploring stroke may extend the entire depth, from the base of the pocket to just beneath the gingival margin.

_____

_____

n. True or False (circle one). In a deep pocket, controlled strokes 2- to 3-mm long, that move gradually deeper into the sulcus can provide more acute sensitivity to the surface and allow improved adaptation of the instrument.

_____

_____

o. True or False (circle one). A deep pocket should be explored in sections. First, explore the apical area next to the base of the pocket, then move up to a higher section, overlapping for full coverage.

_____

_____

p. True or False (circle one). Trauma to the gingival margin caused by repeated withdrawal and reinsertion of an instrument that is not well adapted to the surface of the tooth can cause the patient posttreatment discomfort.

_____

_____

q. True or False (circle one). Roll the explorer instrument handle between the fingers to keep the tip closely adapted as the tooth's contour changes.

_____

_____

r. True or False (circle one). Subgingival calculus is most commonly confined to the lingual surfaces of the mandibular anterior teeth and the facial surfaces of the maxillary first and second molars, opposite the openings to the salivary ducts.

_____

_____

s. True or False (circle one). To determine the width of the total gingiva, place the probe on the external surface of the gingiva and measure from the mucogingival junction to the gingival margin.

_____

_____

t. True or False (circle one). Increased tooth mobility can be an important clinical sign of disease.

_____

_____

u. True or False (circle one). When a pocket extends into a furcation area, special adaptation of the probe is required.

_____

_____

v. True or False (circle one). A double-ended instrument has two working ends.

_____

_____

w. True or False (circle one). A thick explorer usually gives a more acute sense of tactile discrimination to small irregularities than does a fine explorer.

_____

_____

x. True or False (circle one). A rating of + means the tooth displays 1° of fremitus and significant vibration can be felt.

_____

_____

y. True or False (circle one). On a radiograph, the evidence of health can be identified when the crestal lamina dura is indistinct, irregular, radiolucent, and fuzzy.

_____

_____

z. True or False (circle one). Early furcation involvement may appear as a small radiolucent black dot or as a slight thickening of the periodontal ligament space, which can be confirmed by probing.

_____

_____

13. Describe the procedures used to assess the adequacy of the frenal attachment.

_____

_____

_____

_____

_____

_____

_____

_____

_____

14. Match each tooth with the appropriate anatomic features. There are two answers for each type of tooth.

TYPE OF TOOTH	ANATOMIC FEATURES
____ and ____ Mandibular molars	A. Furcation area is accessible from the mesial and distal aspects, under the contact area
____ and ____ Maxillary molars	B. Palatal root and two buccal roots (mesiobuccal and distobuccal); access for probing is from the mesial, buccal, and distal surfaces
____ and ____ Maxillary first premolars	
____ and ____ Maxillary primary molars	C. Bifurcation
____ and ____ Mandibular primary molars	D. Widespread roots
	E. Furcation area is accessible from the facial and lingual surfaces
	F. Trifurcation

15. Fill in the blanks to help you learn about the general purposes and uses of the explorer.

a. An explorer is used to detect, using _____ sense, the character of the tooth surface and to examine the tooth surfaces for _____ and _____ lesions.

b. An explorer is used to locate irregularities on the tooth surfaces and _____ of restorations and other irregularities that are not apparent by direct observation.

c. An explorer is also used to _____ direct observations. It allows the clinician to define the extent of instrumentation that is needed.

d. The explorer is used to _____ the completeness of treatment by identifying a _____ tooth surface or restoration.

16. Match the tooth surface irregularities with the correct tactile sensation. Each answer is used more than once.

TOOTH SURFACE IRREGULARITY	TACTILE SENSATION
Enamel pearl____	A. Normal
Smooth surface of enamel____	B. Irregular: increases or elevations in tooth surface
Carious lesion____	C. Irregular: depressions, grooves
Anatomic configurations, such as cingula, furcations____	
Abrasion____	
Root surface that has been planed____	
Calculus____	
Erosion____	
Irregular margins (overhang) ____	
Pits such as those caused by enamel hypoplasia____	
Areas of cemental resorption on the root surface____	
Unusually pronounced cementoenamel junction____	
Deficient margins____	
Overcontoured restoration____	
Rough surface of a restoration ____	

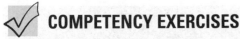

COMPETENCY EXERCISES

Apply information from the chapter and use critical thinking skills to complete the competency exercises. Write responses on paper or create electronic documents to submit your answers.

1. Your employer, Dr. Harriet Golden, asks you put together instrument kits for the office and label them "basic setup." Identify the instruments you have placed in the kit and discuss why you have included each one.

2. Whenever you are using air, you should take care to avoid some very specific situations that may hurt or startle the patient. List some of these situations and describe how you would avoid them.

3. When your instructor verifies your probing, many differences are found. You are having difficulty and need to look at the factors that affect probe determinations and probing procedures. Knowing the right question to ask yourself is a great way to solve a problem. Develop questions that will help you look at these factors and allow you to self-evaluate your own performance.

4. Identify the number on the handle of each explorer in your student kit. Describe the design of the working end, shank, handle, and construction of each one and specify its use.

5. Your patient Tony Wade presents with both mobility (III on teeth 22 to 27) and fremitus (+ on teeth 6 to 11). You note generalized bleeding and probe readings of 5 to 6 mm. The radiographs show horizontal bone loss in all posterior and anterior areas and vertical bone loss on the distal side of tooth 29. The crestal lamina dura is indistinct, irregular, and radiolucent throughout Tony's mouth. There are furcation involvements on teeth 30 and 31. The periodontal ligament spaces are thickened on teeth 28 and 29. Describe how the pocket depth, mobility, and fremitus findings were determined.

6. Label Tony's radiograph in Figure 15-2 with the following findings.

FINDINGS

- Horizontal bone loss
- Vertical bone loss
- Change in crestal lamina dura
- Furcation involvement
- Changes in the periodontal ligament

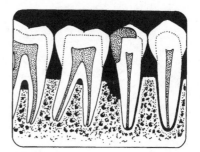

Figure 15-2

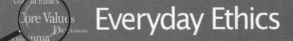

Everyday Ethics

Before completing the learning exercises below, reread and reflect on the Everyday Ethics scenario and Questions for Consideration in this chapter of the textbook. It may also be useful to review the Dental Hygiene Ethics discussion in Chapter 1, the Ethical Applications in the introduction pages for each section in the textbook, as well as the Codes of Ethics in Appendices I, II, and III.

Individual Learning Activity
Imagine that you are the dental hygienist in this scenario. Answer each of the questions for consideration at the end of the scenario.

Collaborative Learning Activity
Work with a small group to develop a 2- to 5-minute role-play that introduces the Everyday Ethics scenario described in the chapter (a great idea is to video record your role-play activity). Then develop separate 2-minute role-play scenarios that provide at least two alternative approaches/solutions to resolving the situation. Ask classmates to view the solutions, ask questions, and discuss the ethical approach used in each. Ask for a vote on which solution classmates determine to be the "best."

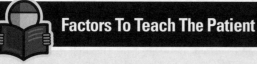

Factors To Teach The Patient

This scenario is related to the following factors listed in this chapter of the textbook:

- The need for a careful, thorough examination if treatment is to be complete and effective
- Information about the instruments and how their use makes the examination complete (e.g., the complete radiographic survey, probing 360° around each tooth, and exploring each subgingival tooth surface)
- Why bleeding can occur when probing. Healthy tissue does not bleed.
- The relation of probing depth measurements to normal sulci
- The significance of mobility

You have completed assessment procedures for Tony Wade (described in Competency Exercise 5). She is very confused about all the tests you have just performed and what all the information means. She wants you to take the time to explain all the data you have collected and the significance of the information you have identified.

Use the examples of patient conversations in Appendix D as a guide to create a conversation to explain to Tony the need for a careful examination, why bleeding can occur, the relationship of probing depth measurements to normal sulci, and the significance of the mobility. Be sure to refer to the figure you labeled in Competency Exercise 6 to illustrate some of your points. You may find it helpful to draw some pictures when discussing probing depths.

CHAPTER 16

Periodontal Disease Development

Upon successful completion of these exercises, you will be able to:

1. Identify and define key terms and concepts related to the development of periodontal disease.

2. Classify and describe periodontal diseases and conditions.
3. Discuss the development of gingival and periodontal infections.
4. Identify risk factors for development of periodontal disease.

 KNOWLEDGE EXERCISES

Write your answers for each question in the space provided.

1. Using the information in Table 16-1, describe each of the four types of biofilm-induced *gingival* diseases.

   _____

   _____

   _____

   _____

   _____

   _____

2. Fill in the blanks to complete the following sentences.

   a. Three bacteria that can lead to gingival lesions are _____, _____, and _____.

   b. Gingival diseases of viral origin are _____ infections, primary _____ gingivostomatitis, recurrent _____ _____, and _____ infections.

   c. Gingival diseases of fungal origin can be the result of _____ species infections, such as generalized gingival _____, _____ gingival erythema, and histoplasmosis.

   d. An example of a gingival lesion of genetic origin is hereditary gingival _____.

   e. Gingival manifestations of systemic conditions include mucocutaneous disorders such as _____, _____, _____ _____, _____ _____, and _____ _____.

   f. Gingival lesions may be caused by allergic reactions to dental restorative materials, such as mercury, _____, and _____.

   g. Gingival lesions can be caused by reactions attributable to dental-care products, such as _____ and _____, as well as chewing gum and food *additives*.

   h. The gingiva may suffer from traumatic lesions (factitious, iatrogenic, accidental) caused by _____, _____, or _____ injury or by reactions to *foreign* bodies.

3. How is the location of chronic and aggressive periodontitis described?

_____

_____

4. Periodontitis as a manifestation of systemic disease can be associated with hematologic disorders. Name some conditions in which you may find this association.

_____

_____

5. Periodontitis can be associated with genetic disorders. Name some conditions in which you may find this association.

_____

_____

_____

_____

6. Name the necrotizing periodontal diseases.

_____

_____

_____

7. List types of abscesses of the periodontium.

_____

_____

_____

8. You may find periodontitis associated with endodontic lesions. What is the term used to refer to these?

_____

_____

9. Periodontitis as a manifestation of systemic disease can be associated with _____ or acquired deformities and conditions.

10. Localized tooth-related factors that modify or predispose the area to biofilm-induced gingival diseases/periodontitis include tooth anatomic factors, dental _____, root fractures, cervical _____ resorption, and cemental tears.

11. Mucogingival deformities and conditions around the teeth that are manifestations of systemic disease include gingival _____, lack of _____ gingiva, _____ vestibular depth, aberrant frenum/muscle position, and gingival excess.

12. Occlusal trauma is classified as _____ or _____ and is noted as a manifestation of periodontitis associated with systemic disease.

13. Match each descriptive statement with the appropriate stage of development of gingivitis and periodontal disease. Each answer may be used more than once.

DEVELOPMENTAL STAGE	DESCRIPTION
A. Initial lesion B. Early lesion	_____ Inflammatory response to biofilm occurs within 2–4 days. _____ Biofilm becomes older and thicker (7–14 days; time reflects individual differences). _____ Migration and infiltration of white blood cells into the junctional epithelium and gingival sulcus _____ Signs of gingivitis become apparent with slight gingival enlargement. _____ No clinical evidence of change _____ Infiltration of fluid, lymphocytes, and neutrophils with a few plasma cells into the connective tissue _____ The gingivitis is reversible when biofilm is controlled and inflammation is reduced; healthy tissue may be restored. _____ Increased flow of gingival sulcus fluid

14. Match each descriptive statement with the appropriate stage of development of gingivitis and periodontal disease. Each answer may be used more than once.

DEVELOPMENTAL STAGE	DESCRIPTION
C. Established lesion D. Advanced lesion	_____ Inflammation spreads through the bone marrow and out into the periodontal ligament. _____ Fluid and leukocyte migration into tissues and sulcus increase; plasma cells are related to areas of chronic inflammation. _____ Exposed cementum where Sharpey fibers were attached becomes altered by inflammatory products of bacteria and the sulcus fluid. _____ Clear evidence of inflammation is present, with marginal redness, bleeding on probing, and spongy marginal gingiva; later, chronic fibrosis develops. _____ Proliferation of the junctional and sulcular epithelium continues in an attempt to wall out the inflammation. _____ Inflammation spreads through the loose connective tissue along (beside) the blood vessels to the alveolar bone. _____ Connective tissue fibers below the junctional epithelium are destroyed; the epithelium migrates along the root surface. _____ Bacteria from supragingival biofilm enter the sulcus and provide the source for subgingival biofilm. _____ Diseased cementum contains a thin superficial layer of endotoxins from the bacterial breakdown. _____ Formation of pocket epithelium

15. In your own words, define and describe a periodontal pocket. Include the following in your description the following:

   ■ What distinguishes a pocket from a sulcus?

   ■ Describe the walls and the base of a pocket.

   ■ Compare the histology of a healthy pocket and the histopathology of a diseased pocket.

   _____

   _____

   _____

   _____

   _____

   _____

   _____

16. Fill in the blanks to complete the following sentences about *gingival* pockets.

   a. A gingival pocket is a pocket formed by gingival _____ without apical migration of the _____ _____.

   b. The margin of the gingiva has moved toward the _____ or _____ direction, without the deeper periodontal structures becoming involved.

   c. The tooth wall is _____. During eruption, the base of the _____ is at various levels along the wall.

   d. The base of the sulcus of a fully erupted tooth is near the _____ junction.

   e. All gingival pockets are _____, that is, the base of the pocket is coronal to the crest of the alveolar bone.

17.

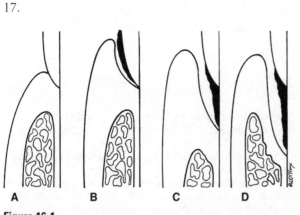

A   **B**   **C**   **D**

Figure 16-1

Use the following terms to label Figure 16-1, which illustrates types of periodontal pockets.

- Normal relationship

- Gingival pocket

- Periodontal pocket

- Suprabony

- Intrabony

- Cementoenamel junction

- Enamel

- Cementum

- Alveolar bone

- Gingival tissue

- Calculus

18. Fill in the blanks to complete the following sentences about *periodontal* pockets.

a. A periodontal pocket is formed as a result of disease or degeneration that caused the _____ _____ to migrate apically along the _____.

b. The periodontal deeper structures (attachment apparatus) involved in periodontal pocketing are the _____, _____ ligament, and _____.

c. The tooth wall is _____ or partly _____ and partly enamel.

d. The _____ of the pocket is on cementum at the level of the attached periodontal tissue.

e. Periodontal pockets may be _____ or intrabony.

f. When the base of the pocket is coronal to the crest of the alveolar bone, the pocket is _____.

g. When the base of the pocket is below or apical to the crest of the alveolar bone, the pocket is _____.

19. Match each of the following definitions with the correct term.

FACTOR	DEFINITION
A. Etiologic factor	_____ A factor that lends assistance to, supplements, or adds to a condition or disease.
B. Predisposing factor	_____ A factor that results from or is influenced by a general physical or mental disease or condition.
C. Risk factor	_____ A factor that is the actual cause of a disease or condition.
D. Contributing factor	_____ A factor in the immediate environment of the oral cavity or specifically in the environment of
E. Local factor	the teeth or periodontium.
F. Systemic factor	_____ A factor that renders a person susceptible to a disease or condition.
	_____ An exposure that increases the probability that disease will occur.

20. Describe in your own words the sequence of natural self-cleaning mechanisms that happen during and after mastication.

_____

_____

_____

_____

_____

_____

_____

_____

_____

COMPETENCY EXERCISES

Apply information from the chapter and use critical thinking skills to complete the competency exercises. Write responses on paper or create electronic documents to submit your answers.

1. After probing, you determine that disease is limited to the gingiva. Discuss the care planning objectives and some questions you may have for your patient.

2. Your next patient presents with apical positioning of the periodontal attachment, with alveolar bone loss and other indications of periodontitis. List some questions, concerns, and general guidelines you consider as you start to plan treatment for this patient.

3. You detect a class II furcation on tooth 30 and a class III furcation involvement on tooth 31 as you collect data for your 10 AM patient, Woody Green. Woody asks many questions and wants to understand what these terms mean. Explain the terms to him, and use drawings of the teeth to help describe the conditions.

4. You are asked to develop patient education materials for the practice you are in. You decide to focus on local contributing factors in disease development. Develop a checklist that can be filled out during a patient education session to identify specific factors relevant for each individual patient.

Everyday Ethics

Before completing the learning exercises below, reread and reflect on the Everyday Ethics Scenario and Questions for Consideration in this chapter of the textbook. It may also be useful to review the Dental Hygiene Ethics discussion in Chapter 1, the Ethical Applications in the introduction pages for each section in the textbook, as well as the Codes of Ethics in Appendices I, II, and III.

Discovery Activity

Ask a dental hygienist who has been practicing for a year or more to read the scenario. Provide them with a copy of the Code of Ethics as well. Share the responses you have made to answer each question and ask that person to discuss the situation with you. What insights did you have or what did you learn during this discussion?

Collaborative Learning Activity

Work with a small group to develop a 2- to 5-minute role-play that introduces the Everyday Ethics scenario described in the chapter (a great idea is to video record your role-play activity). Then develop separate 2-minute role-play scenarios that provide at least two alternative approaches/solutions to resolving the situation. Ask classmates to view the solutions, ask questions, and discuss the ethical approach used in each. Ask for a vote on which solution classmates determine to be the "best."

Factors To Teach The Patient

This scenario is related to the following factors listed in this chapter of the textbook:

- Factors that contribute to disease development and progression
- What a risk factor is and the importance of planning personal and professional care to include risk factor problems

During data collection for your patient, Maria Manuela Rodriguez, you note the following information:

- She smokes two packs of cigarettes per day.
- She takes 10 mg Fosamax (alendronate) per day to prevent/control osteoporosis.
- There is a family history of diabetes.
- She is overweight.
- She takes 10 mg Procardia three times per day to treat her high blood pressure and ventricular arrhythmia (this is nifedipine, which is a calcium channel blocker).
- She tends to have a soft diet.

Use the example of patient conversations in Appendix D as a guide to write a statement explaining Maria's risk factors for periodontal disease.

Use the conversation you created to educate a patient or friend, and then modify it based on what you learned.

WORD SEARCH

```
E K U M F B O L N K W F N G F E E
R J G A G I N G I V I T I S P D P
C G U R R E F R A C T O R Y L E K
O L C P C Y I W N C J R L M X M P
L R F X I H M L D O D X E K N A E
L L E M C E P T E L D D U G T D R
A X N W A Z A I S L X I K S G U I
G G Z R T W C J Q A E A O V L S O
E W Y N R D T C U G R S C S E W D
N U M W I O I R A E O T Y G S H O
Z J E A X U O K M N S E T T I U N
Z N R S F C N N A A T M E O O K T
B O Z H S D U E T S O A S X N Z I
U K V C Y Z Z S I E M V V I I T
G D K Z T R V T O Y I Z U N N E I
P K S W T D K H N U A A A R W Z S
A D X O S J R P E R M E A B L E X
```

WORD SEARCH CLUES

1. Refers to wounds, sores, ulcers, tumors, or any other tissue damage
2. The numbers of these increase inside the diseased pocket as inflammation increases.
3. White fibers of the connective tissue
4. Poison; protein produced by certain animals, higher plants, and pathogenic bacteria
5. Shedding of the outer epithelial layer of the stratified squamous epithelium of skin or mucosa
6. Accumulation of excessive fluid in cells or tissues
7. Not readily responsive to treatment
8. Forceful wedging of food into the periodontium by occlusal forces
9. Inflammation of the gingiva.
10. A space or abnormal opening; in dentistry, a space between two adjacent teeth in the same dental arch
11. Enzyme that contributes to the hydrolysis of collagen
12. Inflammation of the periodontium
13. Protein secreted by body cells that acts as a catalyst to induce chemical changes in other substances
14. Permitting passage of a fluid
15. Dryness of the mouth from a lack of normal secretions
16. Fibrous tissue left after the healing of a wound

CHAPTER 17

The Teeth

Learning Objectives

Upon successful completion of these exercises, you will be able to:

1. Identify and define key terms and concepts related to the teeth.
2. Discuss various types of dental caries in terms of classification, development, and detection.
3. Describe noncarious dental lesions and their causes and appearance.
4. Describe a clinical examination of the teeth.
5. Detail the development and eruption of permanent teeth.
6. Identify various strategies for the recognition of carious lesions and describe tests for vitality.

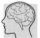

KNOWLEDGE EXERCISES

Write your answers for each question in the space provided.

1. A visual examination can be used to identify dental caries.

   a. Initially, you should dry each tooth or group of teeth with _____ and carefully inspect each surface.

   b. Characteristic changes in the _____ and _____ of tooth structure may be observed.

   c. Such changes may be signs of _____ _____.

   d. Variations in color and translucency include: _____ _____ areas of demineralization, or _____ _____ discoloration of marginal ridges caused by dental caries of the proximal surface underneath.

   e. Grayish-white color spreading from _____ _____ can indicate secondary dental caries.

   f. In relation to an amalgam restoration, dental caries appears _____ in the outer portion and _____ adjacent to the amalgam.

   g. Open carious lesions may vary in color from _____ to _____.

   h. A dark shadow on a proximal surface of anterior teeth may be observed by using _____.

2. An exploratory examination can be used to identify dental caries.

   a. When exploring for smooth surface caries, the clinician adapts the _____ of the tip of the explorer closely to the tooth surface.

   b. Examine for _____ versus softness, for _____ versus smoothness, and for _____ of the tooth surface.

   c. Do not use pressure or attempt to break the surface when checking an area that may be _____.

   d. Chart irregularities of existing restorations. When a _____ or _____ is discolored, it is not possible to determine visually whether dental caries is present, except when a large obvious cavity can be seen.

e. An _____ _____ should not be explored.

3. During the clinical examination, information revealed by radiographs is used for supplementation and confirmation.

a. A few principal items to be seen in a radiographic examination of the teeth are:

_____

_____

b. _____ surface lesions may be missed if radiographs are not used.

c. Bitewing or periapical radiographs made using a _____ _____ with no _____ are most satisfactory for dental caries detection.

d. Mounted radiographs displayed on _____ (multiple words) are necessity during charting and treatment procedures.

e. For the detection of early carious lesions on radiographs, a _____ _____ can be of invaluable assistance.

f. Most root caries lesions occur in the vicinity of the cementoenamel junction and appear in a radiograph as _____ -shaped lesions that undermines the enamel, or may be located beneath an _____ _____.

4. Match the description with the correct term. Each term may be used more than once.

TERMINOLOGY	DESCRIPTION
A. Simple cavity	_____ Involves more than two tooth surfaces
B. Compound cavity	_____ Caries on the occlusal surface of a molar
C. Complex cavity	_____ Covering two surfaces
D. Pit and fissure caries	_____ Closure of the enamel plates is imperfect
E. Smooth surface caries	_____ Occurs in proximal tooth surfaces
	_____ Mesio-occlusal caries, for example
	_____ Involves one tooth surface
	_____ The buccal groove of a mandibular molar, for example
	_____ Distal-occlusal caries
	_____ Irregularity occurs where three or more lobes of the developing tooth join
	_____ Caries in an area where there is no pit, groove, or other fault

5. The standard method for classifying dental caries was developed by Dr. G. V. Black. Match the description with the correct classification. Each classification may be used more than once.

G. V. BLACK CLASSIFICATIONS	DESCRIPTIONS
A. Class I	_____ Cavities in pits or fissures
B. Class II	_____ Cavities in the cervical third of facial or lingual surfaces (not pit or fissure)
C. Class III	_____ Radiographs not useful for detection
D. Class IV	_____ Cavities in proximal surfaces of incisors or canines that involve the incisal angle
E. Class V	_____ Lingual surfaces of maxillary incisors
F. Class VI	_____ Cavities in proximal surfaces of premolars
	_____ Transillumination is useful for detection
	_____ Facial and lingual surfaces of molars
	_____ Early caries detected by radiographs
	_____ Cavities in proximal surfaces of incisors and canines that do not involve the incisal angle
	_____ Cavities on incisal edges of anterior teeth and cusp tips of posterior teeth
	_____ Occlusal surfaces of premolars and molars

6. As you examine your next patient, you note a defect that occurs as a result of a disturbance in the formation of the organic enamel matrix. This hereditary condition is referred to as _____ _____.

7. Factors that may contribute to enamel hypoplasia during tooth development include _____ _____, particularly rickets; or _____ _____, such as measles, chickenpox, and scarlet fever.

8. In your own words, describe the appearance of various types of hypoplasia.

_____

_____

_____

_____

9. List the teeth most frequently affected by enamel hypoplasia. Why are these teeth affected?

_____

_____

10. Complete Infomap 17-1 to help you differentiate among attrition, erosion, and abrasion.

INFOMAP 17-1					
CONDITION	**DEFINITION**	**OCCURRENCE**	**ETIOLOGY**	**PREDISPOSING FACTORS**	**APPEARANCE**
Attrition					
Erosion					
Abrasion					

11. List the relevant findings for each response during an electric pulp test.

RESULT OF VITALITY TEST	FINDING
No response	
Lingering pain after removal of stimulus	
Pain subsides promptly	

12. List and describe the types of thermal tests used to determine pulpal vitality.

_____

_____

_____

_____

13. List and describe the factors that can influence response or reaction to the thermal tests.

_____

_____

_____

_____

_____

_____

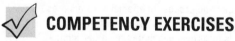 **COMPETENCY EXERCISES**

Apply information from the chapter and use critical thinking skills to complete the competency exercises. Write responses on paper or create electronic documents to submit your answers.

1. Your patient presents with both Class II and Class V dental caries. Describe how you detected each of these lesions.

2. Your patient, Oliver Summerlin, uses a hard tooth-brush and an abrasive nonfluoride-containing dentifrice. He wears a partial denture on the mandible and takes a medication that causes xerostomia. You note abrasion in all four quadrants and root caries on the facial surfaces of teeth 27–30. Differentiate abrasion from root caries, and discuss the prevention of both root caries and abrasion.

3. Your patient at 3 PM is Paulo Jacoby. He is 16 years old, is an avid basketball player, and never wears a mouthguard. Describe potential oral injuries.

4. Clive Williams is 10 years old. He wants to know if he will get "more grown-up teeth." Explain to him the formative stages that his remaining teeth are in and the age at which most children can expect more permanent teeth to erupt.

5. Clive's cousin Jamal is 5 years old. He and Clive have a bet as to who still has the most teeth to erupt. Who will win the bet and why?

6. Jamal's sister wants to get in on the bet. She is 15 years old and says she will not have any more teeth erupt because all of her teeth are in and she is a grown-up. She has never had any teeth extracted. Who will win the bet and why?

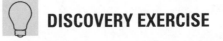

DISCOVERY EXERCISE

Review the data collection forms that are used in your dental hygiene program. What form will you use to document each of the examination features that are listed in Table 17-2 in the textbook?

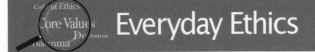

Everyday Ethics

Before completing the learning exercises below, reread and reflect on the Everyday Ethics scenario and Questions for Consideration in this chapter of the textbook. It may also be useful to review the Dental Hygiene Ethics discussion in Chapter 1, the Ethical Applications in the introduction pages for each Section in the textbook, as well as the Codes of Ethics in Appendices I, II, and III.

Individual Learning Activity
Imagine that you are the dental hygienist in this scenario. Answer each of the questions for consideration at the end of the scenario.

Discovery Activity
Ask a friend or relative who is not involved in healthcare to read the scenario and discuss it with you from the perspective of a "patient" who receives services within the healthcare system. Discuss what you learned from the concerns, insights, or difference in perspective that person expressed.

Factors To Teach The Patient

This scenario is related to the following factors listed in this chapter of the textbook:

- The cause and process of enamel or root caries formation and development for the patients at risk
- Methods for prevention of dental caries, such as fluorides, biofilm prevention and control, and control of cariogenic foods in the diet
- Methods for prevention of early childhood caries (Nothing but plain water should be used in bedtime or nap-time nursing bottles. Avoid the use of a sweetener on a pacifier. Use of a cup for milk or juice by the baby's first birthday.)

Andrea Carfagno has arrived in the reception area of the clinic. She is holding her 26-month-old daughter,

Nicole, and her 9-month-old twin boys are in a stroller. Nicole is your patient today. The girl is holding a baby bottle filled with fruit punch. She is a happy, attentive youngster who is anxious to please.

    Use the examples of patient conversations in Appendix D as a guide to write a statement explaining the need to have Nicole switch from a bottle to a cup. Be sure to address the use of fruit juices in a bottle and to explain early childhood caries. These issues pertain to both Nicole and her brothers.

    Use the conversation you create to role-play this situation with a fellow student. If you are the patient in the role-play, be sure to ask questions. If you are the dental hygienist, try to anticipate questions and answer them in your explanation.

CROSSWORD PUZZLE

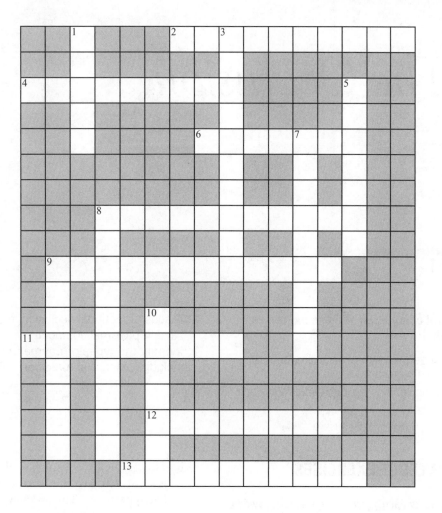

ACROSS

1. Food that promotes dental caries.
4. One of the terms used to refer to the primary teeth.
6. An oral habit of grinding, clenching, or clamping the teeth; involuntary, rhythmic, or spasmodic movements outside the chewing range; may damage teeth and attachment apparatus.
8. Loss of primary teeth following physiologic resorption of root structure.
9. Production and development of enamel.
11. Term used to refer to dental caries that occur on a surface adjacent to a restoration.
12. The tearing away or forcible separation of a tooth from the alveolus.
13. Incomplete or defective formation of the enamel of either primary or permanent teeth. The result may be an irregularity of tooth form, color, or surface.

DOWN

1. A small, flattened surface on a tooth that results from attrition or repeated parafunctional contact.
3. Gradual dissolution of a mineralized tissue.
5. This term is used to describe the widespread formation of dental caries.
7. Refers to very early carious lesion.
8. Without teeth.
9. Refers to carious lesion that has become stationary.
10. One of the terms used to refer to the first teeth; normally will be shed and replaced by permanent teeth.

The Occlusion

Learning Objectives

Upon successful completion of these exercises, you will be able to:

1. Identify and define key terms and concepts related to occlusion.
2. Classify malocclusions for both adult and child patients.

3. Discuss functional occlusion in terms of occlusal and proximal contacts.
4. Identify the types of trauma from occlusion, including clinical and radiographic findings.

KNOWLEDGE EXERCISES

Write your answers for each question in the space provided.

1. Fill in the blanks in the following statements concerning facial profiles.

   a. Your patient presents with a prominent maxilla and a mandible posterior to its normal relationship. This is known as a convex, or _____ profile.

   b. This patient's cousin has slightly protruded jaws, which give the facial outline a relatively flat appearance. This is known as a straight, or _____ profile.

   c. The father of your patient is waiting in the reception area. He has a prominent, protruded mandible and a normal maxilla. This is known as a concave, or _____ profile.

2. Match the following definitions with the correct term from the list.

DEFINITION	TERMS
Consists of all contacts during chewing, swallowing, or other normal action_____	A. Centric relation
Maximum intercuspation or contact of the teeth of the opposing arches; also called habitual occlusion_____	B. Centric occlusion
Any contact of opposing teeth that occurs before the desirable intercuspation_____	C. Static occlusion
Seen when jaws are closed in centric relation_____	D. Normal occlusion
Most unstrained, retruded physiologic relation of the mandible to the maxilla from which lateral movements can be made_____	E. Functional occlusion
Abnormal or deviated function_____	F. Malocclusion
Any deviation from the physiologically acceptable relationship of the maxillary arch and/or teeth to the mandibular arch and/or teeth_____	G. Occlusal prematurity
All teeth in the maxillary arch are in maximum contact with all teeth in mandibular arch in a definite pattern; maxillary teeth slightly overlap the mandibular teeth on the facial surfaces_____	H. Parafunctional

3. Match the following definitions with the correct term from the list.

TERMS	DEFINITION
A. Ankylosis B. Dental ankylosis C. Primate space D. Diastema E. Drifting F. Pathologic migration G. Facet H. Tongue thrust	_____ Rigid fixation of a tooth to the surrounding alveolus as a result of ossification of the periodontal ligament; prevents eruption and orthodontic movement _____ Diastema, or gap, in the tooth row occasionally observed in the human primary dentition _____ Tooth Movement that occurs when disease is present _____ Infantile pattern of suckle–swallow movement in which the tongue is placed between the incisor teeth or alveolar ridges _____ Space between two adjacent teeth in the same arch _____ Union or consolidation of two similar or dissimilar hard tissues previously adjacent but not attached _____ Migration with a healthy periodontium _____ Shiny, flat, worn spot on the surface of a tooth, frequently on the side of a cusp

4. Match the following definitions with the correct term from the list.

TERMS	DEFINITION
A. Orthopedics B. Orthodontic and dentofacial orthopedics C. Cephalostat D. Cephalometer E. Cephalometric analysis F. Occlusal guard	_____ Head-holding instrument used to obtain cephalometric radiographs _____ Orienting device for positioning the head for radiographic examination and measurement _____ Specialty area of dentistry concerned with the diagnosis, supervision, guidance, and treatment of the growing and mature dentofacial structures _____ Process of evaluating dental and skeletal relationships by way of measurements obtained directly from the head or from cephalometric radiographs and tracings made from the radiographs _____ Correction of abnormal form or relationship of bone structures _____ Removable dental appliance usually made of plastic that covers a dental arch and is designed to minimize the damaging effects of bruxism and other oral habits

5. Label each of the following figures (Figures 18-1 to 18-15) with the condition illustrated by the figure; then write a short description of your observations about each condition.

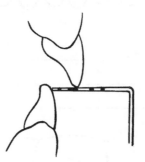

Figure 18-2

_____

_____

_____

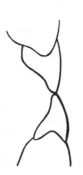

Figure 18-1

_____

_____

_____

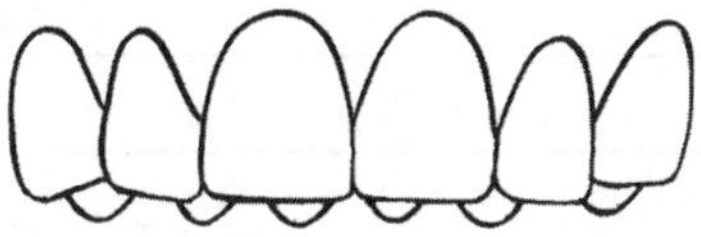

Figure 18-3

_____

_____

_____

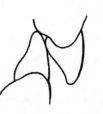

Figure 18-4

_____
_____
_____

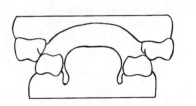

Figure 18-5

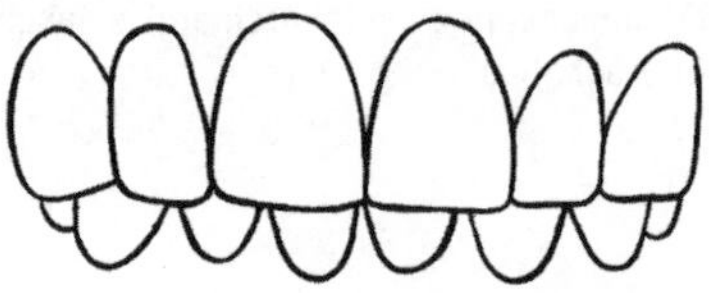

_____
_____
_____

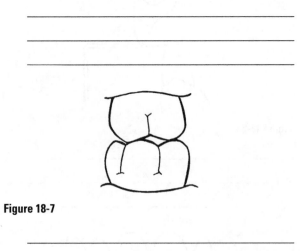

Figure 18-6

_____
_____
_____

Figure 18-7

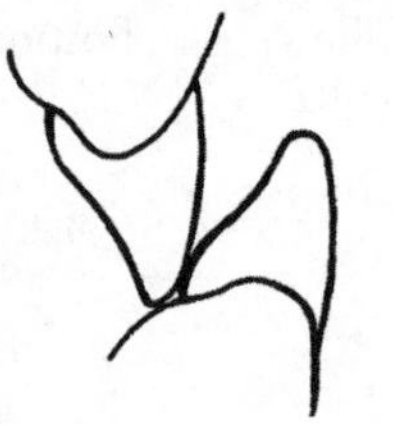

_____
_____
_____

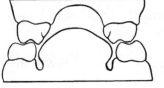

Figure 18-8

_____
_____
_____

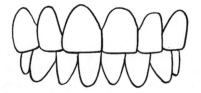

Figure 18-9

_____
_____
_____

Figure 18-10

_____
_____
_____

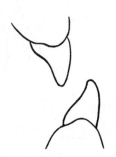

Figure 18-11

_____
_____
_____

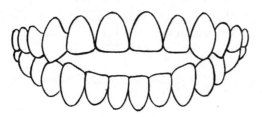

Figure 18-12

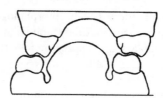

Figure 18-13

_____

_____

_____

_____

_____

_____

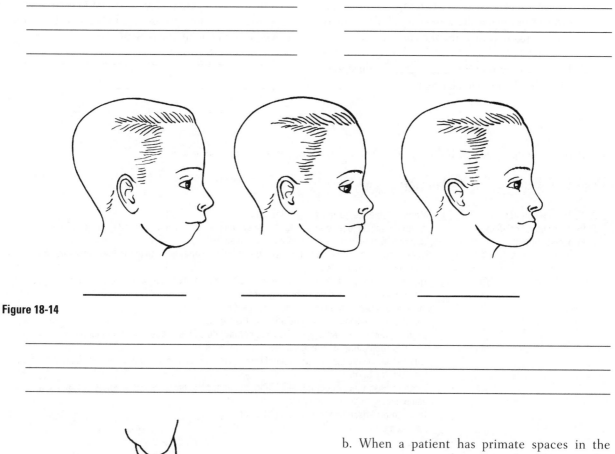

Figure 18-14

_____

_____

_____

Figure 18-15

_____

_____

_____

6. Fill in the blanks as you think about the occlusion of the primary teeth.

   a. The primary canine relation is _____ the permanent dentition.

   b. When a patient has primate spaces in the _____ arch, you see these between the canine and first molar.

   c. In the _____ arch, you see primate spaces between the lateral incisor and canine.

   d. You can expect the second primary molar relation to appear as the _____ cusp of the maxillary second primary molar occluding with the _____ groove of the mandibular second primary molar.

   e. There can be variations in distal surfaces relationships, called terminal steps. An example is when the _____ surface of the mandibular primary molar is _____ to that of the maxillary, thereby forming a mesial step.

f. Although there can be morphologic variation in molar size, maxillary and mandibular primary molars are approximately the same in _____ width.

g. When a patient has a terminal step, the first permanent molar erupts directly into _____ occlusion.

h. A terminal plane occurs when the _____ surfaces of the maxillary and mandibular primary molars are on same vertical plane.

i. The maxillary molar is _____ mesiodistally than the mandibular molar.

j. When a patient has a terminal plane, the first permanent molars erupt _____ to _____.

k. Primate spaces affect the eruption of the _____.

7. Functional occlusion consists of all contacts during chewing, swallowing, and other normal action. Functional occlusion is associated with performance. List some reasons why normal functional occlusion benefits the patient.

_____

_____

_____

8. Match each definition with the correct term. Each term is used more than once.

TERM	DEFINITION
A. Functional contact	_____ Made outside the normal range of function
B. Parafunctional contact	_____ When contact is lost, teeth can drift into spaces created by unreplaced missing teeth.
C. Proximal contact	_____ This results from occlusal habits and neuroses.
	_____ Normal contact that is made between the maxillary teeth and the mandibular teeth during chewing and swallowing
	_____ This is potentially injurious to the periodontal supporting structures, but only in the presence of bacterial plaque and inflammatory factors.
	_____ Attrition or wear of the teeth occurs at this type of contact.
	_____ This creates wear facets and attrition on the teeth.
	_____ Each contact is momentary, so the total contact time is only a few minutes each day.
	_____ Tooth-to-tooth contact; bruxism, clenching, tapping
	_____ This serves to stabilize the position of teeth in the dental arches and to prevent food impaction between the teeth.
	_____ Tooth-to-hard-object contact; nail biting, occupational use (tacks or pins), use of smoking equipment (pipestem or hard cigarette holder)
	_____ Tooth-to-oral-tissues contact; lip or cheek biting
	_____ Pathologic migration

9. Refer to Figure 18-16 when answering the following questions.

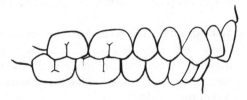

Figure 18-16

a. Using a red pencil, mark the teeth you will evaluate to determine this patient's occlusal classification.

b. Describe the tooth relationships that will influence your decision about the patient's occlusal classification.

_____

_____

_____

_____

_____

_____

c. What is this patient's occlusal classification?

_____

10. Refer to Figure 18-17 when answering the following questions.

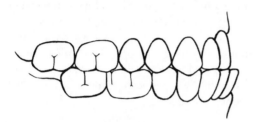

Figure 18-17

a. Using a red pencil, mark the teeth you will evaluate to determine this patient's occlusal classification.

b. Describe the tooth relationships that will influence your decision about the patient's occlusal classification.

_____

_____

_____

_____

_____

_____

c. What is this patient's occlusal classification?

_____

11. Refer to Figure 18-18 when answering the following questions.

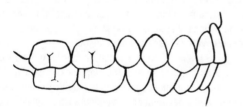

Figure 18-18

a. Using a red pencil, mark the teeth you will evaluate to determine this patient's occlusal classification.

b. Describe the tooth relationships that will influence your decision about the patient's occlusal classification.

_____

_____

_____

_____

_____

_____

c. What is this patient's occlusal classification?

_____

12. Refer to Figure 18-19 when answering the following questions.

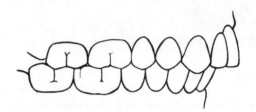

Figure 18-19

a. Using a red pencil, mark the teeth you will evaluate to determine this patient's occlusal classification.

b. Describe the tooth relationships that will influence your decision about the patient's occlusal classification.

_____

_____

_____

_____

_____

_____

c. What is this patient's occlusal classification?

_____

 COMPETENCY EXERCISES

Apply information from the chapter and use critical thinking skills to complete the competency exercises. Write responses on paper or create electronic documents to submit your answers.

1. You are performing an examination to determine if your patient has an overbite. Describe the strategies you will use and how you will elucidate your findings. Which figures from this chapter of the workbook will help you explain an overbite to your patient?

2. You are asked to explain an overjet. Which figure from this chapter of the workbook will help you do this? Describe the procedure for evaluating an overjet, and then go back to the figure you selected and determine the approximate overjet reading for this patient.

3. Your patient, Song Yee, presents with chronic, generalized, moderate periodontal disease. Song just had new restorations placed on teeth 30 and 3. You are concerned about her occlusion because you have seen evidence of both primary and secondary trauma in her mouth. She wants to understand the term you used and to understand these concepts by being given an example of what you saw in her mouth. Explain to Song the clinical and radiographic findings that you have evaluated in order to determine that her occlusion is a factor in her periodontal disease.

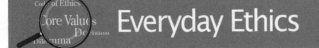

Everyday Ethics

*Before completing the learning exercises below, reread and reflect on the **Everyday Ethics scenario and Questions for Consideration in this chapter of the textbook**. It may also be useful to review the Dental Hygiene Ethics discussion in Chapter 1, the Ethical Applications in the introduction pages for each section in the textbook, as well as the Codes of Ethics in Appendices I, II, and III.*

Collaborative Learning Activity
Work with another student colleague to role-play the scenario. The goal of this exercise is for you and your colleague to work though the alternative actions to come to consensus on a solution or response that is acceptable to both of you.

Discovery Activity
Summarize this scenario for faculty member at your school and ask them to consider the questions that are included. Is their perspective different than yours or similar? Explain.

Factors To Teach The Patient

This scenario is related to the following factors listed in this chapter of the textbook:

- Interpretation of the general purposes of orthodontic care (function and aesthetics) to patients referred by the dentist to an orthodontist
- Dependence of masticatory efficiency on the occlusion of the teeth
- Influence of masticatory efficiency on food selection in the diet
- Influence of masticatory efficiency and diet on the nutritional status of the body and oral health

Your patient, Placido Perez, is a 35-year-old insurance salesman. He is overweight and reports that he can eat only soft foods because of the way he bites. Although Placido admires that famous late-night talk show host that everyone tells him he looks like, he is unhappy with his appearance. He presents with a class III malocclusion.

Use the examples of patient conversations in Appendix D and the figures in this chapter of the workbook as a guide to help you write a statement explaining to Placido what you see in his mouth and what ideal occlusion looks like. Explain why referral to an orthodontist may be recommended.

Use the conversation you create to role-play this situation with a fellow student. If you are the patient in the role-play, be sure to ask questions. If you are the dental hygienist, try to anticipate questions and answer them in your explanation.

CHAPTER 19

Dental Biofilm and Other Soft Deposits

Upon successful completion of these exercises, you will be able to:

1. Identify and define key terms and concepts related to oral soft deposits.
2. Differentiate dental biofilm from pellicle, materia alba, and food debris in terms of composition, significance, and detection.
3. Discuss the implications of dental biofilm in terms of periodontal disease and caries.
4. Describe the essentials for dental caries as well as other contributing factors.

 KNOWLEDGE EXERCISES

Write your answers for each question in the space provided.

1. List and describe the various types of nonmineralized tooth deposits. Be sure to identify the derivation of each.

_____
_____
_____
_____
_____
_____
_____
_____

2. Make a drawing of each of these bacteria.

- Bacillus

- Coccobacilli

- Diplococci

- Filamentous bacilli

- Fusiform bacilli

- Sarcina

- Spirochetes

- Staphylococci

- Streptococci

- Vibrios

3. Label Figure 19-1 to identify the bacteria present. To the right of the figure, indicate the timeframe for the development of the observed changes in the bacteria when the teeth are not cleaned.

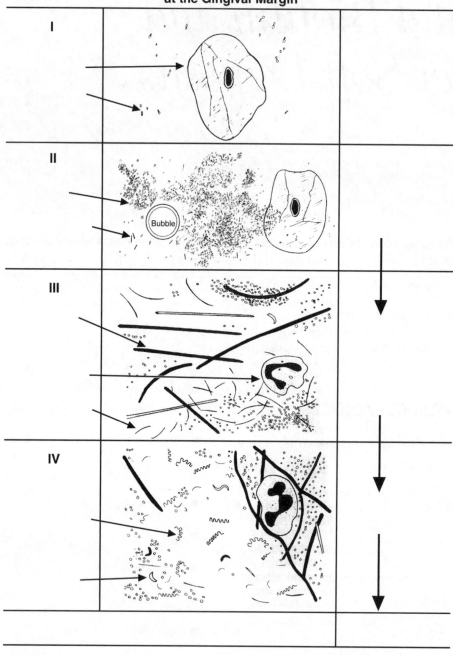

Accumulative Changes in Biofilm Bacteria at the Gingival Margin

Figure 19-1

4. Why is acquired pellicle significant?

_____

_____

_____

_____

5. The interactions involved in the formation of biofilm are listed below. Number the list in the correct order (1 = first interaction; 5 = last interaction).

_____ Matrix formation

_____ Formation of a pellicle

_____ Biofilm growth and maturation

_____ Bacterial multiplication and colonization

_____ Bacteria attach to the pellicle

6. Mark each of the following statements as true or false. If the statement printed here is false, correct it.

a. **True** or **False** (circle one). Dental caries and gingival and periodontal infections are not caused by microorganisms in microbial or dental biofilms.

_____

_____

b. **True** or **False** (circle one). Cleansing of debris from about fixed prostheses and orthodontic appliances is an important part of oral sanitation.

_____

_____

c. **True** or **False** (circle one). The hard deposits are acquired pellicle or cuticle, dental biofilm, materia alba, and food debris.

_____

_____

d. **True** or **False** (circle one). The soft deposits on teeth are dental calculus.

_____

_____

e. **True** or **False** (circle one). The incipient carious lesion begins as visible demineralization.

_____

_____

f. **True** or **False** (circle one). Acquired pellicle is composed primarily of glycoproteins from the saliva, which are selectively adsorbed by the hydroxyapatite of the tooth surface.

_____

_____

g. **True** or **False** (circle one). The unstained pellicle is readily visible.

_____

_____

h. **True** or **False** (circle one). The probability of the development of dental caries and/or gingivitis increases as the number of microorganisms decreases.

_____

_____

i. **True** or **False** (circle one). Gingivitis is clinically evident within 2 to 3 days when biofilm is left undisturbed on the tooth surfaces.

_____

_____

j. **True** or **False** (circle one). Subgingival biofilm results from the apical proliferation of microorganisms from supragingival biofilm.

_____

_____

k. **True** or **False** (circle one). The flora of the subgingival biofilm does not differ from that of the supragingival biofilm.

_____

_____

l. **True** or **False** (circle one). The biofilm attached to the tooth surface is associated with calculus formation, root caries, and root resorption.

_____

_____

m. **True** or **False** (circle one). Between the layers of attached biofilm are many motile, gram-negative organisms. These are considered part of the attached biofilm.

_____

_____

n. **True** or **False** (circle one). Loosely attached to the pocket epithelium are many gram-negative microorganisms and numerous white blood cells. These make up the epithelium-associated biofilm.

_____

_____

o. **True** or **False** (circle one). Microbial biofilm plays a major role in the initiation and progression of both dental caries and periodontal diseases.

_____

_____

p. **True** or **False** (circle one). Surface pellicle is continuous with subsurface pellicle, which is embedded in the tooth structure, particularly where the tooth surface is partially demineralized.

_____

_____

q. **True** or **False** (circle one). The concentration of calcium, phosphorus, magnesium, and fluoride is higher in biofilm than in saliva.

_____

_____

r. **True** or **False** (circle one). Biofilm on the lingual surfaces of the maxillary anterior teeth contains a higher concentration of calcium and phosphate than does biofilm on the other teeth, and the concentration of these minerals is even higher in heavy calculus formers.

_____

_____

s. **True** or **False** (circle one). When stained with a disclosing agent, unstained pellicle appears thin, with a pale staining that contrasts with the thicker, darker staining of dental biofilm.

_____

_____

t. **True** or **False** (circle one). The concentration of fluoride in biofilm is higher when fluoridated water is used, and it increases after professional topical applications of fluoride and the use of fluoride-containing dentifrices and mouthrinses.

_____

_____

u. **True** or **False** (circle one). Carbohydrates contribute to the adherence of the microorganisms to each other and the teeth.

_____

_____

v. **True** or **False** (circle one). The acquired pellicle begins to form within hours after all external material has been removed from the tooth surfaces with an abrasive.

_____

_____

w. **True** or **False** (circle one). Subgingival biofilm contains proteins from gingival sulcus fluid.

_____

_____

x. **True** or **False** (circle one). General oral cleanliness is not influenced by the removal of dental biofilm deposits.

_____

_____

y. **True** or **False** (circle one). Dental caries is a disease of the dental calcified structures (enamel, dentin, and cementum) that is characterized by demineralization of the mineral components and dissolution of the organic matrix.

_____

_____

z. **True** or **False** (circle one). The number of microorganisms is higher in subgingval biofilm than in supragingival biofilm.

_____

_____

7. Match the following descriptions of biofilm with the correct type. Each type is used more than once.

TYPE OF BIOFILM	DESCRIPTION
A. Supragingival biofilm B. Subgingival biofilm	__1__ Shape and size are affected by the friction of tongue, cheeks, and lips __2__ The main source of nutrients for bacterial proliferation is gingival sulcus fluid __3__ Coronal to the margin of the free gingiva __4__ May become thicker as the diseased pocket wall becomes less tight __5__ Early biofilm; primarily gram-positive cocci __6__ Heaviest collection on areas not cleaned daily by patient __7__ Found on the cervical third, especially facial surfaces, the lingual mandibular molars, and proximal surfaces __8__ Down growth of bacteria from supragingival biofilm __9__ Diseased pocket; primarily gram-negative, motile, spirochetes, rods __10__ Sources of nutrients for bacterial proliferation are saliva and ingested food __11__ Made up of three layers __12__ The structure is an adherent, densely packed microbial layer over pellicle on the tooth surface

8. The sequence of events for demineralization and dental caries follows a predictable pattern. Number the list of events in the correct order (1 = first event; 10 = last event).

_____ Demineralization occurs.

_____ Acid forms immediately.

_____ Cariogenic food stuff eaten

_____ Biofilm in the oral cavity

_____ White spot lesions; incipient lesions formed

_____ Frequent exposure of tooth surface to acid

_____ Fermentable carbohydrate taken into biofilm

_____ Caries process initiated

_____ pH of biofilm drops.

_____ Dental caries occurs.

 COMPETENCY EXERCISES

Apply information from the chapter and use critical thinking skills to complete the competency exercises. Write responses on paper or create electronic documents to submit your answers.

1. Your patient, Daron Horwitz, is curious about how to remove the soft deposits in his mouth. He presents with biofilm, materia alba, and food debris. Discuss patient instructions for the removal of all three deposits.

2. As you evaluate Mrs. Eltheia Shore, you note that she presents with a significant amount of supragingival, subgingival, gingival, and fissure biofilm. Educate her about the factors that can contribute to biofilm accumulation and the surfaces most commonly affected. Describe the strategies used for detection of biofilm.

3. You are providing patient education for Alison Alverez and her 10-year-old son, Juan. Juan has multiple carious lesions, and his mother is very interested in preventing more from occurring. Juan drinks soda daily. He purchases a 32-oz. bottle on his way to school and sips the soda every chance he gets. Juan's mother remembers hearing something about acids in the mouth and wants to know more about this.

4. Your patient is Nguyen Tho Phan, a 58-year-old research microbiologist. Her area of research is disease prevention, and she wants to understand the major pathogens that are identified in destructive periodontal disease and caries. If Nguyen presents with mutans streptococci, what disease is she most at risk for? Her brother has periodontal disease, and Nguyen want to know if he would have the same bacteria in his mouth.

5. Specific microorganisms, a susceptible tooth surface, and a diet high in cariogenic foods are essential for caries to develop. List some recommendations you can provide to an adult patient for prevention of dental caries.

Everyday Ethics

Before completing the learning exercises below, reread and reflect on the Everyday Ethics scenario and Questions for Consideration in this chapter of the textbook. It may also be useful to review the Dental Hygiene Ethics discussion in Chapter 1, the Ethical Applications in the introduction pages for each section in the textbook, as well as the Codes of Ethics in Appendices I, II, and III.

Individual Learning Activity

Imagine that you have observed what happened in the scenario, but are not one of the main characters involved in the situation. Write a reflective journal entry that

- describes how you might have reacted (as an observer-not as a participant),
- expresses your personal feelings about what happened, or identifies personal values that affect your reaction to the situation.

Collaborative Learning Activity

Work with another student colleague to role-play the scenario. The goal of this exercise is for you and your colleague to work though the alternative actions in order to come to consensus on a solution or response that is acceptable to both of you.

Factors To Teach The Patient

This scenario is related to the following factors listed in this chapter of the textbook:

- Location, composition, and properties of dental biofilm with emphasis on its role in dental caries and periodontal infections
- Effects of personal oral care procedures in the prevention of dental biofilm
- Biofilm control procedures with special adaptations for individual needs

You have just seated your patient, Mrs. Lorna Patel. Refer to her assessment data in the Section III Summary or her completed care plan in Appendix C to review the assessment findings, concentrating on her dental history and dental findings.

Use the examples of patient conversations in Appendix D as a guide to write a statement explaining to Mrs. Patel the appearance of acute gingivitis and the impact of effective brushing and flossing after a specified period of time. You may also want to refer to the figure in Knowledge Exercise 4 when writing your statement. Compare your conversation with a student colleague to identify any missing information.

CROSSWORD PUZZLE

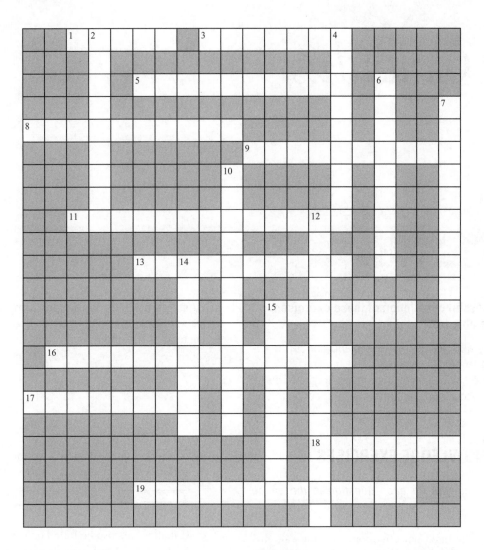

ACROSS

1. The collective organisms of a given locale
3. Organism that is able to live under more than one specific set of environmental conditions
5. The microscopic living organisms of a region
8. The action of a substance in attracting and holding other materials or particles on its surface
9. Conducive to the initiation of dental caries
11. Not self-sustaining; feeding on others
13. Organism that lives upon dead or decaying organic matter
15. Refers to heterotrophic microorganism that can live and grow in the presence of free oxygen
16. Formation of calculus
17. Opposite of facultative
18. Any matrix-enclosed bacterial populations adherent to each other and/or to surfaces or interfaces
19. Minute living organism

DOWN

2. White blood corpuscle capable of ameboid movement; functions to protect the body against infection and disease
4. Refers to heterotrophic microorganism that lives and grows in complete (or almost complete) absence of oxygen
6. Invasion and multiplication of a microorganism in body tissues
7. Pleomorphic, gram-negative bacteria that lack cell walls
10. Development of dental caries
12. Matrix between bacteria in dental biofilm; derived from saliva and gingival exudate
14. Disease-producing agent or microorganism
15. Not made up of or containing cells
10. Development of dental caries
12. Matrix between bacteria in dental biofilm; derived from saliva and gingival exudate
14. Disease-producing agent or microorganism
15. Not made up of or containing cells

Calculus

Learning Objectives

Upon successful completion of these exercises, you will be able to:

1. Identify and define key terms and concepts related to dental calculus.
2. Describe calculus in terms of type, location, distribution, occurrence, appearance, and consistency.
3. Describe calculus formation, composition, and attachment.
4. Discuss the significance of calculus.

 KNOWLEDGE EXERCISES

Write your answers for each question in the space provided.

1. What is the main objective for removing calculus from the surfaces of teeth?

   _____

   _____

2. Fill in the blanks as you learn about supragingival calculus.

   a. Supragingival calculus is located on the _____ crown of the tooth, _____ to the margin of the gingiva.

   b. It is found most frequently on the _____ surfaces of _____ anterior teeth and the _____ surfaces of _____ first and second molars.

   c. Calculus can also be found on surfaces of dental _____ and barbells worn in tongue or lip piercing.

3. Supragingival calculus may be referred to by other names. List some of these other terms.

   _____

   _____

   _____

   _____

4. Match each term with its definition.

TERMS RELATED TO CALCULUS	DEFINITION
_____ Pyrophosphate	A. Mineralized biofilm covered on the external surface with vital, tightly adherent, non-mineralized biofilm
_____ Amorphous	B. Without definite shape or visible differentiation in structure
_____ Germ free	C. Intercellular or intermicrobial substance of a tissue or the tissue from which a structure develops, gains support, and is held together
_____ Matrix	D. Nucleus; focus; point of origin
_____ Calculus	E. Free from microorganisms
_____ Nidus	F. Crystalline mineral component of bones and teeth that contains calcium and phosphate
_____ Apatite	G. Abnormal concretion composed of mineral salts
_____ Saturated	H. Examples are pulp stones, denticles, and salivary calculi
_____ Denture calculus	I. Out of place; arising or produced at an abnormal site or in a tissue where it is not normally found
_____ Supersaturated	J. Addition of mineral elements, such as calcium and phosphorus, to the body or a part thereof with resulting hardening of the tissue
_____ Ectopic oral calcification	K. Inhibitor of calcification that occurs in parotid saliva of humans in variable amounts; anticalculus component of tarter-control dentifrices
_____ Mineralization	L. Holding all of a substance (solute) that can be dissolved in the solution
_____ Ectopic	M. A solution containing more of an ingredient than can be held in solution permanently

5. List the agents that can be used as active ingredients that help control supragingival calculus in "tartar control" mouthrinses and dentifrices.

_____

_____

_____

6. Match the description with the type of calculus deposit. Each type of deposit is used more than once.

TYPE OF CALCULUS DEPOSIT	DESCRIPTION
A. Supragingival calculus	___1___ Light to dark brown, dark green, or black
B. Subgingival calculus	___2___ May be stained by tobacco, food, or other pigments
	___3___ Crusty, spiny, or nodular
	___4___ Shape of calculus mass is determined by the anatomy of teeth; contour of gingival margin; and pressure of tongue, lips, and cheeks
	___5___ Thin, smooth veneers
	___6___ Amorphous, bulky
	___7___ Increased amount in tobacco smokers
	___8___ Newest deposits near bottom of pocket are less dense and hard
	___9___ White, creamy yellow, or gray
	___10___ Brittle, flint-like
	___11___ Finger- and fern-like
	___12___ Slight deposits may be invisible until dried with compressed air
	___13___ Flattened to conform with pressure from the pocket wall
	___14___ Moderately hard
	___15___ Stains derived from blood pigments from diseased pocket
	___16___ Newer deposits less dense and hard

7. Fill in the blanks in the statements below as you read about subgingival calculus.

    a. Subgingival calculus is located apical to the _____ of the gingiva. It extends nearly to the _____ of the pocket.

    b. As the pocket is deepened by _____, calculus forms on the exposed root surface.

    c. This deposit may be _____ on a group of teeth or _____ on a single tooth.

    d. Heaviest deposits are often found on the _____ surfaces.

8. Subgingival calculus may be referred to by other names. List some of these terms.

    _____

    _____

9. Identify some strategies that will help you find supragingival and subgingival calculus in your patient's mouth.

    _____

    _____

    _____

    _____

    _____

    _____

10. List the three basic steps in calculus formation.

    _____

    _____

    _____

11. Mark each of the following statements **true** or **false.** If the statement is false, correct it, and write the true statement in the space provided.

    a. True or False (circle one). The control of biofilm deposits by the patient, supplemented by complete professional calculus removal, can reduce or eliminate gingival inflammation.

    _____

    _____

    b. True or False (circle one). Calculus is a predisposing factor in pocket development because it provides a haven for the collection of bacterial masses on the deposit's rough surface.

    _____

    _____

    c. True or False (circle one). Dental calculus is classified by its location on a tooth surface as related to the cemented-enamel junction; that is, supragingival or subgingival.

    _____

    _____

    d. True or False (circle one). With its rough surface, permeable structure, and porosity, calculus can act as a reservoir for endotoxins and tissue breakdown products.

    _____

    _____

    e. True or False (circle one). Calculus occurs only on the permanent teeth and in patients older than 12 years.

    _____

    _____

    f. True or False (circle one). Subgingival calculus is always covered by masses of active biofilm. The bacterial mass is in contact with the diseased pocket epithelium and promotes gingivitis and periodontitis.

    _____

    _____

    g. True or False (circle one). Subgingival deposits may be seen directly or indirectly, using a mouth mirror.

    _____

    _____

    h. True or False (circle one). Irritation to the pocket lining stimulates greater flow of gingival sulcus fluid, which contains minerals for supragingival calculus formation.

    _____

    _____

    i. True or False (circle one). A gentle air blast can deflect the margin from the tooth for access into the pocket.

    _____

    _____

j. True or False (circle one). Subgingival calculus does not develop by direct extension from supragingival calculus. Subgingival biofilm forms by extension of supragingival biofilm. Each biofilm mineralizes separately.

_____

_____

k. True or False (circle one). Mineralization of supragingival and subgingival calculus is essentially the same, even the source of the elements for mineralization is the same.

_____

_____

l. True or False (circle one). The location of supragingival calculus is related to the openings of the salivary gland ducts, especially the facial surface of mandibular molars and the facial surface of mandibular anterior teeth.

_____

_____

m. True or False (circle one). Pellicle begins to form within hours after all deposits have been removed from the tooth surface.

_____

_____

n. True or False (circle one). The source of elements for subgingival calculus is the saliva.

_____

_____

12. Mark each of the following statements **true** or **false.** If the statement is false, correct it, and write the true statement in the space provided.

a. True or False (circle one). The gingival sulcus fluid and the inflammatory exudate supply the minerals for the supragingival deposits.

_____

_____

b. True or False (circle one). Pyrophosphate is an inhibitor of calcification and is used in anticalculus dentifrices.

_____

_____

c. True or False (circle one). Subgingival biofilm contains pathogenic bacteria that cause inflammation and destruction of the gingival tissue and lead to loss of attachment to the tooth surface and development and deepening of the pocket.

_____

_____

d. True or False (circle one). Dental enamel is the most highly calcified tissue in the body and contains 96% inorganic salts; dentin contains 65%, and cementum and bone contain 45 to 50%.

_____

_____

e. True or False (circle one). Current research studies point to the probability that calcification of calculus may involve the same phenomena as other ectopic calcifications (e.g., urinary or renal calculi) and may be similar to normal calcification of bone, cartilage, enamel, and dentin.

_____

_____

f. True or False (circle one). The biofilm on the calculus surface contains nonviable organisms.

_____

_____

g. True or False (circle one). The surface of a calculus mass is rough and can be detected by use of an explorer. As observed by electron microscope, the surface roughness appears as depressions, ridges, and ledges.

_____

_____

h. True or False (circle one). The ease or difficulty of removal can be related to the manner of attachment of the calculus to the tooth surface.

_____

_____

i. True or False (circle one). Heavy calculus formers have higher levels of parotid pyrophosphate than do light calculus formers.

_____

_____

j. True or False (circle one). Calculus is primarily made up of organic components and water.

_____

_____

k. True or False (circle one). Inorganic components of calculus are mainly calcium (Ca), phosphorus (P), carbonate (CO_3), sodium (Na), magnesium (Mg), and potassium (K).

_____

_____

l. True or False (circle one). The concentration of fluoride in calculus varies and is influenced by the amount of fluoride received from fluoride in the drinking water, topical application, dentifrices, or any form that is received by contact with the external surface of the calculus.

_____

_____

m. True or False (circle one). The surface of the enamel is more permeable than the surface of the cementum and thus has higher fluoride content.

_____

_____

n. True or False (circle one). At least two thirds of the inorganic matter of calculus is crystalline, principally apatite. Predominating is pyrophosphate, which is the same crystal present in enamel, dentin, cementum, and bone.

_____

_____

13. Mark each of the following statements **true** or **false.** If the statement is false, correct it, and write the true statement in the space provided.

a. True or False (circle one). The organic proportion of calculus consists of various types of nonvital microorganisms, desquamated epithelial cells, leukocytes, and mucin from the blood.

_____

_____

b. True or False (circle one). The microorganisms in early biofilm are predominantly filamentous. After 5 days, cocci and rod-shaped organisms are found.

_____

_____

c. True or False (circle one). Most of the organisms within calculus are considered viable.

_____

_____

d. True or False (circle one). Small amounts of calculus that have not been stained are frequently more visible when they are wet with saliva.

_____

_____

e. True or False (circle one). With increased pocket depth, greater amounts of biofilm can accumulate, with increased numbers of pathogenic organisms.

_____

_____

f. True or False (circle one). The incidence of calculus decreases with age.

_____

_____

g. True or False (circle one). Although the proportion varies, depending on the age and hardness of a deposit and the location from which the sample for analysis is taken, mature calculus usually contains between 75 and 85% inorganic components; the rest is organic components and water.

_____

_____

h. True or False (circle one). Calculus is mineralized biofilm. The biofilm next to the tooth surface is mineralized last.

_____

_____

i. True or False (circle one). Various trace elements have been identified in inorganic calculus. These include chlorine (Cl), zinc (Zn), strontium (Sr), bromine (Br), copper (Cu), manganese (Mn), tungsten (W), gold (Au), aluminum (Al), silicon (Si), iron (Fe), and fluorine (F).

_____

_____

j. True or False (circle one). Agents used in "tartar control" dentifrices and mouthrinse act only on calculus and have no effect on oral tissues.

_____

_____

COMPETENCY EXERCISES

Apply information from the chapter and use critical thinking skills to complete the competency exercises. Write responses on paper or create electronic documents to submit your answers.

1. Compare and contrast the distribution of supragingival and subgingival calculus. Discuss how the distribution affects your detection strategies.

2. Discuss the process of calculus formation in your own words. Be sure to address pellicle formation and biofilm maturation. Concentrate on mineralization.

3. Your patient John Weston is wondering about calculus formation. He is trying to understand the exact time frame of the process. Help him understand calculus formation by defining calculus and discussing the influencing factors. Make a list that describes calculus formation in terms of minutes, hours, and days.

4. While scaling in the mandibular right quadrant, you are having varying degrees of difficulty detecting and removing the calculus. Describe the three modes of calculus attachment. Explain how each mode affects detection and removal.

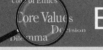

Everyday Ethics

Before completing the learning exercises below, reread and reflect on the Everyday Ethics scenario and Questions for Consideration in this chapter of the textbook. It may also be useful to review the Dental Hygiene Ethics discussion in Chapter 1, the Ethical Applications in the introduction pages for each section in the textbook, as well as the Codes of Ethics in Appendices I, II, and III.

Individual Learning Activity
Imagine that you are the dental hygienist in this scenario. Answer each of the questions for consideration at the end of the scenario.

Discovery Activity
Summarize this scenario for faculty member at your school and ask them to consider the questions that are included. Is their perspective different than yours or similar? Explain.

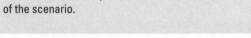

Factors To Teach The Patient

This scenario is related to the following factors:

■ That good oral hygiene and frequent professional care for complete scaling are consistent with low levels of supragingival and subgingival calculus
■ The effect of calculus on the health of the periodontal tissues and, therefore, on the general health of the oral cavity
■ What to expect from use of an anticalculus dentifrice
■ The importance of selecting products with an ADA Seal of Approval

Louisa Gregory, a 53-year-old first-grade teacher, is busy with her two daughters, aged 12 and 14. She does not take time for herself and has come to the dental hygiene clinic after a 5-year absence. She uses any type of toothpaste that is on sale, and her current dentifrice is in a decorative

dispenser; she does not know anything else about it except that it matches her bathroom perfectly! As you examine Louisa's mouth you see generalized heavy supragingival and subgingival calculus. She wants to know what to do about "all this hard stuff" on her teeth.

Use the example of patient conversations in Appendix D as a guide to create a conversation to educate Louisa about the impact of good oral hygiene and frequent professional care for complete scaling on the levels of supragingival and subgingival calculus. Be sure to address product selection criteria and the need for the use of an anticalculus toothpaste.

Use the conversation you create to role-play this situation with a fellow student. If you are the patient in the role-play, be sure to ask questions. If you are the dental hygienist, try to anticipate questions and answer them in your explanation.

Dental Stains and Discolorations

Learning Objectives

Upon successful completion of these exercises, you will be able to:

1. Identify and define key terms and concepts related to dental stains and discolorations.

2. Classify and document various stains according to their location and source.

 KNOWLEDGE EXERCISES

Write your answers for each question in the space provided.

1. Match the following terms with the correct definition.

TERM		DEFINITION
A. Chlorophyll	1	Incomplete development or underdevelopment of an organ or a tissue
B. Endogenous	2	Producing color or pigment
C. Chronologic	3	Imperfect formation of enamel; hereditary condition in which the ameloblasts fail to lay down the enamel matrix properly or at all
D. Chromogenic		
E. Dentinogenesis imperfecta	4	Originating outside or caused by factors outside
	5	Hereditary disorder of dentin formation in which the odontoblasts lay down an abnormal matrix; can occur in both primary and permanent dentitions
F. Amelogenesis imperfecta		
G. Hypoplasia	6	Produced within or caused by factors within
H. Intrinsic	7	Situated entirely within
I. Exogenous	8	Green plant pigment essential to photosynthesis
J. Extrinsic	9	Arranged in order of time
	10	Derived from or situated on the outside; external

2. Stains are classified by location and source.

   a. List examples of extrinsic exogenous stains.

   _____

   _____

   b. List examples of intrinsic endogenous stains.

   _____

   _____

c. List examples of intrinsic exogenous stains.

_____

_____

_____

_____

3. Your patient presents with a stained pulpless tooth. Describe the clinical appearance of the stain and how it was formed. The patient is scheduled for endodontic treatment on another tooth and wants to know if that tooth will also stain. What would you tell this patient?

_____

_____

_____

_____

4. Clinically you observe enamel that is partially or completely missing because of a generalized disturbance of the ameloblasts. Teeth are yellowish-brown or gray-brown. What is this condition is called?

_____

5. Your patient was born with erythroblastosis fetalis (Rh incompatibility). This condition may a leave the teeth with a _____, _____, or _____ hue.

6. Complete Infomap 21-1 to help you organize information about extrinsic stains.

INFOMAP 21-1					
TYPE OF STAIN	**APPEARANCE**	**DISTRIBUTION**	**OCCURRENCE**	**CAUSE/ORIGIN**	**CLINICAL ISSUES**
Yellow					
Green					
Other Green					
Black Line					
Tobacco					
Other Brown					
Orange and Red					
Metallic—Industrial					
Metallic—Drugs					

✓ COMPETENCY EXERCISES

Apply information from the chapter and use critical thinking skills to complete the competency exercises. Write responses on paper or create electronic documents to submit your answers.

1. Your 1:30 PM patient, Fawez Sadarage, 47 years old, presents with a stain on the second and third molars caused by tetracycline. Describe the stain that you see and list some follow-up questions you will ask Mr. Sadarage. Approximately how old was Mr. Sadarage when he took this antibiotic?

2. Several strategies will help you recognize and identify stains that you observe during assessment of the oral cavity. Explain the types of stains (color and cause) that can be identified using each of the strategies listed below.

   ■ Medical history

   ■ Questions about industrial occupation

■ Questions about dietary habits

■ Dental history

■ Dental charting (e.g., endodontic therapy, restorative materials)

Everyday Ethics

Before completing the learning exercises below, reread and reflect on the Everyday Ethics scenario and Questions for Consideration in this chapter of the textbook. It may also be useful to review the Dental Hygiene Ethics discussion in Chapter 1, the Ethical Applications in the introduction pages for each section in the textbook, as well as the Codes of Ethics in Appendices I, II, and III.

Collaborative Learning Activity
Answer each of the questions for consideration at the end of the scenario in the textbook. Compare what you wrote with answers developed by another classmate and discuss differences/similarities.

Discovery Activity
Summarize this scenario for faculty member at your school and ask them to consider the questions that are included. Is their perspective different than yours or similar? Explain.

Factors To Teach The Patient

This scenario is related to the following factors listed in this chapter of the textbook:

■ Predisposing factors that contribute to stain accumulation
■ Personal care procedures that can aid in the prevention or reduction of stains
■ Advantages of starting a smoking-cessation program
■ Reasons for not using an abrasive dentifrice with vigorous brushing strokes to lessen or remove stain accumulation
■ The need to avoid tobacco, coffee, tea, and other beverages or foodstuffs that can stain to prevent discoloration of new restorations

Your patient, Shaneeka Harris, is a 21-year-old college student. She has recently started to smoke cigarettes and marijuana and drink a lot of coffee and tea. Her last blood test showed that she was anemic, and her physician has prescribed daily oral doses of iron. Shaneeka is finding college overwhelming and very stressful. The reason she made an appointment in the dental hygiene clinic is because she has noticed that her teeth have a brown and gray-green stain, and she is really unhappy with how they look. She does not remember having all these stains before.

Use the example of patient conversations in Appendix D as a guide to write a statement to help Shaneeka understand the factors affecting stain accumulation and the removal and prevention strategies.

Use the conversation you create to role-play this situation with a fellow student. If you are the patient in the role-play, be sure to ask questions. If you are the dental hygienist, try to anticipate questions and answer them in your explanation.

CHAPTER 22

Indices and Scoring Methods

Upon successful completion of these exercises, you will be able to:

1. Identify and define key terms and concepts related to dental indices and scoring methods.
2. Identify the purpose, criteria for measurement, scoring methods, range of scores, and reference or interpretation scales for a variety of dental indices.
3. Select and calculate dental indices for a use in a specific patient or community situation.

KNOWLEDGE EXERCISES

Write your answers for each question in the space provided.

DENTAL INDICES INFOMAPS

Infomaps are tables that place related information about different factors of one topic on a single page. This method of organizing not only allows you to learn information as you transfer key points from the textbook but also provides a study guide that lets you visually compare and contrast the different dental indices easily and effectively.

Transfer enough basic information about each index from the textbook to the appropriate Infomap so that you can use the collected data to complete the Competency Exercises for this chapter. The blank Infomaps, 22-1 to 22-5, are located on the next few pages.

INFOMAP 22-1 | ORAL HYGIENE STATUS INDICES

INDEX	WHAT IS MEASURED?	TEETH AND/OR SURFACES SCORED	CRITERIA USED FOR MEASUREMENT	SCORING/ CALCULATION OF INDEX	REFERENCE SCALES, RANGE OF SCORES, AND ADDITIONAL INFORMATION
PL I					
"Plaque-Control Record"					
"Plaque-Free Score"					
PHP					
OHI-S					

INFOMAP 22-2 | GINGIVAL HEALTH INDICES

INDEX	WHAT IS MEASURED?	TEETH AND/ OR SURFACES SCORED	CRITERIA USED FOR MEASUREMENT	SCORING/ CALCULATION OF INDEX	REFERENCE SCALES, RANGE OF SCORES, AND ADDITIONAL INFORMATION
SBI					
GBI					
EIBI					
GI					

INFOMAP 22-3	INDIVIDUAL AND COMMUNITY PERIODONTAL INDICES				
INDEX	WHAT IS MEASURED?	TEETH AND/ OR SURFACES SCORED	CRITERIA USED FOR MEASUREMENT	SCORING/ CALCULATION OF INDEX	REFERENCE SCALES, RANGE OF SCORES, AND ADDITIONAL INFORMATION
PSR					
CPI					

INFOMAP 22-4	DENTAL CARIES INDICES				
INDEX (AND AUTHOR)	WHAT IS MEASURED?	TEETH AND/ OR SURFACES SCORED	CRITERIA USED FOR MEASUREMENT	SCORING/ CALCULATION OF INDEX	ADDITIONAL INFORMATION
DMFT					
DMFS					
dft and dfs					
deft and defs					
dmft and dmfs					
ECC and S-ECC					
RCI					

INFOMAP 22-5	FLUOROSIS INDICES				
INDEX (AND AUTHOR)	**WHAT IS MEASURED?**	**TEETH AND/ OR SURFACES SCORED**	**CRITERIA USED FOR MEASUREMENT**	**SCORING/ CALCULATION OF INDEX**	**ADDITIONAL INFORMATION**
Dean's Fluorosis Index					
TSIF					

COMPETENCY EXERCISES

Apply information from the chapter and use critical thinking skills to complete the competency exercises. Write responses on paper or create electronic documents to submit your answers.

COMMUNITY CASE SCENARIO

Answer the following questions based on this community case scenario.

You, several student colleagues, and some of the faculty members at your school are asked to be part of a statewide, community-based oral health surveillance project conducted by your local Department of Community Health. The project requires that you collect data during the local Toothtown Activity Center Health Fair for young adults ages 17–25.

You are excited that you will be participating in calibration exercises, collecting data with other members of your school team, and then actually calculating and interpreting the results of your own data collection. What a great way to learn about the dental indices you have just been studying!

1. Determine the index (or identify a group of indices) that will provide the most comprehensive information about this population. What are the advantages or disadvantages of the indices you have selected?

2. The Department of Community Health has decided to use the DMFT index to collect data about the caries experience of the group of individuals at the activity center. Discuss the advantages and disadvantages of using this index instead of the DMFS index for community screening.

3. After participating in the screening day at the Toothtown Activity Center, you feel quite confident about using the DMFT index and OHI-S to score individuals as well as the GI that your team decided to use. Now it is time to calculate the results and practice interpreting your findings.

   Using the information in Table 22-1, calculate the individual DMFs, the total group DMF, and the group average DMF.

4. Using the data in Table 22-1, calculate the percentage of DMF teeth in this group that currently have decay.

5. Using the data in Table 22-1, calculate the percentage of DMF teeth that have been restored.

6. Using the data in Table 22-1, calculate the percentage of individuals in this group who have at least one decayed tooth.

7. Using the data in Table 22-1, calculate the percentage of individuals in this group who have treatment needs.

TABLE 22-1	CALCULATING DMF DATA			
INDIVIDUAL	**D**	**M**	**F**	**INDIVIDUAL DMF**
Abbe	12	0	14	
Bill	0	0	6	
Charlie	4	2	0	
David	1	0	6	
Edwin	3	0	0	
Frank	0	1	1	
Grace	4	0	6	
Harry	6	0	7	
Ida	18	2	0	
Joe	2	0	5	
Total				
Group Average DMF				

8. Use Tables 22-2 and 22-3 to calculate a gingival index (GI) score for Grace and an average GI score for all the individuals in the group.

TABLE 22-2	CALCULATING GI DATA: AREA SCORES FOR GRACE			
Tooth	**M**	**F**	**D**	**L**
3 (16)	2	0	2	0
9 (21)	0	0	0	0
12 (24)	1	0	1	0
19 (36)	2	0	2	0
25 (41)	0	0	0	0
28 (44)	1	0	1	0
Total				
GI score				

TABLE 22-3	CALCULATING THE GROUP AVERAGE GI SCORE
NAME	**GI SCORE**
Charlie	2.9
Harry	1.0
Ida	1.7
Joe	2.6
Grace	?_____
Total	
Group Average GI	

TABLE 22-4	OHI-S DATA FOR BILL	
TOOTH	**DI**	**CI**
3 (16)	3	0
8 (11)	3	0
14 (26)	3	2
19 (36)	3	0
24 (31)	3	0
30 (46)	2	0
Total		
Scores		
OHI-S score		

9. What does Grace's GI score mean?

10. What is your interpretation of the average gingival health of the group?

11. Imagine that you have calculated GI scores for more than 150 individuals who were screened at the Activity Center Health Fair. You calculate that this group's average score is 2.78. How can you use this *group average score* as baseline data to evaluate the effect of oral hygiene presentations that you and your students will provide at a later time?

    In other words, explain how you might use this baseline average GI score to determine whether the people in this community were motivated to better oral health because of your education project.

12. Use Table 22-4 to calculate a DI score, a CI score, and an OHI-S score for Bill.

13. Use Table 22-5 to calculate a group OHI-S score. Make sure to include Bill's score.

TABLE 22-5	CALCULATING GROUP OHI-S DATA
INDIVIDUAL	**OHI-S SCORE**
Abbe	4.33
Bill	
Charlie	1.20
David	1.03
Edwin	1.00
Group OHI-S	

14. What does each individual person's OHI-S score indicate about his or her oral cleanliness? What does the average group score indicate?

15. You and your classmates had so much fun and learned so much at the Toothtown Activity Center screening that you want to do some more community-based screenings. You find out that the Department of Community Health is planning to set up a mobile clinic to provide dental services for a group of 3000 homeless individuals in your city. There is not enough money to offer all possible services for this group of people, but the health department is hoping to provide enough care to meet most of the people's needs.

    Your class decides to visit with the Director of Community Health to explain how the results of a Basic Screening Survey that you and your classmates plan to conduct can help to identify and prioritize the oral health services that are needed by this population. Present your ideas for class discussion and compare them with the ideas of your other classmates.

16. As part of the screening you conduct among the homeless population, you also provide individualized oral hygiene instructions and free oral health products to everyone who agrees to participate in the screening. One person, Mrs. Combs, is missing teeth 1, 2, 16, 17, and 32. The others are all present. When you disclose her teeth before providing oral hygiene instructions, you note that there is significant biofilm on every single proximal surface, the facial surfaces of 3 and 4, and the lingual surfaces of all four mandibular molars.

    Use the patient biofilm recording form that your clinic recommends (or make up one of your own using the models provided in the textbook) and color in all the areas with biofilm with a red pen or pencil.

    Using the information from this form, calculate both the plaque-control record and the plaque-free scores for biofilm on Mrs. Combs' teeth.

💡 DISCOVERY EXERCISES

Explore the Association of State and Territorial Dental Directors Web site (http://www.astdd.org) to locate information about the *Basic Screening Surveys: An Approach to Monitoring Community Oral Health* community data collection system. Many states in the U.S. use this system to gather oral health surveillance data. Download and study all of the components that are available on the Web site to help you learn about how this oral health surveillance system works. Consider purchasing the training videotape so you and your classmates can be trained to use the system in a future community screening.

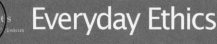

Everyday Ethics

Before completing the learning exercises below, reread and reflect on the Everyday Ethics scenario and Questions for Consideration in this chapter of the textbook. It may also be useful to review the Dental Hygiene Ethics discussion in Chapter 1, the Ethical Applications in the introduction pages for each section in the textbook, as well as the Codes of Ethics in Appendices I, II, and III.

Individual Learning Activity
Identify a situation you have experienced that presents a similar ethical dilemma. Write about you would do differently now than you did at the time the incident happened—support your discussion with concepts from the dental hygiene codes of ethics.

Collaborative Learning Activity
Answer each of the questions for consideration at the end of the scenario in the textbook. Compare what you wrote with answers developed by another classmate and discuss differences/similarities.

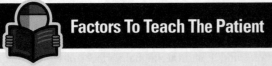

Factors To Teach The Patient

This scenario is related to the following factors listed in this chapter of the textbook:

- How an index is used and calculated and what the scores mean
- Correlation of index scores with current oral health practices and procedures
- Procedures to follow to improve index scores and bring the oral tissues to health

As you are marking the areas of biofilm on the patient form, Mrs. Combs (from Competency Exercise 16) asks why dental hygienists always bother to do all that "extra work" just to provide oral hygiene instructions. Apparently no one had ever explained it to her before.

Using the examples of patient conversations in Appendix D as a guide, write a statement explaining these dental indices to your patient.

Use the conversation you create to role play this situation with a fellow student. If you are the patient in the role play, be sure to ask questions. If you are the dental hygienist, try to anticipate questions and answer them in your explanation.

CROSSWORD PUZZLE

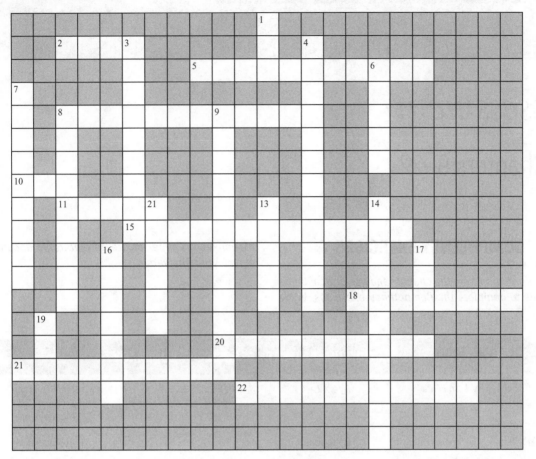

ACROSS

2. An index that combines a debris score and a calculus score using specific surfaces of six teeth.
5. A determination of accuracy and consistency between examiners; affects the reliability of data collection.
8. An index that measures conditions that are not able to be changed; in other words, evidence of the condition will remain even after treatment; example is dental caries.
10. Periodontal screening index used for community oral health surveillance that can be used in conjunction with a code related to loss of attachment.
11. Index that measures fluorosis using six categories.
15. A sweeping motion of the dental probe determines bleeding evaluation when this index is used (two words)
18. Refers to index teeth numbers 3, 9, 12, 19, 25, and 28; teeth used for classic epidemiological studies of periodontal disease.
20. A type of index that measures all the evidence of a condition, past and present.
21. The total number of cases of some disease or condition in a given population.
22. Index that is used to assesses thickness of dental biofilm at the gingival area (two words).

DOWN

1. This index uses unwaxed dental floss to determine areas of interproximal gingival bleeding.
3. Refers to a brief initial exam for an individual or an assessment of many individuals to determine a certain characteristic in a population.
4. Type of index that measures a condition that can be changed and no evidence of the condition will remain; example is dental biofilm.
6. An expression of clinical observations in numerical values.
7. A factor that is measured and analyzed to describe health status.
8. Refers to the number of new cases of a disease that occur during a certain period of time.
9. The systematic collection of oral health data for use in planning public health programs.
12. A category of indices that measures only the presence or absence of a condition.
13. Measures what it is intended to measure.
14. Consistency of measurement; enhanced by calibration of examiners.
16. This index uses a triangular wooden interdental cleaner to identify areas of interproximal bleeding.
17. Index used to determine caries experience.
19. Index similar to the Community Periodontal Index that is used to screen individual patients in a private practice setting.

Assessment

■ Chapters 9–22

 COMPETENCY EXERCISES

Apply information from the chapter and use critical thinking skills to complete the Competency exercises. Write

responses on paper or create electronic documents to submit your answers.

SECTION III – PATIENT ASSESSMENT SUMMARY

Patient Name: *Mrs. Lorna Patel* Age: *49* Gender: M F √ Initial Therapy

☐ Maintenance

Provider Name: *D.H. Student* Date: *Today* ☐ Re-evaluation

Chief Complaint:

Gum tissues bleed when brushing and flossing. Mouth is dry all the time.

ASSESSMENT FINDINGS

Health History At Risk For:

- History of high blood pressure managed by medication
- Cholesterol managed by medication
- Mitral valve prolapse
- Allergy to penicillin
- Zocar 20 mg/1 per day
- Caltrate 1 per day
- Enapril 10 mg/hydrochlorothiazide 15 mg/1 per day
- Multiple vitamin 1 per day
- Clindamycin 20.0 g taken 1 hour before appointment
- ASA Classification—11
- ADL level—0

Social and Dental History At Risk For:

- 1.5 years since last recall
- Localized 4–5 mm probing depths
- Flosses daily
- Rinses with Listerine
- Mouth dry all the time
- Uses mints and candy for dry mouth
- Uses bottled water with no fluoride content

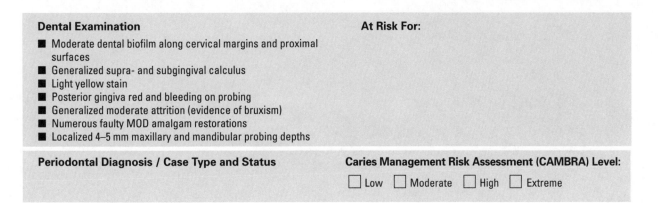

Dental Examination

- Moderate dental biofilm along cervical margins and proximal surfaces
- Generalized supra- and subgingival calculus
- Light yellow stain
- Posterior gingiva red and bleeding on probing
- Generalized moderate attrition (evidence of bruxism)
- Numerous faulty MOD amalgam restorations
- Localized 4–5 mm maxillary and mandibular probing depths

At Risk For:

Periodontal Diagnosis / Case Type and Status

Caries Management Risk Assessment (CAMBRA) Level:

☐ Low   ☐ Moderate   ☐ High   ☐ Extreme

Read the Section I Patient Assessment Summary to help you answer the following questions.

1. Identify follow-up questions to ask Mrs. Patel that will help you determine any additional information you will need to complete this patient's dental hygiene care plan.

2. When you question her, Mrs. Patel states that she has been taking clindamycin, as prescribed by her physician, prior to each dental appointment for many years. Would you request a medical consultation with her physician prior to scheduling a scaling and root planing appointment for Mrs. Patel? Explain why or why not.

3. Use the assessment findings information you have for Mrs. Patel to complete the "At Risk For" sections of her Patient Assessment Summary.

4. Complete the Periodontal Diagnosis and CAMBRA sections of the Assessment Summary form. What assessment information was available on the form that helped you to make those decisions? What additional information would be helpful as you completed those sections of the Assessment Form?

DISCOVERY EXERCISES

1. Collect samples of the worksheets that are used for patient assessment record keeping from several dental practices in your community. Compare these systems with those used in your school clinic. Discuss the advantages and disadvantages of each system with your student colleagues.

2. Many patients you provide dental hygiene care for will not speak English (or the language that most people in your country speak) as their first language. Those patients can often have a more difficult time accurately completing health history information.

Explore the Internet to discover health history forms that are translated into other languages. A fine place to start is at the MetDental.com Web site https://www.metdental.com/prov/execute/Content This Web page includes a link leading you to a site where you can download and print health history forms in a variety of languages. Click on the RESOURCE CENTER tab at the top of the page and then scroll down to find the link to Multi-Language Health History forms.

3. Look through the scientific literature to find periodontal disease studies that use some of the dental indices you learned about in Chapter 22 to collect data on periodontal disease status.

4. Explore the Internet to find oral health surveillance statistics for your community, state, or country. Analyze the statistics to describe the oral health status, and write a description of specific ways in which the oral health status of the population in your community might be improved by community-based dental hygiene interventions.

FOR YOUR PORTFOLIO

1. Include your personal written responses to the questions in the Everyday Ethics section from any of the chapters.

2. Complete patient assessment summaries for several patients who are scheduled with you in your clinic.

3. Demonstrate your interest and the development of your skills in providing culturally competent care by including any patient data collection or patient education materials that you discover for patients who are culturally different from yourself. Include a reflective journal entry describing ways that you can use these materials to enhance the quality of dental hygiene care you provide.

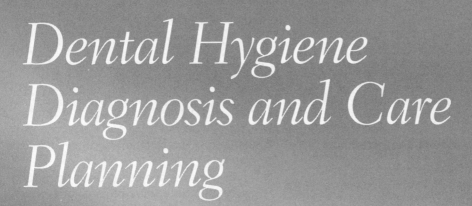

Dental Hygiene Diagnosis and Care Planning

Chapters 23–24

■ LEARNING OBJECTIVES

Completing the exercises in this section of the workbook will prepare you to:

■ Use assessment data to write dental hygiene diagnostic statements.

■ Develop a formal dental hygiene care plan based on the dental hygiene diagnosis that sequences evidence-based dental hygiene interventions in order to address identified patient needs.

■ Identify and apply procedures for obtaining informed consent.

■ Document all aspects of informed consent and the plan for patient care.

■ COMPETENCIES FOR THE DENTAL HYGIENIST (APPENDIX A)

Competencies supported by the learning in Section IV:

Core Competencies: C3, C4, C5, C7, C9, C10, C11, C12, C13

Health Promotion and Disease Prevention: HP1, HP2, HP4, HP5

Patient/Client Care: PC1, PC2, PC3, PC4, PC5, PC6, PC7, PC8, PC9, PC11, PC13

Planning for Dental Hygiene Care

Upon successful completion of these exercises, you will be able to:

1. Identify and define key terms and concepts related to planning dental hygiene care.
2. Identify and explain assessment findings and individual patient factors that affect patient care.

3. Identify additional factors that can influence planning for dental hygiene care.
4. Apply the evidence-based decision-making process to determine patient care recommendations.

KNOWLEDGE EXERCISES

Write your answers for each question in the space provided.

1. Supply the term or concept that matches each of the following descriptions:

   a. Measure of ability to perform self-care.

   _____

   b. A measure that integrates a combination of physical and cognitive ability.

   _____

   c. Statements that identify a problem.

   _____

   d. An outcome that can be expressed as "excellent," "poor," or "guarded,"

   _____

   e. Diagnostic model that uses the phrase "related to" to link identified patient problems with risk factors or etiology.

   _____

   f. Systemic conditions, behavioral factors, or environmental factors that can lead to increased probability of oral disease.

   _____

2. Identify factors from the patient assessment that are analyzed and considered when planning dental hygiene care.

   _____

   _____

   _____

   _____

   _____

3. Identify and briefly describe the issues indicated by the mnemonic OSCAR:

   O: _____

   S: _____

   C: _____

   A: _____

   R: _____

4. Briefly define each of the five ASA classification levels.

   _____

   _____

   _____

   _____

   _____

5. Define dental hygiene diagnosis in your own words.

   _____

   _____

6. List the factors that determine prognosis after dental hygiene interventions.

   _____

   _____

   _____

   _____

   _____

7. In your own words, define anticipatory guidance.

   _____

   _____

8. Summarize the factors that affect treatment outcomes (prognosis) following periodontal treatment interventions.

   _____

   _____

   _____

   _____

9. What is the role of the patient in determining outcomes following dental hygiene care?

   _____

   _____

10. What is the purpose of preprocedural tissue conditioning with antimicrobials?

    _____

11. The need for anesthetic during dental hygiene procedures is determined by:

    _____

    _____

    _____

12. Your patient's clinical diagnosis, provided by the periodontist, is "Chronic Periodontitis." List the therapeutic goals of treatment for this patient.

    _____

    _____

 COMPETENCY EXERCISES

Apply information from the chapter and use critical thinking skills to complete the competency exercises. Write responses on paper or create electronic documents to submit your answers.

1. At which ASA classification levels would you be most likely to consider contacting the patient's physician prior to planning for dental hygiene care? Provide a rationale for your answer.

2. Table 23-5 in the textbook contains a list of diagnostic models used in planning dental hygiene care along with a description of how diagnostic statements are constructed within the model. Which model seems closest to the approach your school clinic uses for planning individualized patient care? Explain.

3. For each of patient scenarios described below:

   a. Identify the OSCAR issue(s) that need to be evaluated.

   b. Determine the ASA classification you will assign when assessing the patient during planning of dental hygiene care.

   c. Write a justification for your selection.

   Scenario A: Mrs. Kujath is 90 years old and in very good physical and mental health. She has chronic arthritis, which is managed very well with daily pain medication, and only has minor problems with mobility, including sitting still for long. She doesn't really like the way her old denture looks, and she desires a new one.

She states that there is no problem about having the money to pay for the new denture.

Scenario B: Mr. Diamond has type I diabetes. His blood sugar levels indicate that his diabetes is not well controlled. Mr. Diamond has numerous posterior teeth that present with significant bone loss, generalized mobility, and class II or III furcations. Moreover, he is not particularly compliant with your recommendations for self-care for those furcation areas.

Scenario C: Mrs. Abdul must make a decision about treatment options for several teeth with severe periodontal involvement. Her health history indicates mild hypertension that is well controlled by medication. It has been many years since she has been to the dentist because of an extremely unpleasant dental experience in childhood. She squirmed and protested when you measured her probing depths and, in general, had a very difficult time cooperating during the collection of assessment data. She says that she must talk with her son, as he will be bringing her for her appointments and also be paying for whatever treatment is decided on.

Scenario D: Ms. Anitha Jones has cerebral palsy. She arrives at the dental office in a wheelchair and is accompanied by an attendant. Because of extreme muscle spasticity caused by her condition, her arms and legs are in constant motion, sometimes lashing out unexpectedly, and she must have a variety of pads and restraints to maintain her position and safety in her wheelchair chair. You and her caregiver plan to transfer her from her wheelchair to the dental chair for treatment. Her health history indicates that she is NOT mentally disabled.

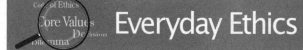

Everyday Ethics

Before completing the learning exercises below, reread and reflect on the Everyday Ethics scenario and Questions for Consideration in this chapter of the textbook. It may also be useful to review the Dental Hygiene Ethics discussion in Chapter 1, the Ethical Applications in the introduction pages for each Section in the textbook, as well as the Codes of Ethics in Appendices I, II, and III.

Individual Learning Activity
Imagine that you have observed what happened in the scenario, but are not one of the main characters involved in the situation. Write a reflective journal entry that

■ describes how you might have reacted (as an observer-not as a participant),

■ expresses your personal feelings about what happened, or
■ identifies personal values that affect your reaction to the situation.

Discovery Activity
Ask a friend or relative who is not involved in healthcare to read the scenario and discuss it with you from the perspective of a "patient" who receives services within the healthcare system. Discuss what you learned from the concerns, insights, or difference in perspective that person expressed.

Factors To Teach The Patient

This scenario is related to the following factors listed in this chapter of the textbook:

■ Why disease control measures are learned before and in conjunction with scaling
■ Facts of oral disease prevention and oral health promotion relevant to the patient's current level of health-care knowledge and individual risk factors

Your next patient, Jonathon Meyers, is a 26-year-old graduate student. He has not seen a dentist since he was a child. When his girlfriend told him about his bad breath, he decided to take advantage of the services offered at the dental clinic.

He presents with an aggressive periodontal condition in the lower anterior sextant of his mouth. Because he was not

exposed to much dental education in his life, Jon has a low dental IQ and doesn't understand the cause and progression of dental disease. He smokes, demonstrates poor biofilm control, and states that he wants you to just "fix him up" with your treatments.

Using the example of a patient conversation from Appendix D as a guide, write a statement explaining why disease control measures must happen before and in conjunction with scaling. Explain *his role* in attaining and maintaining oral health.

Use the conversation you create to role-play this situation with a fellow student. If you are the patient in the role-play, be sure to ask questions. If you are the dental hygienist, try to anticipate questions and answer them in your explanation.

CHAPTER 24

The Dental Hygiene Care Plan

Upon successful completion of these exercises, you will be able to:

1. Identify and define key terms and concepts related to the written dental hygiene care plan.
2. Identify the components of a dental hygiene care plan.
3. Write dental hygiene diagnostic statements on the basis of assessment findings.
4. Prepare a written dental hygiene care plan.
5. Apply procedures for discussing a care plan with the dentist and the patient.
6. Identify and apply procedures for obtaining informed consent.

KNOWLEDGE EXERCISES

Write your answers for each question in the space provided.

1. Define the following terms in your own words.

■ Dental hygiene intervention: _____
_____
_____

■ Informed consent: _____
_____
_____

■ Implied consent: _____
_____
_____

■ Informed refusal: _____
_____
_____

2. Identify and define the three parts of a dental hygiene care plan.
_____
_____
_____
_____
_____
_____
_____

3. List the 10 components of a written care plan.
_____
_____
_____
_____
_____
_____
_____
_____
_____

4. List three individual patient requirements that can require significant adaptations in the written dental hygiene care plan.

_____

_____

_____

5. Circle the factor in the list below that might affect the SEQUENCE you select for quadrant scaling and root planing in a dental hygiene care plan.

   a. availability of a power-driven scaler

   b. patient complaint of pain associated with a periodontal abscess

   c. the amount of calculus in the lower anterior sextant

   d. chronic systemic disease

6. What is the purpose for explaining the entire treatment plan to the patient?

_____

_____

7. What are some important points to consider when explaining the dental hygiene care plan to the patient?

_____

_____

_____

_____

_____

_____

_____

8. Identify five areas of information that you will discuss with the patient when you are obtaining informed consent.

_____

_____

_____

_____

_____

COMPETENCY EXERCISES

Apply information from the chapter and use critical thinking skills to complete the competency exercises. Write responses on paper or create electronic documents to submit your answers.

1. Explain the role of the patient in developing a plan for care that prioritizes the patient's needs.

2. Explain the relationship between the master treatment plan and the dental hygiene care plan.

3. Why are medical, personal, and clinical findings linked to actual or potential risk factors in the assessment findings section of a written dental hygiene care plan?

4. Using your institution's guidelines for writing in patient records, document that the dental hygiene care plan was presented to the supervising dentist prior to explaining the plan to the patient.

5. Use the following information from the case of Jonathon Meyers to answer the questions below. Jon has not seen a dentist since he was a child. When his girlfriend told him about his bad breath, he decided to take advantage of the services offered at the dental clinic in your school.

   Jon presents with an aggressive periodontal condition in the lower anterior sextant of his mouth. He has a low dental IQ and doesn't understand the cause and progression of dental disease. He smokes, demonstrates poor biofilm control, and states that he wants you to just "fix him up" with your treatments.

   a. Write at least one dental hygiene diagnosis statement related to the information provided about the patient in this scenario.

   b. What interventions will you plan to target the problem(s) you identified?

   c. Write a goal for each problem you identified. Include a time frame for meeting the goal. How will you measure whether or not Jon met the goal?

Everyday Ethics

Before completing the learning exercises below, reread and reflect on the Everyday Ethics scenario and Questions for Consideration in this chapter of the textbook. It may also be useful to review the Dental Hygiene Ethics discussion in Chapter 1, the Ethical Applications in the introduction pages for each Section in the textbook, as well as the Codes of Ethics in Appendices I, II, and III.

Individual Learning Activity
Imagine that you have observed what happened in the scenario but are not one of the main characters involved in the situation. Write a reflective journal entry that

■ describes how you might have reacted (as an observer-not as a participant),

■ expresses your personal feelings about what happened, or

■ identifies personal values that affect your reaction to the situation.

Discovery Activity
Ask a friend or relative who is not involved in healthcare to read the scenario and discuss it with you from the perspective of a "patient" who receives services within the healthcare system. Discuss what you learned from the concerns, insights, or difference in perspective that person expressed.

Factors To Teach The Patient

This scenario is related to the following factors listed in this chapter of the textbook:

■ Why patient input into the final care plan is important

■ The patient's rights and responsibilities regarding informed consent

Using the examples of patient conversations from Appendix D as a guide, write a statement explaining to Mrs. Kwan, the patient in the Everyday Ethics scenario provided in Chapter 24 of the textbook, what informed consent means.

Dental Hygiene Diagnosis and Care Planning

■ Chapters 23–24

 COMPETENCY EXERCISES

Apply information from the chapter and use critical thinking skills to complete the competency exercises. Write responses on paper or create electronic documents to submit your answers.

SECTION IV—PATIENT ASSESSMENT SUMMARY

Patient Name: *Mrs. Diane White*	Age: *27*	Gender: M [F]	☐ Initial Therapy
			☑ Maintenance
Provider Name: *D.H. Student*	Date: *Today*		☐ Re-evaluation

Chief Complaint:

Presents for routine maintenance appointment. Gum tissues bleed when brushing and flossing.

ASSESSMENT FINDINGS

Health History

- First trimester of first pregnancy; experiences significant nausea daily and occasional morning vomiting
- Husband smokes cigarettes in house and car; patient does not smoke.
- ASA Classification—II and ADL level—0

At Risk for:

- Enamel erosion and increased dental caries risk
- Infant at risk for second-hand smoke exposure

Social and Dental History

- 9 months since previous recall appointment; missed her 6-month appointment.
- Infrequent flossing
- Uses bottled water with no fluoride content; smell of fluoridated toothpaste makes her feel nauseated.
- Frequent high-carbohydrate snacks (graham crackers) to help control nausea

At Risk for:

- Increased risk for periodontal disease
- Increased caries risk and risk for enamel erosion
- Increased caries risk

Dental Examination	At Risk for:
■ No current cavitated lesions; a small number of occlusal surface restorations are all in good repair. ■ Moderate biofilm along cervical margins and on proximal surfaces ■ Generalized 4 mm probing depths; no radiographic indication of bone loss ■ Generalized red, bulbous tissue and generalized bleeding on probing	■ Increased risk for caries and periodontal infection ■ Oral infection, increased risk for periodontal/gingival infection ■ Increased risk for periodontal/gingival infection and pyogenic granuloma

Periodontal Diagnosis / Case Type and Status	Caries Management Risk Assessment (CAMBRA) Level:
Gingivitis	☐ Low ☑ Moderate ☐ High ☐ Extreme

Read the Section I Patient Assessment Summary to help you answer questions 1 and 2.

1. Use a copy of the dental hygiene care plan template in Appendix B, or use the care plan format your school provides to write dental hygiene diagnosis statements for Mrs. White's care plan.

2. Use the care plan template in Appendix B or your school format to write a plan for clinical, education/counseling, and oral hygiene instruction/home care interventions for Mrs. White.

3. Use the care plan template in Appendix B of the workbook, or the care plan form used in your clinic to write a formal care plan from assessment data collected during an initial appointment of a patient you are providing care for in your school clinic.

4. Write an outline of important points to address when presenting the care plan to the patient to obtain informed consent to proceed with the dental hygiene interventions you have planned.

5. Present the care plan to the patient.

6. Write a progress note documenting that you have presented the care plan and obtained informed consent.

 ## DISCOVERY EXERCISES

1. Remember Jonathon Meyers, the graduate student from the Competency Exercises in Chapter 24? Imagine that you have now completed his initial therapy plan and are evaluating the results. He has reached most of the goals you set together in the plan, and his oral health status has much improved.

You recommend a 3-month periodontal maintenance interval, but he wants to wait at least 6 months before coming to see you again. He cites recent toothpaste television commercials that recommend seeing a dentist every 6 months. You know that patients with a history of periodontal infection need to be seen more often.

Conduct a brief review of recent literature to determine what scientific evidence supports a shorter periodontal maintenance interval. Write an outline of points you will cover when you explain to Jon why those research findings influence your recommendations for his continuing care plan.

2. Develop a PICO question related to determining the best **fluoride regimen** to recommend for a preschool-aged child with extreme caries risk.

3. Select two or three current articles from your literature search that seem as if they would be useful for helping you decide which fluoride therapies you will recommend for this preschool-aged patient. Either go to the library to find the paper journal or use online full-text sources to read the articles you have selected. Read the articles and evaluate the strength and usefulness of the information that is in them.

 ## QUESTIONS PATIENTS ASK

What sources of information can you identify that will help you answer your patient's questions in this scenario?

"I saw something on the Internet recently about new research that proves that a certain new kind of treatment is more effective than the recommendations you have made in my dental hygiene care plan. Can we change my dental hygiene care plan?"

FOR YOUR PORTFOLIO

1. Using the patient-specific dental hygiene care plan template in Appendix B or the care-plan format used in your dental hygiene program, complete comprehensive dental hygiene care plans for a variety of patients you have assessed in your school clinic. Demonstrate your ability to plan for a diverse selection of patients by selecting care plans prepared for patients with a variety of systemic conditions, risk factors, and levels of dental disease.

2. In your portfolio, include a care plan prepared at the beginning of your education and one for a similar patient prepared near the end of your education. Provide a written statement that reflects on and analyzes the ways in which a comparison of the two care plans demonstrates what you have learned about planning patient care.

WORD SEARCH

```
G  C  R  H  H  W  E  Z  P  C  F  W  N  I  N  A  W
Z  A  L  T  C  U  Y  Z  O  Y  W  O  X  A  P  S  M
D  P  Q  J  I  N  I  A  S  F  I  M  L  U  K  S  O
P  U  C  J  K  L  A  I  S  T  P  P  K  E  K  E  D
M  Q  O  H  G  Y  S  B  A  K  T  E  D  F  I  S  I
F  Q  U  B  I  O  S  U  S  N  Q  E  E  E  N  S  F
J  L  L  Z  N  E  L  V  E  C  S  V  Z  L  T  M  I
K  C  O  G  P  A  F  M  J  A  E  I  L  Y  E  E  A
W  T  A  S  V  Z  T  C  B  I  T  S  C  Q  R  N  B
P  I  K  E  S  N  S  E  O  I  A  N  S  A  V  T  L
D  B  E  E  I  I  C  I  R  M  E  K  R  V  E  A  E
J  R  T  O  I  N  N  O  K  G  P  B  A  F  N  V  I
Y  N  P  D  E  E  I  G  R  L  M  L  Y  Z  T  G  L
B  P  O  D  M  R  R  U  S  A  O  U  A  B  I  G  V
A  Q  I  P  P  W  H  B  C  W  F  K  A  I  O  W  H
O  V  C  K  A  O  T  O  B  A  C  C  O  N  N  M  D
E  V  I  D  E  N  C  E  B  A  S  E  D  M  J  T  H
```

WORD SEARCH CLUES

1. One type of acute gingival or periodontal condition.
2. A critical analysis and evaluation or judgment related to patient's medical, dental, and personal health-related data.
3. Patient care interventions supported by relevant, scientifically sound research.
4. A significant risk factor for poor periodontal outcomes, certain systemic conditions, and oral cancer.
5. A dental related example of "activities of daily living."
6. The patient's statement regarding the reason for seeking dental care (two words).
7. Risk factors influenced by dental hygiene interventions that change health behavior.
8. A statement that identifies a patient problem.
9. To arrange in order of importance.
10. Refers to a dental hygiene treatment or recommendation that is intended to improve a patient's oral health.
11. Acronym that refers to a protocol used to determine caries risk level and select interventions based on risk level.
12. Discomfort or pain that requires first attention when planning dental hygiene care.
13. Treatment that is based on documented evidence of success (two words).
14. Assessment to determine whether expected outcomes of treatment have been met.
15. The section of the dental hygiene care plan that outlines the sequence of interventions planned in a series of appointments (two words).

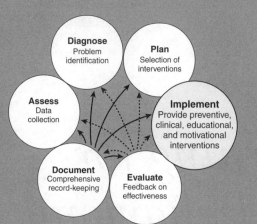

Diagnose
Problem
identification

Plan
Selection of
interventions

Assess
Data
collection

Implement
Provide preventive,
clinical, educational,
and motivational
interventions

Document
Comprehensive
record-keeping

Evaluate
Feedback on
effectiveness

Implementation: Prevention

Chapters 25–36

■ LEARNING OBJECTIVES

Completing the exercises in this section of the workbook will prepare you to:

1. Educate patients regarding the prevention of oral disease.
2. Promote patient behaviors and practices that enhance oral health.
3. Select patient-specific dental hygiene interventions that will prevent oral disease and promote oral health.
4. Document prevention interventions and recommendations.

■ COMPETENCIES FOR THE DENTAL HYGIENIST (APPENDIX A)

Competencies supported by the learning in Section V:

Core Competencies: C3, C4, C5, C7, C9, C10, C11, C12.

Health Promotion and Disease Prevention: HP1, HP2, HP4, HP5.

Patient/Client Care: PC10, PC11, PC33.

Patient Learning for Health and Behavioral Change

Upon successful completion of these exercises, you will be able to:

1. Identify and define key terms and concepts related to health promotion and disease prevention.
2. List and describe the steps in a preventive program.

3. Describe key factors and procedures that enhance successful patient learning and motivation.
4. Identify and describe disclosing agents.
5. Identify the causes, effects, and management of xerostomia and halitosis.

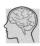 **KNOWLEDGE EXERCISES**

Write your answers for each question in the space provided.

1. Your skills in communication and marketing will have an effect on patient motivation and compliance with oral health recommendations. In your own words, define these concepts.

   ■ Communication _____
   _____

   ■ Marketing _____
   _____

   ■ Motivation _____
   _____

   ■ Compliance _____
   _____

2. In your own words, define *behavior modification*.
   _____
   _____

3. Patients who desire to attain and maintain their own oral health will often increase their knowledge or skills in all three learning domains. Define the three domains of learning.
   _____
   _____
   _____

4. Read the definitions of *dental health education, health education, health promotion,* and *preventive dental hygiene* in Box 25-1 in the textbook. Combine these definitions to write a brief definition of your role as a health educator during each patient's dental hygiene appointment.
   _____
   _____

5. In your own words, briefly describe each of the steps in a preventive program.

_____

_____

_____

_____

_____

6. In your own words, briefly summarize or restate the principles of learning.

_____

_____

_____

_____

_____

_____

_____

7. Why is it important to provide initial oral hygiene instructions for your patient before any clinical treatment is started?

_____

_____

_____

8. Patient education is not provided in a rote, unchanging manner, but rather is adapted to individual patient needs, readiness to practice new health behaviors, and current health status. Oral disease prevention programs are usually more successful if a series of lessons are planned and coordinated to build and reinforce patient knowledge and skills. State the objective and briefly describe what is included in each lesson of a series of patient education sessions in biofilm control.

■ Lesson 1 _____

_____

_____

■ Lesson 2 _____

_____

_____

■ Additional lessons _____

_____

_____

9. Identify the general characteristics that determine the value of teaching aids and health education reading materials that you select for patient education.

_____

_____

_____

_____

_____

10. Models and toothbrushes are commonly used to teach brushing methods to patients. What factors limit this method of teaching oral hygiene measures for individual patients?

_____

_____

11. In what ways does a disclosing agent help you provide patient instruction?

_____

_____

12. List the properties of an acceptable disclosing agent.

_____

_____

_____

_____

_____

_____

13. Identify the major types of disclosing agents that are available for use. Be sure to ask your instructor how much detail you will be expected to know about the composition of each formula.

_____

_____

_____

_____

_____

14. List the steps for direct application of a disclosing agent.

_____

_____

_____

_____

_____

_____

15. What steps will you take after you have applied the disclosing solution to your patient's teeth?

_____

_____

_____

_____

16. The best prevention programs help your patients increase their knowledge about all aspects of their oral health. During oral hygiene instructions, you will teach your patients much more about oral disease prevention than just biofilm removal. For example, saliva has numerous functions relating to the maintenance of oral health. List the functions of saliva that help protect your patients' oral health.

_____

_____

_____

_____

_____

_____

17. What are the oral effects of xerostomia?

_____

_____

_____

_____

18. Dental hygienists are often the first to recognize or hear patient complaints of oral dryness. What recommendations can you make to help your patient overcome and manage the effects of xerostomia?

_____

_____

_____

_____

_____

19. Halitosis can be described as the _organoleptic_ recognition of _putrefaction_ or _volatile sulfur compounds_. Use the definitions of the italicized terms to explain halitosis in your own words (see Box 25-1 in the textbook).

_____

_____

20. Identify the oral and non-oral factors that you will investigate if your patient complains of halitosis.

■ Oral factors

_____

_____

_____

_____

_____

_____

_____

■ Non-oral factors

_____

_____

_____

_____

_____

COMPETENCY EXERCISES

Apply information from the chapter and use critical thinking skills to complete the competency exercises. Write responses on paper or create electronic documents to submit your answers.

1. Compare the steps in a preventive program with the dental hygiene process of care.

2. When you complete your assessment for Patrick Callaghan, who has presented for a 6-month maintenance appointment, you conclude that overall he has very good oral hygiene and periodontal health. You notice only very slight biofilm and slightly enlarged and reddened interproximal papilla in the maxillary right molar area. You note a slight coating on his tongue and think that this may be related to his comment that he sometimes feels like he has bad breath, especially in the morning when he wakes up.

   Write a dental hygiene diagnosis statement for Mr. Callaghan's care plan.

3. You decide Mr. Callaghan needs very little reinforcement for his toothbrushing techniques, as his biofilm levels are very low. You spend the available patient education time concentrating on his flossing technique in the upper right side of his mouth, where you noticed the biofilm on the proximal surfaces. You also spend a few minutes demonstrating tongue cleaning with a scraper to help him learn how to remove the biofilm accumulating there. Using your institution's guidelines for writing in patient records, document the oral hygiene instructions you provided for Mr. Callaghan during his appointment.

4. To answer this question, first review the information related to Motivational Interviewing found in Chapter 2 in the textbook and also the example patient conversations in Appendix D in this workbook).

   It has been slightly more than 1 year since you last saw Melina for a dental hygiene maintenance appointment. As you update her health history, Melina impresses you with a description of her school science fair project, which focuses on the effects of different diseases on the quality of life. She talks to you for a long time about her discovery, from reading the surgeon general's *Report on Oral Health* and other documents, that the effects of oral diseases, especially dental caries and periodontal infections, can cause children and adults to miss millions of hours of work and school. She accurately discusses the concept that oral diseases are directly related to general health status. She excitedly gives you examples of how oral diseases are completely preventable by limiting sucrose in the diet, taking adequate oral hygiene measures, using fluorides, and having regular access to preventive dental services. However, after you collect assessment data for Melina, you discover that her own daily brushing and flossing are inadequate for biofilm removal and, like many other teenagers, she often drinks carbonated beverages and juice several times during the day.

   Using information in the patient scenario above, compare Melinda's apparent level on the learning ladder with what you determine might be her current Stage of Change level.

5. Describe how you can use Motivational Interviewing techniques to approach Melina, during this and subsequent dental hygiene appointments, and help her climb each remaining step of the learning ladder.

Everyday Ethics

Before completing the learning exercises below, reread and reflect on the Everyday Ethics scenario and Questions for Consideration in this chapter of the textbook. It may also be useful to review the Dental Hygiene Ethics discussion in Chapter 1, the Ethical Applications in the introduction pages for each section in the textbook, as well as the Codes of Ethics in Appendices I, II, and III.

Individual Learning Activity
Identify a situation you have experienced that presents a similar ethical dilemma. Write about you would do differently now than you did at the time the incident occurred—support your discussion with concepts from the dental hygiene codes of ethics.

Collaborative Learning Activity
Answer each of the questions for consideration at the end of the scenario in the textbook. Compare what you wrote with answers developed by another classmate and discuss differences/similarities

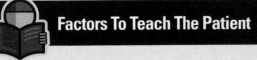

Factors To Teach The Patient

This scenario is related to the following factors listed in this chapter of the textbook:

■ The relationship between preventive measures and clinical services
■ Why particular preventive measures are selected for a particular patient

Mr. Callaghan (presented in Competency Exercise question 2) compliments you on your oral hygiene instructions and says he remembers that the other dental hygienist, Patty, whom he saw 6 months ago, told him exactly the same things. He wonders if you two have a memorized script that you each simply repeat every time a patient comes in.

Use the examples of patient conversations in Appendix D as a guide to write a statement explaining your patient-education procedures to Mr. Callaghan.

CHAPTER 26

Protocols for Prevention and Control of Dental Caries

 KNOWLEDGE EXERCISES

Write your answers for each question in the space provided.

1. In your own words, describe how the metabolic action of *Streptococcus mutans* and *Lactobacillus* bacteria contributes to the destruction of tooth structure and causes dental caries.

   _____

   _____

   _____

2. A child can be at risk for dental caries as soon as tooth eruption begins. Why?

   _____

   _____

3. List the types of fermentable carbohydrates.

   _____

   _____

   _____

   _____

4. Identify the acids produced during the metabolic process of the bacteria in dental biofilm.

   _____

   _____

   _____

   _____

5. The _____ of carbohydrate ingestion in your patient's diet has a strong influence on the amount of acid produced and the extent of tooth destruction.

6. In what ways does the presence of adequate saliva protect your patient against dental decay?

_____

_____

_____

7. In your own words, describe how fluoride protects your patient against dental decay.

_____

_____

_____

8. Although the incidence of dental caries in the general population has declined in recent years, dental caries is still a major problem that affects the health and welfare of adults and children alike. The dental hygienist's focus in caries detection has changed from identifying only end-stage dental caries that require restoration to identifying patient risk factors and the earliest stages of dental caries. At this point, dental hygiene interventions can help remineralize the natural tooth structure. What tools will you use to identify dental caries at very early stages during an oral examination of your patient?

_____

_____

_____

_____

_____

9. In your own words, describe what you will observe during a visual examination at each of the stages of dental caries on a tooth surface.

■ Initial infection _____

_____

■ Early subsurface infection _____

_____

■ Early white spot lesion _____

_____

■ Later white spot lesion _____

_____

■ Cavitation _____

_____

■ Radiographic (proximal surface) early dental caries _____

_____

■ Large proximal surface dental caries _____

10. In your own words, outline the dental hygienist's role (objectives and interventions) in planning patient care for caries management.

_____

_____

_____

_____

_____

11. What is the purpose of discussing individualized caries risk assessment with each patient?

_____

_____

_____

_____

12. List the 5 risk factor categories associated with the CAMBRA guidelines for caries management.

_____

_____

_____

_____

_____

13. List the 4 CAMBRA risk levels.

_____

_____

_____

_____

14. List the four prevention interventions that are identified in the CAMBRA management guidelines.

_____

_____

_____

_____

15. How can you best gather data to assess your patient's individual caries risk factors?

_____

_____

_____

_____

_____

16. Outline a protocol for remineralization that you can initiate when your patient has evidence of early carious lesions that do not yet require restorative treatment.

_____

_____

_____

_____

_____

✓ COMPETENCY EXERCISES

Apply information from the chapter and use critical thinking skills to complete the competency exercises. Write responses on paper or create electronic documents to submit your answers.

1. Seventeen-year-old Tren Nguyen emigrated to the United States with his family about 6 years ago. Since he arrived, Tren has embraced all things American and spends his free time playing computer games, snacking on fast food, and hanging out with friends. Tren's history of dental visits has been infrequent. He has been seen in your office only twice before—right after he arrived in the United States and then again about 3 years ago for a prophylaxis. No significant dental findings were charted at either of those visits. He has no history of previous dental restorations. He came to the clinic today because a dental checkup is required as part of his physical examination to play sports when he goes off to college next fall.

   When you examine Tren's mouth today, you find significant early and late white spot lesions on the facial surfaces of almost all of his teeth. It is interesting that there are no observable caries in the pits and fissures on the occlusal surfaces of any of his teeth and the surfaces are not deeply grooved. Make a list of the questions you will ask Tren as you gather caries risk assessment data before you write his dental hygiene care plan.

2. Now comes the fun part. You don't usually get to make up answers for all the questions that you ask your patients, but this time we can't go any further with these exercises unless we have some data. In the interest of your own learning, make up reasonable-sounding answers for each of the questions you asked Tren during your discussion of caries risk factors.

   Using the data you have collected from Tren's caries risk assessment, determine his CAMBRA level.

3. Write two dental hygiene diagnosis statements for Tren's care plan.

4. List the dental hygiene interventions you will plan to help Tren *arrest or control* disease and *regenerate, restore, or maintain* his oral health.

Everyday Ethics

Before completing the learning exercises below, reread and reflect on the Everyday Ethics scenario and Questions for Consideration in this chapter of the textbook. It may also be useful to review the Dental Hygiene Ethics discussion in Chapter 1, the Ethical Applications in the introduction pages for each section in the textbook, as well as the Codes of Ethics in Appendices I, II, and III.

Individual Learning Activity

Imagine that you have observed what happened in the scenario, but are not one of the main characters involved in the situation. Write a reflective journal entry that:

- describes how you might have reacted (as an observer-not as a participant),
- expresses your personal feelings about what happened,

or

- identifies personal values that affect your reaction to the situation.

Collaborative Learning Activity

Work with a small group to develop a 2 to 5-minute role-play that introduces the Everyday Ethics scenario described in the chapter (a great idea is to video record your role-play activity). Then develop separate 2-minute role-play scenarios that provide at least two alternative approaches/solutions to resolving the situation. Ask classmates to view the solutions, ask questions, and discuss the ethical approach used in each. Ask for a vote on which solution classmates determine to be the "best."

Factors To Teach The Patient

This scenario is related to the following factors listed in this chapter of the textbook:

- What causes cavities and how they develop
- That early dental caries is not a cavity; what demineralization means
- How remineralization can be accomplished using fluoride toothpaste and drinking fluoridated water daily
- That the use of fluorides is necessary throughout life

Use the example of patient conversations in Appendix D as a guide to write a conversation explaining the components of Tren's care plan to him in such a way that you will motivate him to comply with your recommendations. (This patient was introduced in the Competency Exercises for this chapter.)

CROSSWORD PUZZLE

ACROSS

3. A species of bacteria that is more active in the later stages (progression) of decay.
5. Describes rapidly progressing caries in many teeth; an acute condition as opposed to a chronic condition.
8. Refers to management of dental caries risk through use of fluoride preparations.
11. Describes the caries process that has been halted.
12. Process in which minerals are removed from the tooth structure by acids.
14. Aided by sufficient saliva and by the action of topical fluorides.
15. Habits, behaviors, lifestyles, or conditions that increase the probability of a disease occurring (two words).
17. Refers to bacteria that are capable of turning fermentable carbohydrates into acid.
18. Ingredient in chewing gum that reduces levels of *Streptococcus mutans* and promotes remineralization.
19. Type of radiograph that can reveal caries on proximal surfaces of teeth.
20. A protocol for caries management.

DOWN

1. Capable of neutralizing acid in a solution; one function of saliva.
2. Designates the highest level of risk for determining dental caries management protocols.
4. Identifies to two specific types of bacteria that predominate in the initial stages of the caries process.
6. This lesion gives evidence of subsurface demineralization (two words).
7. The final stage in the process of caries formation.
9. Professional term for dental decay.
10. Another term for secondary caries.
13. The science and study of dental decay.
16. Buffers acids in the mouth and supplies minerals to replace the calcium and phosphate ions dissolved during demineralization.

Oral Infection Control: Toothbrushes and Toothbrushing

Learning Objectives

Upon successful completion of these exercises, you will be able to:

1. Identify and define key terms and concepts related to toothbrushes and toothbrushing.
2. Describe the characteristics, factors influencing selection, and proper care of manual toothbrushes.
3. Describe indications, procedures, and limitations for a variety of toothbrushing methods and select appropriate toothbrushing methods for individual patients.
4. Discuss indications for use of power toothbrushes and identify important design, technique, and patient instruction factors.
5. Identify indications and methods for supplemental brushing.
6. Select toothbrushing techniques for special conditions.

 KNOWLEDGE EXERCISES

Write your answers for each question in the space provided.

1. Define toothbrush abrasion.

   _____

   _____

2. In your own words, describe an effective toothbrush handle.

   _____

   _____

3. Describe a tuft in the head of a toothbrush.

   _____

   _____

4. List four factors that affect the stiffness or firmness of toothbrush filaments.

   _____

   _____

   _____

   _____

5. List four factors that influence the type of toothbrush selected for an individual patient.

   _____

   _____

   _____

   _____

6. In your own words, describe the procedure for holding a toothbrush and positioning it in the mouth for effective removal of dental biofilm.

_____

_____

_____

_____

7. Identify methods you can suggest to your patient for timing brushing in order to enhance effectiveness.

_____

_____

_____

_____

8. The Bass method of brushing is widely taught by dental hygienists to enhance effectiveness of their patients' oral cleaning. What problems are sometimes encountered as patients try to learn this technique?

_____

_____

_____

9. Which two methods of toothbrushing are sometimes taught to young children when they have difficulty mastering a sulcular brushing technique?

_____

_____

10. Describe the procedure for the modified Stillman method of toothbrushing.

_____

11. Which toothbrushing methods instruct the patient to direct the brush filaments at a 45° angle toward the gingival margin?

_____

_____

12. Which toothbrushing method instructs the patient to direct the brush filaments at a 45° angle toward the occlusal plane?

_____

13. What are the problems with biofilm removal when the patient uses the method described in question 12?

_____

_____

_____

14. What three factors in toothbrushing are most likely to contribute to gingival recession or tooth abrasion?

_____

_____

_____

15. List two methods for brushing occlusal surfaces.

_____

_____

16. What two anatomic features contribute to retention of dental biofilm on a patient's tongue?

_____

_____

17. Identify two methods for cleaning the tongue.

_____

_____

18. List alterations in the appearance of gingival tissues that require you to recommend a different toothbrushing technique in order to correct or reduce gingival damage.

_____

_____

19. Identify at least three special circumstances in which the use of a powered toothbrush can enhance the removal of bacterial biofilm.

_____

_____

_____

_____

20. In your own words, describe the motion of an oscillating power toothbrush head. (*Hint:* Use your hand to demonstrate the motion described in Table 27-3 in the textbook.)

_____

_____

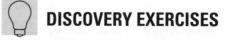

COMPETENCY EXERCISES

Apply information from the chapter and use critical thinking skills to complete the competency exercises. Write responses on paper or create electronic documents to submit your answers.

1. Nicholas Bean, a 12-year-old who is your first patient of the day, is going right from his prophylaxis appointment to the orthodontist's office, where they will be placing full-mouth bands and brackets on his teeth. You know that the best toothbrush to recommend for him to use is a bilevel orthodontic toothbrush, but you do not happen to have a sample to give him. You decide to tell his mother what it looks like so she can get one. Using terminology that describes the parts of a toothbrush from Figure 27-1 in the textbook and the pictures from Figure 27-2 in the textbook, develop a brief description of this type of toothbrush.

2. Mr. Gabriel Chin is one of your favorite patients, and he loves to share stories of his travels around the world. Today, when he presents for his recall appointment, he shows you some toothbrushes that he recently brought back from a trip to visit relatives in his native country. The toothbrush, he states proudly, is the type his family has been using for many years and is made from the hairs of wild boars. You want to educate him without belittling his enthusiasm for his family's history. To help him understand about a better alternative, list three reasons why nylon or synthetic filaments are used today for toothbrushes instead of natural bristles.

3. Mrs. Janette Evans has been diagnosed with active periodontal disease. You will be working closely with her once a week for the next 2 months to control oral disease and obtain periodontal health because she will soon be going into the hospital for open-heart surgery. What important information should you give her about how to care for her toothbrush?

4. As you are providing oral hygiene instructions using the Bass method for Mrs. Evans, she asks you how much time she should spend brushing her teeth to thoroughly remove all of the biofilm, as you are recommending. Explain one of the methods she can use to monitor her toothbrushing.

5. When you are showing Mrs. Evans how to brush, you note that she needs some extra help with the distal surfaces of tooth 19, the most posterior tooth in that arch. Explain how she should position her toothbrush.

6. How can Mrs. Evans effectively use her toothbrush to clean the mesial surface of tooth 7, which is extremely rotated and tilted in a labial direction.

7. Using your institution's guidelines for writing in patient records, document the oral hygiene instructions you provided for Mrs. Evans. Be sure to include enough detail so that you can use the comments at a subsequent visit to reinforce the information you provided.

8. When you see Mrs. Evans a week later, her biofilm scores are a bit lower but still not at the levels you would like to see after your extensive oral hygiene instructions. When you do your intraoral examination, you notice a scuffed epithelial surface, several red pinpoint spots, and some generalized redness along the lingual gingival margin of teeth 13–15 and the facial margins of teeth 29–31. You determine that these acute lesions may be the result of toothbrushing activity during the previous week. Identify three possible precipitating factors and explain measures that or Mrs. Evans can take to eliminate the problems.

9. What are some reasons you might recommend a power toothbrush for Mrs. Evans instead of the manual toothbrushing technique you originally taught her?

DISCOVERY EXERCISES

Collaborate with your classmates to gather samples of a variety of different power toothbrushes. (Hint: Contacting dental product companies is one way to do this, or you can use models that you, your classmates, or your faculty already own.)

1. Examine several different brands or models of power toothbrushes to determine the following information:

   ■ Motion

   ■ Brush head shape

   ■ Filaments

   ■ Handle size and shape

   ■ Overall weight

   ■ Power source

   ■ Speed

2. Discuss which model would be best for a variety of situations—for example, which one would you recommend for a child; for a caregiver to use when brushing someone else's teeth? Think of other situations and types of patients.

3. Conduct a PubMed search and review professional literature to evidence to support the recommendation of the type of power toothbrush you like best.

? QUESTIONS PATIENTS ASK

What sources of information can you identify that will help you answer your patient's questions in this scenario?

"What toothbrush is right for me?" "Is a power toothbrush really worth buying? Will it help keep my teeth cleaner and my gums healthier?" How do you know that the toothbrushing method you are teaching me is right for me?" You will hear these types of questions from your patients many, many times.

Everyday Ethics

Before completing the learning exercises below, reread and reflect on the Everyday Ethics scenario and Questions for Consideration in this chapter of the textbook. It may also be useful to review the Dental Hygiene Ethics discussion in Chapter 1, the Ethical Applications in the introduction pages for each section in the textbook, as well as the Codes of Ethics in Appendices I, II, and III.

Collaborative Learning Activity
Work with a small group to develop a 2- to 5-minute role-play that introduces the Everyday Ethics scenario described in the chapter (a great idea is to video record your role-play activity). Then develop separate 2-minute role-play scenarios that provide at least two alternative approaches/solutions to resolving the situation. Ask classmates to view the

solutions, ask questions, and discuss the ethical approach used in each. Ask for a vote on which solution classmates determine to be the "best."

Discovery Activity
Ask a friend or relative who is not involved in healthcare to read the scenario and discuss it with you from the perspective of a "patient" who receives services within the healthcare system. Discuss what you learned from the concerns, insights, or difference in perspective that person expressed.

Factors To Teach The Patient

This scenario is related to the following factors listed in this chapter of the textbook:

■ How dental biofilm forms and its effects on the teeth and gingiva
■ Why it is necessary to remove dental biofilm from the teeth daily, especially before going to sleep

Thomas Ravelli, 18, is home for the holiday from his first term at college, and his mother has insisted that he keep his appointment with you for his regular 6-month cleaning. As you collect assessment data before providing dental hygiene care, you become very aware that his overall oral status is not the same as it has been at previous visits. You note generalized bleeding on probing and overall red and inflamed gingiva. Fortunately, there is no radiographic evidence of bone level changes.

Further questioning reveals that his overall home-care routine has not been adequate and his eating patterns

include frequent snacking because he doesn't particularly like the regular meals served in his dorm. He tells you about how hard it is to keep a regular schedule when he is so stressed by his college workload. He comments that it has been especially tough during the last several weeks when he was writing final exams. That's when he started noticing that his gums were bleeding every time he brushed his teeth! It hurt to brush, so he admits that he has been neglectful of his daily oral care.

Use the examples of patient conversations in Appendix D to write a statement explaining how using the proper brushing techniques can help prevent future problems for Thomas.

Use the conversation you create to role-play this situation with a fellow student. If you are the patient in the role-play, be sure to ask questions. If you are the dental hygienist, try to anticipate questions and provide evidence-based answers for them in your explanation.

WORD SEARCH

```
S  O  Y  A  R  V  J  I  U  S  A  R  K  S  V
K  R  R  O  L  L  I  Y  Z  T  K  C  N  U  W
G  V  L  B  A  S  S  J  V  I  A  K  F  L  O
L  E  H  F  H  L  Q  P  S  L  R  D  O  C  N
E  R  N  O  F  H  G  H  K  L  O  M  N  U  G
O  T  S  A  R  G  T  Y  M  M  U  S  E  L  H
N  I  M  J  S  I  C  S  S  A  V  B  S  A  Y
A  C  O  F  M  C  Z  I  O  N  W  Y  O  R  C
R  A  D  S  C  I  O  O  N  M  H  Q  T  P  H
D  L  I  K  W  R  L  L  N  N  B  F  T  V  A
N  Z  F  U  S  C  X  O  E  T  W  S  Y  B  R
V  T  I  Y  C  U  U  G  Z  N  A  N  U  K  T
L  K  E  T  R  L  P  I  C  Z  O  L  I  Q  E
C  A  D  U  U  A  U  C  A  L  I  A  Z  Y  R
N  P  W  A  B  R  L  T  Z  Y  Q  T  V  F  S
```

There are a variety of different toothbrushing methods you can teach your patients. Some are better than others for maximizing biofilm removal and minimizing damage to oral tissues. But all of them, listed below, are included in this word search puzzle.

Bass
Charters
Circular
Fones
Horizontal
Leonard
Modified
Physiologic
Roll
Scrub
Smith's
Stillman
Sulcular
Vertical

Interdental Care

Upon successful completion of these exercises, you will be able to:

1. Identify and define key terms and concepts related to interdental care.
2. Describe the interdental embrasures.
3. Describe the characteristics, indications, and procedures for use of a variety of interdental cleaning devices.
4. Include individualized recommendations for interdental care in dental hygiene care plans.

KNOWLEDGE EXERCISES

Write your answers for each question in the space provided.

1. Posterior teeth have _____ papillae with a col, and anterior teeth have _____ papilla that forms a small col under the contact area.

2. Identify tissue and anatomic characteristics of the col, the adjacent teeth, and the surrounding papillae that contribute to the increased risk of gingivitis in the interdental area.

   _____

   _____

   _____

   _____

3. Identify the different types of floss that you and your patient can select, based on individual preference and needs.

   _____

   _____

4. Complete Infomap 28-1 to compare the benefits and limitations of waxed (or PTFE) and unwaxed floss, as noted in the textbook.

INFOMAP 28-1		
FLOSS TYPE	**BENEFITS**	**LIMITATIONS**
Waxed or expanded PTFE		
Unwaxed floss		

5. Identify the location, cause of, and methods for preventing floss cuts and clefts.

_____

_____

_____

6. List additional flossing aides you can recommend for a patient and identify indications for recommending each one?

_____

_____

_____

_____

_____

7. What kind of flossing motion can be applied with tufted floss, knitting yarn, or gauze strips that is not typically applied with regular floss?

_____

8. Describe the shapes of interdental brushes.

_____

_____

9. Describe a situation in which the interdental brush is a better choice than dental floss for complete biofilm removal or for application of chemotherapeutic agents on proximal surfaces of teeth.

_____

_____

10. End-tuft brushes are usually recommended for a single area that is difficult to reach with a regular toothbrush. In what specific situations can you recommend the use of an end-tuft brush?

_____

_____

_____

11. In your own words, describe a wooden interdental cleaner, state how it is used, and identify factors

you must consider when recommending it for a patient.

_____

_____

_____

_____

12. Describe an interdental tip and a toothpick in holder and explain how they are used.

■ Interdental tip

_____

_____

■ Toothpick in holder

_____

_____

13. Describe oral irrigation.

_____

_____

14. List the three delivery method categories for oral irrigation.

_____

_____

15. List the advantages of patient-applied daily irrigation measures.

_____

_____

_____

16. List the patient assessment factors that provide information to help you assess your patient's individual needs before recommending a specific device for his or her interdental care.

_____

_____

_____

_____

COMPETENCY EXERCISES

Apply information from the chapter and use critical thinking skills to complete the competency exercises. Write responses on paper or create electronic documents to submit your answers.

1. The best way to learn how to teach a patient about flossing is to practice doing it. Apply knowledge gained from reading this textbook chapter to teach a family member or friend (but not one of your student colleagues, because he or she has already read this chapter) about how and when to floss.

2. After careful assessment of his current oral hygiene measures, you find that your patient, Mr. Adamson, has very large hands and has a great deal of difficulty maneuvering dental floss in his posterior teeth. He also has an orthodontic band on tooth 3, which posi-tions a temporary appliance being used to maintain an open space for the later placement of a permanent bridge. He has high levels of biofilm on all proximal areas and along the gingival margin of the orthodontic band. Write two dental hygiene diagnosis statements related to these issues.

3. Write a goal for the problems you identified in the dental hygiene diagnoses in question 2. Include a time frame for meeting the goal. How will you measure whether or not your patient met the goal?

4. You decide to recommend a floss holder for regular floss as well as the use of a "Perio-Aid" for Mr. Adamson. Obtain samples of these interdental devices, if you can, to help you with this exercise (they will also help with the Factors to Teach the Patient section). Write a progress note documenting your recommendations and the oral hygiene instructions that you provided for Mr. Adamson.

Everyday Ethics

Before completing the learning exercises below, reread and reflect on the Everyday Ethics scenario and Questions for Consideration in this chapter of the textbook. It may also be useful to review the Dental Hygiene Ethics discussion in Chapter 1, the Ethical Applications in the introduction pages for each section in the textbook, as well as the Codes of Ethics in Appendices I, II, and III.

Individual Learning Activity
Imagine that you are the dental hygienist in this scenario. Answer each of the questions for consideration at the end of the scenario.

Discovery Activity
Ask a friend or relative who is not involved in healthcare to read the scenario and discuss it with you from the per-spective of a "patient" who receives services within the healthcare system. Discuss what you learned from the concerns, insights, or difference in perspective that person expressed.

Factors To Teach The Patient

This scenario is related to the following factors listed in this chapter of the textbook:

- By demonstration with disclosing agent, how the tooth-brush doesn't clean the interdental area thoroughly
- Dental biofilm and how it collects on the proximal tooth surfaces when left undisturbed
- How vulnerable the interdental area is to gingival infection

- How to use each recommended interdental aid to clean the proximal tooth surfaces

  Use the examples of patient conversations in Appendix D as a guide to develop a conversation explaining to Mr. Adamson (introduced in question 2 of the Competency Exercises) how to assemble and use the interdental devises you are recommending.

Dentifrices and Mouthrinses

Learning Objectives

Upon successful completion of these exercises, you will be able to:

1. Identify and define key terms and concepts related to dentifrices and mouthrinses.
2. Describe the components, action, and therapeutic or cosmetic benefits of a dentifrice.
3. Describe the purpose of, procedure for, and ingredients used in oral rinses.
4. Identify the considerations in selecting patient-specific dentifrices and oral rinses.
5. Define the purpose, requirements, and use of the revised ADA Seal Program.

 KNOWLEDGE EXERCISES

Write your answers for each question in the space provided.

1. What are the beneficial effects of the active ingredients in dentifrices?

   _____

   _____

2. Identify the three purposes of a dentifrice.

   _____

   _____

   _____

3. What is the purpose of the humectants in a dentifrice?

   _____

   _____

4. List at least three types of abrasives used as polishing agents in a dentifrice.

   _____

   _____

   _____

5. What are the purposes of sorbitol or glycerol as an ingredient in a dentifrice?

   _____

   _____

6. What is the purpose of essential oils (e.g., peppermint) used in dentifrices?

   _____

   _____

7. The amount of therapeutic agent in a dentifrice is about _____.

8. Which therapeutic ingredient in a dentifrice is related to prevention of dental caries?

   _____

9. Identify four therapeutic ingredients in a dentifrice that are related to reduction of supragingival calculus formation?

   _____

   _____

   _____

   _____

10. What is the most common ingredient used in dentifrices to aid in reducing sensitivity?

    _____

11. List the six basic ingredients in commercial mouthrinses.

    _____

    _____

    _____

    _____

    _____

    _____

12. List at least three general types of chemotherapeutic agents found in mouthrinses and identify the purpose of each.

AGENT	PURPOSE
_____	_____
_____	_____
_____	_____

13. List at least three characteristics of an effective mouthrinse.

    _____

    _____

    _____

14. Which therapeutic agent available in mouthrinses has the greatest substantivity?

    _____

15. Which therapeutic agent available in mouthrinses acts by causing bacteriolysis?

    _____

16. Which therapeutic agent available in mouthrinses acts by inhibiting bacterial enzymes?

    _____

17. Which therapeutic agent available in mouthrinses is inactivated by a foaming agent frequently contained in commercial dentifrices?

    _____

18. Which two therapeutic agents available in mouthrinses are associated with the adverse effect of staining?

    _____

    _____

19. Describe the action and use of a mouthrinse containing peroxide.

    _____

    _____

20. Explain why rinsing with a mouthwash that contains an effective therapeutic agent may not be effective for a patient with deep periodontal pockets?

    _____

    _____

21. List patient characteristics that are considered when you recommend a dentifrice or mouthrinse.

    _____

    _____

    _____

    _____

22. Which mouthrinse agents have no clinical evidence to support their use for reducing gingivitis or biofilm?

    _____

23. What is the web site for the ADA Seal Program?

    _____

24. List the items that should be documented in the patient's chart concerning dentifrices and mouthrinses.

_____

_____

_____

_____

_____

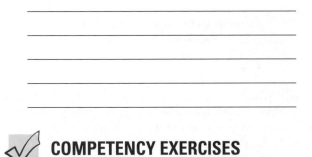

COMPETENCY EXERCISES

Apply information from the chapter and use critical thinking skills to complete the competency exercises. Write responses on paper or create electronic documents to submit your answers.

1. Using the information in the textbook, compare effectiveness, adverse effects, availability to the patient, and any other factors about therapeutic agents that might affect patient acceptance. (*Hint:* Use a separate piece of paper to make a one-page Infomap, or table, to aid in your comparison.) What additional information would you like to have about each of these agents that might help you inform your patients about using them?

2. Evan, a 7-year-old, has been prescribed a fluoride mouthrinse by Dr. Leiberman. Evan demonstrates a rinsing technique in which he fills his mouth with the liquid and rotates his head in all directions and then dribbles the rinse out of his open mouth into the sink.

    You plan to teach him how to rinse using the steps outlined in Box 29-4 of the textbook. Write a dental hygiene diagnosis statement that identifies a problem related to Evan's current rinsing technique.

3. Write a goal for the problem identified in the dental hygiene diagnosis in question 2. How will you measure whether or not Evan met the goal? Include a time frame for meeting the goal.

4. Ms. Greene is a 45-year-old periodontal patient who develops a moderate amount of supragingival calculus. What type of dentifrice might you consider recommending to her?

5. Using your institution's guidelines for writing in patient records, document the recommendation of a toothpaste containing pyrophosphate during patient education.

Everyday Ethics

Before completing the learning exercises below, reread and reflect on the Everyday Ethics scenario and Questions for Consideration in this chapter of the textbook. It may also be useful to review the Dental Hygiene Ethics discussion in Chapter 1, the Ethical Applications in the introduction pages for each Section in the textbook, as well as the Codes of Ethics in Appendices I, II, and III.

Collaborative Learning Activities
- Answer each of the questions for consideration at the end of the scenario in the textbook. Compare what you wrote with answers developed by another classmate and discuss differences/similarities.
- Work with a small group to develop a 2- to 5-minute role-play that introduces the Everyday Ethics scenario described in the chapter (a great idea is to video record your role-play activity). Then develop separate 2-minute role-play scenarios that provide at least two alternative approaches/solutions to resolving the situation. Ask classmates to view the solutions, ask questions, and discuss the ethical approach used in each. Ask for a vote on which solution classmates determine to be the "best."

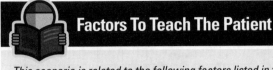

Factors To Teach The Patient

This scenario is related to the following factors listed in this chapter of the textbook:

■ Significance of American Dental Association product acceptance seal (especially because it is a voluntary program, and no seal on a product does not signify that it is unsafe or not effective).

Ms. Cerene Leffler usually prefers to use all-natural products. She has noticed that the dentifrice she likes does not display the ADA seal on the package. She asks you during her dental hygiene appointment if that indicates that the toothpaste is not a good choice. Using patient-appropriate language, write a statement explaining to Ms. Leffler what the ADA seal means.

? QUESTIONS PATIENTS ASK

What sources of information can you identify that will help you answer your patient's questions in this scenario?

After you answer her questions about the ADA seal, Ms. Leffler is very impressed with your knowledge, and she clearly believes that YOU are the expert to ask about dental products. Like many of your patients, she has questions about all kinds of oral-care products that she has heard or read about. "Does it really matter which toothpaste I use?" "There are so many different kinds with different ingredients that claim to do different things—which one is really the best?" "Are there any negative side effects that go along with any of those extra ingredients and chemicals?" "Which mouthrinse do you recommend?"

CROSSWORD PUZZLE

ACROSS

1. A broad-spectrum antibacterial agent that has the ability to bind and remain in the oral cavity over a period of time
3. A substance that causes contraction or shrinkage and arrests discharges
5. A Chemical that impacts the immune- inflammatory process (two words)
7. A type of activity relating to motions of fluids or the forces that produce or affect such motion
11. Treatment of disease by means of chemical substances or pharmaceutical agents
12. A chemical with a bacteriostatic or bacteriocidal effect
14. Added to a dentifrice to prevent separation of the solid and liquid ingredients during storage
15. Description of the amount of toothpaste dispensed on the toothbrush of a 2- to 5-year-old child (two words)
16. Ability of an agent to bind to the pellicle and tooth surface to be released and to retain potency over an extended period of time
17. Reduces oral acidity
18. A chemotherapeutic substance usually used with a toothbrush
19. This flavoring agent in dentifrices has been shown to provide anti-caries benefits.
20. An action in which one agent or drug enhances the effect of another

DOWN

2. Restoration of mineral elements
3. The term that means acid forming
4. This agent has been shown to have a beneficial effect on reducing the bacteria associated with VSC production
6. Added to a dentifrice as a caries prevention agent
7. Substance in a dentifrice that retains moisture and prevents hardening on exposure to air
8. A substance with a high molecular weight that results from chemically combining two or more monomers
9. Type of fluoride that has been shown to help reduce oral biofilm
10. Refers to an ingredient added to a dentifrice to produce a specific preventive or treatment outcome
13. Indicates that efficacy claims of a product have been tested by research studies and are valid (two words)

CHAPTER 30

The Patient With Orthodontic Appliances

Upon successful completion of these exercises, you will be able to:

1. Identify and define key terms and concepts related to the care of patients with orthodontic appliances.
2. Identify appliances and instruments used in orthodontic treatment.
3. Describe procedures for placing and removing orthodontic appliances.
4. Provide oral hygiene instructions for a patient before, during, and following orthodontic treatment.

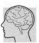 **KNOWLEDGE EXERCISES**

Write your answers for each question in the space provided.

1. A _____ orthodontic appliance is bonded or banded to individual teeth or groups of teeth.

2. A _____ is bonded to the surface of a tooth to hold an arch wire.

3. _____ refers to removal of orthodontic appliances and residual adhesive.

4. A _____ is used to secure arch wires to orthodontic brackets.

5. A space _____ prevents closure, and a space _____ corrects closure of a gap in the dentition that has resulted from a prematurely lost tooth.

6. What is the purpose of an orthodontic retainer?

_____

_____

7. List the advantages of bonded brackets.

_____

_____

_____

_____

_____

8. List the disadvantages of bonded brackets.

_____

_____

_____

_____

9. What materials are bonded brackets commonly made from?

_____

_____

_____

10. What is the bonding pad?

    _____

11. Elastomers hold the arch wire to the bracket. The purpose of the arch wire is to:

    _____

12. How do you condition the enamel surface of teeth before bonding the orthodontic brackets?

    _____

    _____

13. The procedure for applying the bonding agent is similar to the procedure for placing a dental _____.

14. After you etch a tooth before bonding the bracket, microclefts in the enamel are formed that range from _____ μm to _____ μm deep.

15. The use of filler particles in bonding resin increases _____; therefore, heavily filled resins are used for brackets placed on _____ teeth, which are subject to high forces of mastication.

16. A patient with orthodontic appliances is at risk for a higher incidence of which two oral diseases?

    _____

    _____

17. What two factors contribute to the demineralized areas (white spots) commonly found on a patient's teeth after removal of orthodontic brackets and bands?

    _____

    _____

18. List two advantages of recommending a power toothbrush for your patient with orthodontic appliances.

    _____

    _____

19. Describe how a regular toothbrush is adapted on the facial surface of teeth with an orthodontic appliance?

    _____

    _____

    _____

20. Explain how an orthodontic toothbrush, such as that pictured in Figure 30-3 in the textbook, is used.

    _____

    _____

    _____

21. Along with careful periodontal examination, examination for demineralized areas, and removal of leftover composite resin, what other professional intervention is required after debonding orthodontic appliances.

    _____

✓ COMPETENCY EXERCISES

Apply information from the chapter and use critical thinking skills to complete the competency exercises. Write responses on paper or create electronic documents to submit your answers.

1. Ms. Anna Moyer, a real estate agent who really relies on her smile as she interacts with the public in her job, is very excited and yet extremely nervous on the day the brackets that have hidden her smile for so long are being removed. After the brackets and arch wires are removed from Ms. Moyer's teeth, it is important to remove all residual adhesive. Discuss the steps you will take to ensure that all areas of each tooth are thoroughly free from adhesive.

2. Discuss the purpose of post-debonding preventive care that you, the dental hygienist, will provide for Ms. Moyer.

3. Two weeks after her fixed orthodontic appliances are removed, the orthodontist delivers a Hawley appliance to Ms. Moyer. You are responsible for educating and instructing her about the purpose and care of her retainer. What important points will you cover in your discussion?

4. Your next patient is Missy Breckenridge. She has had her fixed orthodontic appliances almost a year and you notice that her gingiva is not as healthy as it was when you saw her 6 months ago. When you disclose her mouth, there is a large accumulation of dental biofilm between the brackets and her gingival margins. What topics will you be sure to include in your discussion with Missy as you provide oral hygiene instructions that address her need to ensure cleanliness on all surfaces.

Everyday Ethics

Before completing the learning exercises below, reread and reflect on the Everyday Ethics scenario and Questions for Consideration in this chapter of the textbook. It may also be useful to review the Dental Hygiene Ethics discussion in Chapter 1, the Ethical Applications in the introduction pages for each section in the textbook, as well as the Codes of Ethics in Appendices I, II, and III.

Individual Learning Activity
Identify a situation you have experienced that presents a similar ethical dilemma. Write about what you would do

differently now than you did at the time the incident happened. Support your discussion with concepts from the dental hygiene codes of ethics.

Discovery Activity
Ask a dental hygienist who has been practicing for a year or more to read the scenario. Provide them with a copy of one of the Codes of Ethics as well. Share your responses for each question and ask that person to discuss the situation with you. What insights did you have or what did you learn during this discussion?

Factors To Teach The Patient

This scenario is related to the following factors listed in this chapter of the textbook:

- The significance of biofilm around orthodontic appliances and teeth
- How, when, and why to use fluoride rinses, toothpastes, and brush-on gels
- The frequency for professional follow-up during and after orthodontic therapy

Nicholas Bean is a 12-year-old patient. He is going directly from his prophylaxis appointment with you to the orthodontist's office, where they will be placing full-mouth bands/brackets and arch wires on his teeth. As they arrive

for the appointment, Nicholas's mother comments that they won't be seeing you again until the braces come off. You want to begin to educate Nicholas and his mother right away about the importance of the use of fluorides, thorough daily oral hygiene measures, and especially why regular maintenance appointments are necessary during orthodontic treatment.

Using the information you learned from reading this chapter and the examples of patient conversations from Appendix D as a guide, prepare an outline for a conversation with Nicholas' mother that provides anticipatory guidance about ways to maintain good oral health status while her son is undergoing orthodontic care.

Care of Dental Prostheses

Learning Objectives

Upon successful completion of these exercises, you will be able to:

1. Identify and define key terms and concepts related to care of dental prostheses.
2. Identify the components and characteristics of a variety of dental prostheses.
3. Describe the cleaning and care of dental prostheses.
4. Identify procedures to care for the remaining natural teeth, implants, and underlying oral tissues.

KNOWLEDGE EXERCISES

Write your answers for each question in the space provided.

1. List the components of a fixed partial denture prosthesis.

   _____

   _____

2. List the criteria for an acceptable fixed partial denture prosthesis.

   _____

   _____

   _____

   _____

3. In your own words, describe the procedures for oral cleansing of a fixed dental prosthesis.

   _____

   _____

   _____

   _____

   _____

4. What characteristic of a removable partial denture prosthesis can negatively affect your patient's gingival health?

   _____

   _____

5. If your patient is unable to remove his or her own partial denture prosthesis, how do you help the patient remove it?

   _____

   _____

6. In your own words, describe an obturator.

   _____

   _____

7. Label Figure 31-1 with the following components.

■ Denture border

■ Impression surface

■ Occlusal surface

■ Polished surface

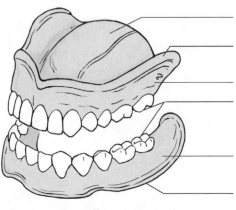

Figure 31-1

8. Identify two kinds of liners that may be present on the impression surface of a complete denture prosthesis.

_____

_____

9. Identify two kinds of complete overdenture prostheses.

_____

_____

10. What are the advantages of a complete overdenture prosthesis?

_____

_____

_____

_____

11. List the criteria that contribute to the success of an overdenture prosthesis.

_____

_____

_____

12. What dental hygiene interventions can provide an added measure of protection for the oral health of a patient with a partial denture, single arch complete denture with natural teeth remaining in the opposite arch, or an overdenture supported by natural teeth?

_____

_____

_____

13. What are the two procedures that can be used to clean an oral prosthesis?

_____

_____

14. Describe the process you will use to remove your patient's complete denture if, for some reason, your patient is not able to remove it himself or herself.

■ Maxillary complete denture

_____

_____

■ Mandibular complete denture

_____

_____

15. Identify two oral conditions that can be prevented with proper cleansing and care of dental prostheses and underlying tissues.

_____

_____

16. What is the purpose of instructing your patients to remove and properly store their dental prosthesis in liquid while sleeping at night?

_____

_____

17. What are the requirements for a denture cleanser you will recommend to your patient?

_____

_____

_____

_____

18. Complete Infomap 31-1 to compare the various types of cleansers that you can recommend for the care of full and partial dentures.

INFOMAP 31-1			
TYPE	**ACTIVE INGREDIENT**	**CLEANSER ACTION**	**DISADVANTAGES**
Immersion Type			
Alkaline hypochlorite (household bleach)			
Alkaline peroxide (commercial powder or tablet)			
Dilute acids (commercial ultrasonic solutions)			
Enzymes (in various cleansers)			
Abrasive Type			
Pastes and powders (various commercial products)			
Household agents (salt, bicarbonate of soda, hand soap, scouring powders)			

 COMPETENCY EXERCISES

Apply information from the chapter and use critical thinking skills to complete the competency exercises. Write responses on paper or create electronic documents to submit your answers.

1. Imagine that you have just joined the onsite dental team at a long-term care facility or nursing home. A short time after you begin your position, you discover that many of the residents wear full or partial dentures and that that those dentures are not being cleaned regularly by the nurses' aides responsible for providing daily care for the residents. Most of the dentures worn by the residents are complete arch dentures made of acrylic resins. Many are old and stained, and some have calculus buildup on the surfaces of the denture. The dentures are seldom removed from the patients' mouths, and when they are, they are often just placed on the bedside table or in the drawer until family members come for a visit and decide that the patient looks better with the denture back in place.

You plan to provide an in-service presentation for the caregivers about the importance of denture care, and you also plan to provide hands-on training in denture-cleaning techniques for the caregiver staff.

■ List the information that you will include in your in-service presentation about denture care.

■ Create a step-by-step checklist that the aides can use at the bedside to document daily cleaning of each resident's removable prosthesis as well as his or her oral tissues.

2. During a dental hygiene appointment, you carefully and completely clean and disinfect your patient's removable maxillary complete denture and mandibular partial denture before returning it to the patient's mouth at the end of the visit. Using your school's guidelines for writing patient progress notes, document the service you provided for this patient.

DISCOVERY EXERCISE

Investigate commercially available denture cleaners so that you can make a recommendation to the long-term care center or nursing home staff. What is the active ingredient in each one? What is the relative cost of each type? Which type might be easiest for the caregivers to use in the nursing home setting? Which one (or ones) will you recommend in your in-service presentation? Provide a rationale for your choice(s).

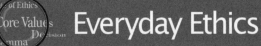

Everyday Ethics

Before completing the learning exercises below, reread and reflect on the Everyday Ethics scenario and Questions for Consideration in this chapter of the textbook. It may also be useful to review the Dental Hygiene Ethics discussion in Chapter 1, the Ethical Applications in the introduction pages for each section in the textbook, as well as the Codes of Ethics in Appendices I, II, and III.

Individual Learning Activity
Imagine that you are the dental hygienist in this scenario. Answer each of the questions for consideration at the end of the scenario.

Discovery Activity
Ask a dental hygienist who has been practicing for a year or more to read the scenario. Provide them with a copy of one of the Codes of Ethics as well. Share your responses to each question and ask that person to discuss the situation with you. What insights did you have, or what did you learn during this discussion?

Factors To Teach The Patient

This scenario is related to the following factors listed in this chapter of the textbook:

■ How to make a self-examination of the oral tissues
■ Why all prostheses need cleaning more than once a day
■ The need to adapt toothbrushing, flossing, and use of other aids to the care of the abutment teeth
■ How tongue cleaning contributes to complete oral health
■ The significance of regular maintenance appointments to have the oral tissues checked and the prostheses professionally cleaned

Evangeline Dada has just received her brand new six-unit anterior bridge, which spans her entire smile from abutment tooth 6 to abutment tooth 11. Before placement of the fixed prosthesis, she had a removable temporary appliance made of plastic. She had no trouble cleaning her teeth when she could remove the old appliance, and she has done a good job of keeping all her oral tissues healthy. She states she is completely at a loss as to how she must take care of this beautiful new smile of hers and asks you to spend some extra time providing oral-hygiene instructions for her today.

Use the example of patient conversations in Appendix D as a guide to develop a conversation to educate Evangeline about her new bridge, the abutment teeth that support it, and maintaining the health of the oral tissues around and underneath this new fixed prosthesis.

Use the conversation you create to role-play this situation with a fellow student. If you are the patient in the role-play, be sure to ask questions. If you are the dental hygienist, try to anticipate questions and answer them in your explanation.

WORD SEARCH

```
A  R  P  R  O  S  T  H  E  S  I  S  O
A  B  U  T  M  E  N  T  M  E  W  S  B
O  C  C  L  U  S  A  L  L  Y  E  T  T
P  P  G  V  V  J  I  B  N  R  H  O  U
O  O  B  J  I  F  A  O  U  S  E  M  R
L  N  J  U  O  V  I  T  N  G  C  A  A
I  T  F  I  O  S  N  E  D  F  O  T  T
S  I  B  M  I  E  S  I  V  I  M  I  O
H  C  E  C  D  A  R  A  K  X  P  T  R
E  R  E  R  B  B  X  I  B  E  L  I  U
D  R  E  F  L  U  O  R  I  D  E  S  M
P  V  P  A  R  T  I  A  L  Z  T  U  C
O  X  R  E  T  A  I  N  E  R  E  L  O
```

WORD SEARCH CLUES

1. Often placed on teeth that support an overdenture prosthesis to aid in caries prevention.
2. The surface of the dental prosthesis that makes contact with teeth in the opposing arch.
3. Can build up on surfaces of a denture the same way it can build up on natural dentition.
4. An artificial replacement for a body part.
5. A type of oral prosthesis that is cleaned and cared for outside of the oral cavity.
6. Component of a fixed partial denture that replaces a missing natural tooth.
7. A type of partial denture prosthesis that is secured to natural teeth or dental implants and must be cleaned and cared for inside the oral cavity.
8. The type of dental prosthesis that replaces one or more teeth, but not all of the teeth in an arch.
9. The clasp that holds a partial denture around abutment teeth.
10. A type of removable dental prosthesis that is supported by both retained natural teeth or implants and the soft tissue of the alveolar ridge.
11. A type of dental prosthesis that replaces the dentition and associated structures in an entire oral arch.
12. The part of a dental prosthesis that rests on the oral mucosa and to which teeth are attached.
13. A dental prosthesis that closes a congenital or acquired opening in oral tissues.
14. A type of connector that attaches a removal prosthesis to a metal receptacle included within a restoration of an abutment tooth.
15. A tooth or implant used to support a fixed or removable dental prosthesis.
16. A term commonly used to refer to a fixed partial denture prosthesis.
17. The external or outer surface of a dental prosthesis is highly _____, whereas the occlusal and impression surfaces are not.
18. An infection of the oral mucosa that can occur under a removable dental prosthesis.

CHAPTER 32

The Patient With Dental Implants

Learning Objectives

Upon successful completion of these exercises, you will be able to:

1. Identify and define key terms and concepts related to care of the patient with implants.
2. Discuss characteristics and factors that influence self-care or dental hygiene care of the rehabilitated mouth.

3. Discuss types, preparation and placement, and maintenance care for dental implants.
4. Discuss the components of a post-restorative evaluation of a dental implant.
5. Identify the factors that contribute to implant failure.

KNOWLEDGE EXERCISES

Write your answers for each question in the space provided.

1. In your own words, briefly describe each of the three types of dental implants.

    _____

    _____

    _____

    _____

    _____

    _____

2. The most common type of dental implant is the _____ type that has a _____ shape.

3. Identify two biological tissues that interface with a dental implant.

    _____

    _____

4. What is the permucosal seal?

    _____

    _____

5. Identify factors that can increase a patient's risk for poor outcomes if dental implants are placed.

    _____

    _____

    _____

    _____

    _____

    _____

    _____

    _____

    _____

    _____

6. Each time the patient with dental implants is scheduled for routine dental hygiene maintenance care, you will examine the implant area carefully. List the basic criteria that indicate a healthy implant.

_____

_____

_____

_____

_____

7. Identify two prominent contributing factors in the breakdown of the peri-implant environment.

_____

_____

8. Identify oral conditions that indicate that the dental implant may be ailing and should be evaluated by the oral surgeon who placed the implant.

_____

_____

_____

9. Explain why it is important to instruct a patient with dental implants to select self-cleaning implements and agents carefully.

_____

_____

10. What types of instruments are used for removing calculus from titanium surfaces of dental implants?

_____

_____

11. What are the components of a post-restorative evaluation for a patient with dental implants?

_____

_____

_____

_____

_____

12. During the calculus removal phase of a professional implant maintenance appointment, what instrument choices are available for the dental hygienist to select?

_____

_____

13. What instrumentation decision is critical when using an ultrasonic instrument for debridement of an implant?

_____

_____

14. What are some of the systemic factors that can contribute to implant failure?

_____

_____

15. What are some of the surgical issues that can contribute to implant failure?

_____

_____

✓ COMPETENCY EXERCISES

Apply information from the chapter and use critical thinking skills to complete the competency exercises. Write responses on paper or create electronic documents to submit your answers.

1. Describe the dental hygienist's role in collaborative treatment planning and preparing the patient for dental implant procedures.

2. Matthew Glenn, aged 45 years, is scheduled today for a periodontal maintenance appointment. You are very excited and anxious to check the area of his dental implant–supported bridge. The prosthesis he received 6 months ago is a 3-unit replacement for teeth 3, 4, and 5, with each pontic supported by an individual dental implant. You provided oral hygiene instructions for him both before and after his implant procedure, but you haven't seen him since.

During your assessment today, you find out that he is not having any oral problems, and the implants have been comfortable and feel just fine. In fact, he is delighted with the implants. His daily oral care is generally very good, but you notice small areas of biofilm in the hard-to-reach areas of the prosthesis, such as the embrasure between teeth 4 and 5 and the distal surface of tooth 3. To your surprise, there is also significant calculus buildup on the facial and mesial surfaces of tooth number 2.

The gingival tissue around the implant looks generally healthy. Mr. Glenn also exhibits some very slight calculus buildup on the facial surfaces of the left side maxillary molars and on the lingual surfaces of his lower anterior teeth. You find no other significant medical history, dental history, or dental examination findings for Mr. Glenn today.

Use a copy of the Individualized Patient Care Plan template (Appendix B) to develop a care plan for Mr.

Glenn that emphasizes daily care techniques to ensure long-term success for his implants and prosthesis.

DISCOVERY EXERCISES

- Research Web sites for viewing a dental implant procedure.
- Research implant manufacturers and supply companies to discover the cost of the instruments.
- Research the CDT codes from the American Dental Association to identify the correct insurance billing codes for implant maintenance procedures.
- Go to the American Association of Periodontolgy (AAP) Web site to find more information about dental implants.

Everyday Ethics

Before completing the learning exercises below, reread and reflect on the Everyday Ethics scenario and Questions for Consideration in this chapter of the textbook. It may also be useful to review the Dental Hygiene Ethics discussion in Chapter 1, the Ethical Applications in the introduction pages for each Section in the textbook, as well as the Codes of Ethics in Appendices I, II, and III.

Individual Learning Activity
Identify a situation you have experienced that presents a similar ethical dilemma. What did you learn from how the situation was (or was not) resolved at the time it happened?

Collaborative Learning Activity
Work with a small group to develop a 2- to 5-minute role-play that introduces the Everyday Ethics scenario described in the chapter (a great idea is to video record your role-play activity). Then develop separate 2-minute role-play scenarios that provide at least two alternative approaches/solutions to resolving the situation. Ask classmates to view the solutions, ask questions, and discuss the ethical approach used in each. Ask for a vote on which solution classmates determine to be the "best."

Factors To Teach The Patient

- How to care for implants: special needs related to titanium surfaces
- How the health of the periodontal tissues and the duration of the implants and prostheses depend on meticulous daily self-care by the patient and regular professional maintenance
- The role of biofilm in periodontitis and peri-implantitis; vulnerability of the implant to infection from periodontal pathogens that may be present on adjacent natural teeth

- How cleaning a mouth with complex restorations takes longer
- How important a healthy diet and lifestyle is to the long-term success of an implant

Use the Individualized Patient Care Plan you developed for Mr. Glenn (introduced in Competency Exercise question 2) and the example conversation in Appendix D as a guide to prepare a conversation to provide oral hygiene instructions for Mr. Glenn during his dental hygiene appointment today.

CROSSWORD PUZZLE

ACROSS

3. A layer of connective tissue between a dental implant and surrounding bone that is indicative of failed osseointegration (two words)
7. Another name for a transosseous implant
10. An oral antimicrobial rinse prescribed for daily use for ailing implants
11. A type of dental implant that penetrates through the full thickness of the alveolar bone
12. Iatrogenic peri-implantitis due to retained cement at the implant–abutment interface
13. Reversible, first-stage infection of the soft tissue surrounding a dental implant
14. The direct attachment of bone and alloplastic material that is required for the success of a dental implant

DOWN

1. Prevents microorganisms from entering the soft tissues around a dental implant (two words)
2. A dental implant that is placed within the alveolar bone
4. A dental implant in which the metal framework rests on top of the alveolar bone but under the periosteum
5. Refers to either the connection between the dental implant and bone or between the dental implant and soft tissue
6. A unique characteristic of the metal titanium that makes it capable of existing in harmony with the biologic environment of the human body
8. An early form of blade- or plate-shaped endosseous implants
9. A metal that is commonly combined with aluminum and vanadium for use in dental implants

CHAPTER 33

The Patient Who Uses Tobacco

Upon successful completion of these exercises, you will be able to:

1. Identify and define key terms and concepts related to the use of tobacco.
2. Explain the systemic and oral effects of tobacco use.
3. Describe the effects of nicotine addiction.
4. Describe strategies for tobacco cessation.
5. Plan dental hygiene care and tobacco cessation interventions for patients who use tobacco.
6. Identify the role of the community-based dental hygienist in tobacco-free initiatives.

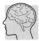

KNOWLEDGE EXERCISES

Write your answers for each question in the space provided.

1. Tobacco contains many components that are _____ to humans. Tobacco use is the single most _____ cause of disease and premature death in the world.

2. **True or False:** Tobacco use with a water-cooled hookah device is a safe alternative to traditional smoking.

   _____

3. Through which tissues can nicotine in **cigarette smoke** be absorbed into the bloodstream?

   _____

   _____

4. List the factors that affect the amounts of nicotine and other tobacco components that are absorbed into the bloodstream.

   _____

   _____

   _____

   _____

   _____

5. Through which tissues can nicotine from **smokeless tobacco** be absorbed into the bloodstream?

   _____

6. To which tissues does nicotine spread through the bloodstream?

   _____

7. Match each of the following descriptive statements with the appropriate tobacco-related term.

TOBACCO-RELATED TERMS	DESCRIPTIVE STATEMENTS
A. Tolerance B. Dependence C. Abuse D. Addiction E. ETS F. TSNAs	_____ The use of any drug in a way that causes harm to the person or other persons who are affected by the user's behavior _____ Refers to the user's need for increased tobacco use over time to create the desired feeling of well-being _____ Loss of control over the amount and frequency of use of tobacco and withdrawal symptoms occur when use of tobacco is discontinued _____ Formed by tobacco smoke reaction with nitrous acid on indoor surfaces. _____ Chronic, progressive, relapsing disease characterized by compulsive use of a substance _____ Refers to passive exposure to second- or third-hand tobacco smoke

8. Match each of the following descriptive statements with the appropriate component of tobacco. Each term may be used more than once.

TOBACCO-RELATED TERMS	DESCRIPTIVE STATEMENTS
E. Cotinine F. Nicotine G. Nitrosamines H. Pyrolysis I. Thiocyanate	_____ By-product of nicotine in found in body fluids _____ The chief psychoactive ingredient in tobacco _____ The chief addictive agent in tobacco _____ Refers to a group of cancer-causing chemicals found in tobacco _____ The process of breaking down chemicals contained in tobacco by heat created at the end of a burning cigarette _____ and _____ Substances measured to determine recent use of nicotine-containing products _____ By-product of hydrogen cyanide that is found in tobacco smoke _____ Substance found in the various aids used for smoking cessation _____ Intensifies the release of dopamine by the brain _____ Although addictive, this chemical is NOT the most physically harmful substance found in tobacco _____ Released with other substances when the tobacco is ignited

9. How is nicotine eliminated from the body?

_____

10. List as many negative health effects of tobacco use and/or exposure to second-hand ETS as you can.

_____

_____

_____

_____

_____

_____

_____

_____

11. Identify as many potential oral health consequences of tobacco use as you can.

_____

_____

_____

_____

_____

_____

_____

12. Peak concentration of nicotine in the blood plasma occurs approximately _____ minutes after the onset of smoking and _____ declines over the next 20 to 30 minutes.

13. Why are children of parents and/or caregivers who use tobacco also at higher risk for disease?

_____

_____

_____

14. As you are providing dental hygiene care for your patient who uses tobacco, you can identify the negative effects of tobacco use that are specific to that patient. In your own words, explain each of the following terms as they relate to your role during the dental hygiene care for each patient.

Detect _____

_____

Explain _____

_____

Relate _____

_____

Motivate _____

_____

Refer _____

_____

Ascertain _____

_____

Consult _____

_____

Document _____

_____

15. Your patient who is dependent on nicotine may still continue to use tobacco, even though you have spent considerable time during a dental hygiene appointment educating him or her about the personal oral health effects of tobacco use. You can inform and advise your patient, but you must wait to provide support until he or she can articulate reasons for quitting and is ready to take that step. Explain two types of treatment programs that can provide support for your patient who is now ready to quit using tobacco.

_____

_____

_____

_____

_____

16. The 5 *A*'s provide the basis for a simple but effective tobacco dependence–intervention approach. Number the 5 *A*'s in the appropriate order (from 1 to 5) and then *briefly* outline the basic premise of each.

_____ Advise

_____

_____

_____ Arrange

_____

_____

_____ Ask

_____

_____

_____ Assess

_____

_____

_____ Assist

_____

_____

17. You use a motivational interviewing technique to determine that your patient is currently in the contemplation stage related to tobacco cessation. Identify the 5 *R*'s that you will use as the basis for a continuing discussion with your patient about tobacco use.

_____ Tailoring advice to each patient

_____ Potential for increased problems

_____ Identifying benefits of quitting

_____ Barriers to quitting

_____ Reinforcing at every visit

18. **True or False:** The electronic nicotine delivery device is an approved method of smoking cessation that can be recommended for a patient by a dental hygienist.

_____

19. List the methods that are available for delivering nicotine-replacement therapy if your patient is considering pharmacotherapy as a treatment for nicotine addiction.

_____

_____

_____

_____

_____

20. Identify non-nicotine pharmacotherapies approved by the FDA for tobacco cessation.

_____

_____

21. In your own words, state the objectives and rationale for using pharmacotherapies to help your patient stop using tobacco.

    _____

    _____

22. What factors should be considered when recommending pharmacotherapies to help your patients stop using tobacco?

    _____

    _____

    _____

23. What are the contraindications for use of pharmacotherapy-assisted tobacco cessation?

    _____

    _____

    _____

    _____

24. What are the most common *oral* side effects of the pharmacotherapies used for the treatment of nicotine addiction?

    _____

    _____

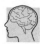

COMPETENCY EXERCISES

Apply information from the chapter and use critical thinking skills to complete the competency exercises. Write responses on paper or create electronic documents to submit your answers.

1. Each of the following statements expresses a concept that some of your patients may believe. But each statement is *false*. Create a true statement and provide an explanation/rationale for each, which you could use to convince your patient that the original statement is not true.

    a. The use of spit tobacco is a safe alternative to smoking tobacco.

    b. It is fairly easy for smokers to stop using tobacco once they decide that they are going to do so.

    c. There is no way to relieve nicotine withdrawal symptoms experienced while trying to quit tobacco use.

2. Use the Tobacco Use Assessment Form (Figure 33-4 in the textbook) to assess the tobacco-using habits of a friend or relative. Use the methods outlined in the Tobacco Cessation Flow Chart to encourage your friend or relative to quit.

3. The Section IV summary exercises section of this workbook, contains a Patient Assessment Summary for Mrs. Diane White, who is in her first trimester of pregnancy. Although Mrs. White does not smoke, her husband does. Describe the tobacco use and cessation information you will want to be sure to cover as you talk to Mrs. White during her dental hygiene and re-evaluation appointments.

4. Using your institution's guidelines for writing in patient records, document that you have provided education and counseling related to the health effects of tobacco use during Mrs. White's appointment.

5. As a dental hygienist, your role in addressing the oral and systemic health damage of tobacco use is more than simply providing assessment, information, motivation, and guidance to individual patients in your clinical practice. Discuss your role in tobacco education and cessation from a personal and community-based or advocacy perspective.

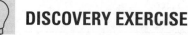

DISCOVERY EXERCISE

Collect a variety of patient education materials—such as brochures, posters, or videotapes—that address the health and/or oral health effects of tobacco use. Encourage each of your student colleagues to collect as many materials as possible from a variety of different sources. Get together in small groups to discuss the materials.

- Determine the scientific accuracy of the information included in the patient-education materials.
- Determine which type of patient each of the materials is best suited for.
- Determine how each of the materials might best be used as part of tobacco-cessation initiatives in your clinic.

Everyday Ethics

Before completing the learning exercises below, reread and reflect on the Everyday Ethics scenario and Questions for Consideration in this chapter of the textbook. It may also be useful to review the Dental Hygiene Ethics discussion in Chapter 1, the Ethical Applications in the introduction pages for each section in the textbook, as well as the Codes of Ethics in Appendices I, II, and III.

Collaborative Learning Activity
Answer each of the questions for consideration at the end of the scenario in the textbook. Compare what you wrote

with answers developed by another classmate and discuss differences/similarities.

Discovery Activity
Summarize this scenario for faculty members at your school and ask them to consider the questions that are included. Is their perspective different than yours or similar? Explain.

Factors To Teach The Patient

This scenario is related to the following factors listed in this chapter of the textbook:

■ Nonsmokers who breath ETS can incur the same serious health problems as smokers. Children are especially susceptible.

Mrs. White's husband (see Competency Question #3 above and the Section IV summary exercises in this workbook) arrives to pick up his wife following her dental hygiene appointment. He wants to discuss their insurance coverage with the office manager, but she is on the telephone, so he must wait for a few minutes to speak with her. He sits down

in a chair and immediately takes out a pack of cigarettes and some matches. He asks you for an ashtray.

Use the example conversations provided in Appendix D as a guide to prepare an outline for explaining the tobacco-free policy in your office to Mr. White. Mr. White is not your patient—how far can you go in approaching him about the dangers of his tobacco use for his unborn child or providing recommendations for smoking cessation measures?

Use the conversation you create to role-play this situation with a fellow student. If you are the patient in the role-play, be sure to ask questions. If you are the dental hygienist, try to anticipate questions and answer them in your explanation.

Diet and Dietary Analysis

Upon successful completion of these exercises, you will be able to:

1. Identify and define key terms and concepts related to providing a dietary assessment.

2. Identify vitamins and minerals relevant to oral health.

3. Plan and provide dietary assessment and patient counseling for caries control.

 KNOWLEDGE EXERCISES

Write your answers for each question in the space provided.

1. List the major food categories included in the MyPlate Food Guide (Figure 34-1 in the textbook).

   _____

   _____

   _____

   _____

   _____

2. Identify two other food categories listed in the Food Intake Patterns table (Figure 34-3 in the textbook) that contribute to an individual's caloric intake.

   _____

   _____

3. The Food Intake Patterns sheet contains a table that outlines daily amount of food that is appropriate on the basis of 12 different _____ levels.

4. Use information on the second page of Figure 34-3 to identify the three characteristics used to determine the appropriate calorie intake level for an individual person's diet.

   _____

   _____

   _____

5. Look at Figure 34-2 in the textbook to find the appropriate calorie level for yourself. Then identify the daily amount of food from the vegetable group that is suggested to meet your nutritional needs.

   _____

   _____

6. What amount of food from the dark green vegetable subgroup is suggested for your diet?

   _____

   _____

7. Table 34-1 in the textbook provides a comprehensive list of nutrients with their functions, associated disease states, and food sources. Your

instructor will let you know the level of detail you are expected to recall from the information in that table. It is most important for you to be able to link deficiencies in nutritional intake with oral manifestations you may observe while providing dental hygiene care for your patients. Table 34-2 provides some oral manifestations that are associated with nutritional deficiencies.

Infomap 34-1 reorganizes information from the textbook to help you associate nutrient deficiencies with specific intraoral findings. Use information throughout Chapter 34 of the textbook to help you complete the Infomap with (a) the oral findings you might observe if your patient is deficient in each listed nutrient and (b) food sources for that nutrient that you can recommend to your patient.

INFOMAP 34-1

NUTRIENT	ORAL MANIFESTATIONS OF DEFICIENCY	FOOD SOURCES
Vitamin A		
Thaimin (Vitamin B$_1$)		
Niacin (Vitamin B$_3$)		
Riboflavin (Vitamin B$_2$)		
Pyridoxine (Vitamin B$_6$)		
Cobalamin (Vitamin B$_{12}$)		
Ascorbic Acid (Vitamin C)		
Vitamin D		
Calcium		
Fluoride		
Foliate		
Iron		
Magnesium		
Phosphorus		
Zinc		
Protein		

8. Which vitamins and minerals are associated with healthy skin and the mucous membrane?

_____

_____

_____

_____

9. Which nutrients are important for healthy wound healing and tissue repair?

_____

_____

_____

10. Which nutrients are essential for the development of healthy tooth structure?

_____

_____

_____

_____

_____

11. Dental caries is the result of intake of _____ foods and is not due to nutrient deficiency.

12. Identify four factors that interact to result in dental caries.

_____

_____

_____

_____

13. Any incident of sucrose intake lowers the pH in the dental biofilm. But what two major factors interact to enhance cariogenic exposure and increase your patient's risk for developing dental caries?

_____

_____

14. In your own words, discuss the purposes of a dietary assessment.

_____

_____

_____

15. Summarize the information you will provide for your patient when you are explaining your dietary assessment intervention before asking the patient to complete a food diary.

_____

_____

_____

16. Identify some common dietary omissions that you will want to be sure to review with your patient as you explain the food diary form.

_____

_____

17. In your own words, explain how to calculate a patient's caries risk using the Sweet Score. (*Hint:* Use the information in Figure 34-7 in the textbook to guide your answer.)

_____

_____

_____

18. If, after calculating the Sweet Score, you determine that your patient is at moderate or high risk for dental caries, what recommendations will you be sure to provide during your oral health education session with that patient?

_____

_____

_____

19. Identify *patient* factors that can affect your success in providing nutritional counseling for your patients.

_____

_____

_____

_____

20. Identify *communication* factors that can affect your success in providing nutritional counseling for your patients.

_____

_____

_____

_____

21. For a patient who is especially caries susceptible, what ingredient in chewing gum will help promote remineralization if chewed immediately after each meal?

_____

 COMPETENCY EXERCISES

Apply information from the chapter and use critical thinking skills to complete the competency exercises. Write responses on paper or create electronic documents to submit your answers.

1. Make a Food Diary Table similar to Figure 34-5 in the textbook and create a food diary for everything you ate yesterday. (No cheating, now; no one will ever see this but you.) What nutrients are missing from your diet?

2. Make a copy of the Scoring the Sweets form (Figure 32-7 in the textbook). Use the information in your 24-hour food diary to calculate your personal risk for dental caries. What recommendations will you give yourself to reduce your caries risk?

3. Ask a student colleague, friend, or member of your family to complete a 3- or 5-day food diary. Make a copy of the Dietary Analysis Recording Form (Figure 34-6 in the textbook) to complete a dietary analysis for that person.

4. Identify topics you would include in a patient education program on the basis of the dietary analysis you completed for question 3.

5. Use the Intereactive Tools link on the USDA MyPlate Web site (available at: http://www.choosemyplate.gov/tools.html) to develop a personalized daily food plan for yourself. Compare your personal food plan with those developed by student colleagues.

6. Discuss and compare food preferences, cultural food choices, and personal eating preferences with your student colleagues. What does this exercise help you realize about possible barriers when you are providing diet counseling for your diverse, individual patients?

7. Because individualized dental hygiene care plans are based on individualized patient needs determined by assessment data, not every dental hygiene care plan you write will include dietary assessment or dietary counseling. Discuss patient assessment findings that would indicate the need to include a 24-hour or 3- to 7-day dietary assessment as part of your patient's dental hygiene care plan.

Everyday Ethics

Before completing the learning exercises below, reread and reflect on the Everyday Ethics scenario and Questions for Consideration in this chapter of the textbook. It may also be useful to review the Dental Hygiene Ethics discussion in Chapter 1, the Ethical Applications in the introduction pages for each section in the textbook, as well as the Codes of Ethics in Appendices I, II, and III.

Individual Learning Activity
Imagine that you are the dental hygienist in this scenario. Answer each of the questions for consideration at the end of the scenario.

Discovery Activity
Ask a dental hygienist who has been practicing for a year or more to read the scenario. Provide them with a copy of one of the Codes of Ethics as well. Share your responses for answer each question and ask that person to discuss the situation with you. What insights did you have or what did you learn during this discussion?

Factors To Teach The Patient

This scenario is related to the following factors listed in this chapter of the textbook:

- Reasons to avoid frequent daily use of medications with sucrose
- Reasons for rinsing with water after a medication contained in a syrupy sucrose mixture
- How dental caries on the tooth surface starts and progresses
- How the interaction of cariogenic foods, tooth surface, saliva, and microorganisms act together in the dental caries process
- How repeated, frequent acid production and the pH in the dental biofilm adversely affect the teeth

Your next patient Nathan is a 7-year-old with a lot of serious medical health issues. Because he often has a queasy stomach, his mother fixes him many small meals each day and states that mostly all he will eat are high-carbohydrate foods. In addition, Nathan is frequently placed on a (sucrose-enhanced) antibiotic liquid preparation prescribed by his physician. He absolutely refuses to take any medication in a pill form, so the antibiotic syrup is the only answer.

Use the example conversations in Appendix D as a guide to prepare an outline for a conversation with Nathan's mother explaining his risk for caries and the importance of changing the boy's daily dietary habits. Make sure to adapt your recommendations for the barriers to behavior change that have been identified in the scenario.

Use the conversation you create to role-play this situation with a fellow student. If you are Nathan's mother in the role-play, be sure to ask questions and try to identify additional real-life barriers to behavior change. If you are the dental hygienist, try to anticipate questions and answer them in your explanation.

CROSSWORD PUZZLE

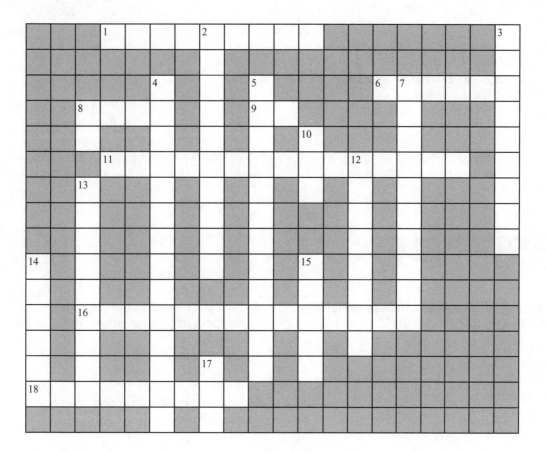

ACROSS

1. Listing of various foods and measurements of amounts eaten during a specific time period (two words).
6. Lifestyle that includes an increased amount of physical activity.
8. Agency that developed the food pyramid.
9. Recommendations for adequate intake of essential nutrients.
11. Refers to comparing the nutrient content of a food with the amount of energy it provides (two words).
16. Foods that do not lower the pH of biofilm or that encourage remineralization.
18. Lifestyle that includes only light physical activity on a day-to-day basis.

DOWN

2. Term that refers to nutritional inadequacy of specific nutrients in body tissues.
3. A factor in exposure to cariogenic food that is very significant for increasing risk for dental caries.
4. Carbohydrate, protein, and fat are examples.
5. Poor nourishment resulting from improper food intake.
7. Foods that lower the pH of oral biofilm and increase risk for dental caries.
8. Maximum intake of a specific nutrient that is unlikely to create adverse health risks for an individual.
10. Average amounts of nutrients that should be consumed daily by healthy individuals.
12. Chemical substance in foods that is needed by the body for building and repair.
13. Developed by the USDA to illustrate the five important food groups important in a balanced diet.
14. United States Department of Health and Human Services.
15. Diet consisting only of plant foods.
17. Comprehensive term that encompasses all categories of dietary reference guidelines.

Fluorides

Learning Objectives

Upon successful completion of these exercises, you will be able to:

1. Identify and define key terms and concepts related to the use of fluorides.
2. Explain fluoride metabolism, mechanism of action, and effect/benefits of fluoride on pre-eruptive and posteruptive teeth.
3. Describe historical aspects, water supply components, and effects/benefits of water fluoridation.
4. Describe topical fluoride compounds and application methods.
5. Discuss fluoride safety.
6. Plan individualized fluoride prevention interventions.

 KNOWLEDGE EXERCISES

Write your answers for each question in the space provided.

1. Fluoride is made available to the tooth surface in two ways. Which method has the primary beneficial effect throughout life?

_____

2. **True or False** Fluoride can slowly be removed from the teeth over time due to resorption or remodeling.

_____

3. Describe how dietary fluoride is absorbed by and distributed to body tissues.

_____

_____

4. Dietary fluoride is excreted mostly through the _____.

5. Approximately 99% of fluoride in the body is located in _____ tissues, such as _____ and _____.

6. During the formation of enamel, fluoride is deposited starting at the _____ _____.

7. Fluoride concentration in the dentin is greatest near the _____. (*Hint:* See Figure 35–1 in the textbook.)

8. Too much fluoride ingested during tooth development can result in _____.

9. Fluoride, from drinking water or from topical fluoride treatments, continues to be deposited on the surface of the tooth after the tooth has _____.

10. When is topical fluoride uptake on the tooth surface most rapid? _____

11. Topical fluoride concentration in the enamel is highest at the _____ of the enamel.

12. Fluoride level in cementum is high and increases with _____.

13. In your own words, describe demineralization.

_____

_____

14. Where does demineralization occur?

_____

_____

_____

15. In early stages of demineralization, which area of the enamel has the greatest fluoride concentration?

_____

_____

16. In your own words, describe remineralization.

_____

_____

17. What is the role of fluoride in the demineralization–remineralization process?

_____

_____

18. What is the effect of fluoride on bacteria?

_____

_____

19. What is dental fluorosis?

_____

_____

_____

20. Who pinpointed fluorine as the element related to the observed changes in tooth enamel and risk for dental caries?

_____

21. Who was Dr. H. Trendley Dean?

_____

_____

22. What is the optimal level of fluoride concentration in community drinking water currently advised by the US Department of Health and Human services for caries prevention?

_____

_____

23. Adding fluoride to the school water supply in communities that do not have access to a fluoridated community water system is one way to benefit children in rural areas. Why is the concentration of fluoride increased from the optimum levels when fluoride is added to only the school water supply?

_____

_____

_____

24. When fluoride is removed from the water in a community, one of two possible effects is noted. What are the two possible effects?

_____

_____

_____

25. What compounds are used to fluoridate water supplies?

_____

_____

26. List factors to investigate when you are trying to determine whether a child needs dietary fluoride supplements.

_____

_____

_____

27. What level of fluoride is typically found in ready-to-feed and reconstituted infant formulas?

_____

_____

28. In what forms can supplementary fluoride be given?

_____

_____

29. If the fluoride water concentration in the community is 0.45 ppm and there is no additional fluoride in the water supply at school, what is the dose of supplemental fluoride that is recommended for a 5-year-old child and her 12-year-old brother?

_____

_____

30. The ideal fluoride regimen for most patients is high frequency, low concentration. That is why fluoridated water is so effective in preventing dental decay for most people. What factors indicate the need for you to include a professionally applied fluoride treatment in your patient's care plan?

_____

_____

_____

_____

_____

_____

_____

_____

31. What are the objectives for a professionally applied topical fluoride?

_____

_____

_____

32. What is the concentration of fluoride ions in a 1.23% acidulated phosphate gel, which you apply to your patient's teeth using a tray?

_____

33. Which professional fluoride preparation contains the highest concentration of fluoride ions?

_____

34. What professionally applied solution is recommended for infants and small children who are at high risk for dental caries?

_____

35. Which type of fluoride application is considered effective to reduce dentinal hypersensitivity?

_____

36. If your patient presents with a four-unit porcelain anterior bridge, which fluoride preparation is *not* appropriate for you to recommend and why?

_____

_____

37. How are the patient's teeth prepared before painting on a fluoride solution, applying a fluoride varnish, or placing the trays during a professional fluoride application?

_____

_____

38. Briefly list the steps for applying a fluoride varnish.

_____

_____

_____

_____

39. Briefly describe the techniques for using self-applied fluorides.

_____

_____

_____

40. Match each of the following descriptions with the appropriate self-applied fluoride *mouthrinse* preparation. Each type of mouthrinse is described more than once in the description column.

DESCRIPTION	MOUTHRINSE TYPE
_____ Once per week use	A. Low potency/high frequency
_____ Recommended for daily use	B. High potency/low frequency
_____ Available only as a sodium fluoride preparation	
_____ Available as a sodium fluoride, acidulated phosphate fluoride, or a stannous fluoride preparation	
_____ Can be purchased as an over-the-counter preparation	
_____ Is available in a 0.5% solution	
_____ Is available in a high-potency solution that is commonly diluted with water before use	
_____ Is sometimes used in school-based fluoride rinse programs	
_____ Has been shown to reduce the incidence of dental caries by 30–40% with reports of a 42.5% reduction in caries in primary teeth	

41. Complete Infomap 35-1 to help you compare type of fluoride ion and concentrations available in each type of preparation available for recommendation to patients who are at risk for dental caries.

INFOMAP 35-1

PREPARATION TYPE	TYPE OF FLUORIDE ION	RANGE OF FLUORIDE ION CONCENTRATION AVAILABLE
Professional Topical Fluoride Foam or Gel Preparations		
Self-Applied Fluoride Gel Preparations		
Self-Applied Fluoride Rinse Preparations		
Fluoride Dentifrice Preparations		
Fluoride Varnish Preparations		
Optimally Fluoridated Water		

42. In your own words, briefly list important safety measures to discuss with your patient when educating him or her about the use of home fluorides.

_____

_____

_____

_____

43. Briefly describe the signs and symptoms of a toxic dose of fluoride.

_____

_____

_____

44. If your patient feels nauseated and has stomach pain after receiving a professional fluoride treatment in your clinic, what is the first thing you should do?

_____

45. What tooth-related, observable symptom is linked to a larger-than-safe dose of systemic fluoride ingested over a long period?

    _____

46. Supply the acronym or chemical formula that can be used to document each type of fluoride preparation in a patient progress note—just one more time to help you remember!

    ■ Acidulated phosphate fluoride

    _____

    ■ Sodium fluoride

    _____

    ■ Stannous fluoride

    _____

✓ COMPETENCY EXERCISES

Apply information from the chapter and use critical thinking skills to complete the competency exercises. Write responses on paper or create electronic documents to submit your answers.

1. Refer to the Patient Assessment Summary for Melody Crane (aged 15 months). Use the information in the summary to develop dental hygiene diagnosis statements and a plan for interventions related to her risk for Early Childhood Caries (ECC).

CHAPTER 35—PATIENT ASSESSMENT SUMMARY

Patient Name: Melody Crane   Age: 15 months   Gender: M [F]   [√] Initial Therapy

    [ ] Maintenance

Provider Name: D.H. Student   Date: Today   [ ] Re-evaluation

Chief Complaint:

Toothache and swollen area in lower left jaw. Ulcerated lesion on upper left lip.

ASSESSMENT FINDINGS

Health History

■ Frequent ear infections—three since birth
■ Frequent use of liquid antibiotics—contain sweeteners
■ ASA classification—II
■ ADL level—3

At Risk For:

■ Early childhood caries

Social and Dental History

■ Initial dental visit—first teeth present at 6 months
■ Family drinks mostly bottled or filtered water.
■ Fluoride toothpaste used 4× per week—unspecified amount of paste
■ Bottle used two times daily at naptime and bedtime, at-will use of "sippy-cup" for juice
■ Five-year-old brother with restorations on all primary molars and some anterior teeth

At Risk For:

■ Early childhood caries

Dental Examination

■ Moderate dental biofilm along cervical margins of maxillary incisors
■ White-spot lesions at cervical of four maxillary incisors
■ Red maxillary anterior gingiva

At Risk For:

Periodontal Diagnosis/Case Type and Status

Gingivitis

Caries Management Risk Assessment (CAMBRA) Level:

[ ] Low   [ ] Moderate   [ ] High   [√] Extreme

DENTAL HYGIENE DIAGNOSIS	
Problem	Related to (Risk Factors and Etiology)

PLANNED INTERVENTIONS
(To arrest or control disease and regenerate, restore or maintain health)

Clinical	Education/Counseling	Oral Hygiene Instruction/Home Care

2. A dental hygienist experienced an unfortunate incident a few days ago when she was preparing a fluoride treatment for a 6-year-old patient in her clinic. She filled a set of trays with the the same amount of neutral sodium fluoride gel that would usually be used for an adult patient. (*Hint:* Consult Figure 35-5 in the textbook.) She left the trays sitting on the counter while she exited the room briefly to get permission for the fluoride treatment from the child's mother. She returned moments later to find that the child had picked up the trays and licked every bit of the fluoride foam out of both the upper and the lower tray. *Calculate the dose of fluoride that the child received in this incident.*

3. Is the child described in question 1 in danger of an acute reaction?

4. A 10-year-old mentally challenged child who weighs 50 lb accidentally ingested 200 mL of fluoridated toothpaste that contained 0.8% Na_2PO_3F. Is this child in danger of an acute toxic reaction?

5. Give an example of a situation that could lead to chronic fluoride toxicity and discuss what you would include in an education presentation for your patient (or patient's parent) to prevent this from happening.

Everyday Ethics

Before completing the learning exercises below, reread and reflect on the Everyday Ethics scenario and Questions for Consideration in this chapter of the textbook. It may also be useful to review the Dental Hygiene Ethics discussion in Chapter 1, the Ethical Applications in the introduction pages for each section in the textbook, as well as the Codes of Ethics in Appendices I, II, and III.

Individual Learning Activity
Imagine the scenario from the patient's perspective. How might the patient's response to the questions following the scenario be different from those of the dental hygienist involved?

Collaborative Learning Activity
Work with another student colleague to role-play the scenario. The goal of this exercise is for you and your colleague to work though the alternative actions to come to consensus on a solution or response that is acceptable to both of you.

Factors To Teach The Patient

This scenario is related to the following factors listed in this chapter of the textbook:

- Personal use of fluorides
- Need for parental supervision
- Determining need for fluoride supplements
- Fluorides being a part of the total preventive program
- Fluoridation
- Bottled drinking water

In Competency Exercise question 1, you developed a plan for a patient specific fluoride intervention for Melody Crane. Use the plan you developed and the example conversations in Appendix D as a guide to prepare a conversation that you might use to educate Melody's mother about the fluoride intervention you have planned and about her role in preventing further caries activity for her children.

WORD SEARCH

```
R  E  M  I  N  E  R  A  L  I  Z  A  T  I  O  N  H
X  R  D  C  A  R  I  O  S  T  A  T  I  C  Z  N  Y
F  L  U  O  R  A  P  A  T  I  T  E  M  U  O  A  P
D  G  H  Y  D  R  O  X  Y  A  P  A  T  I  T  E  O
B  E  W  H  I  T  E  S  P  O  T  E  S  P  J  R  C
C  D  F  Y  V  A  R  N  I  S  H  E  X  J  Z  X  A
I  I  F  L  U  O  R  I  D  E  L  F  Z  B  D  Q  L
C  X  O  R  U  H  A  L  O  E  F  F  E  C  T  G  C
I  D  P  T  P  O  R  A  C  M  C  K  A  Y  G  E  I
D  E  M  I  N  E  R  A  L  I  Z  A  T  I  O  N  F
K  L  J  L  I  A  F  I  E  F  F  I  C  A  C  Y  I
I  D  R  J  F  R  O  L  D  O  T  C  Y  R  G  T  E
D  G  H  A  U  J  T  R  M  A  A  A  E  M  J  N  D
N  N  C  S  G  K  C  T  T  C  T  T  P  B  E  T  R
E  T  B  C  F  L  U  O  R  O  S  I  S  F  M  F  W
Y  U  N  T  O  X  C  I  C  I  T  Y  O  P  J  M  L
S  T  H  I  X  O  T  R  O  P  I  C  P  N  I  X  W
```

WORD SEARCH CLUES

1. Refers to a fluoride preparation with a pH of 3.5 that may etch porcelain (acronym).
2. The researcher who associated Colorado brown stain with drinking water.
3. The result, in an unfluoridated community, of consuming fluoride that has been incorporated into food or beverages during processing (two words).
4. Over the counter (acronym).
5. A small area on the tooth that may be the first clinically detectable caries lesion or an area of demineralization (two words).
6. An area of demineralization below the enamel surface that can become remineralized with fluoride application (two words).
7. $Ca_{10}(PO_4)_6OH_2$.
8. Inhibiting dental caries.
9. The removal of fluoride from a water supply that has a naturally occurring higher-than-optimum fluoride level.
10. Breakdown of the tooth structure with a loss of calcium and phosphorus.
11. Term referring to the ability of clinically tested products to produce a significant health benefit.
12. A less-soluble apatite that is more resistant to acids.
13. A systemic nutrient that enhances tooth remineralization.
14. Small white spots to severe brown staining and pitting of the enamel caused by pre-eruptive ingestion of excessive amounts of fluoride.
15. Most fluoride is excreted from the body through this organ.
16. Refers to enamel with deficient calcification.
17. Parts per million (abbreviation).
18. Fluoride enhances this process, which returns minerals to the tooth.
19. A type of gel that becomes fluid under stress to permit flow.
20. This can occur as a result of a rapid intake of high concentration fluoride over a short period of time.
21. A form of professional topical fluoride application that is easily applied to root surfaces and sets up in the presence of saliva.

Sealants

Upon successful completion of these exercises, you will be able to:

1. Identify and define key terms and concepts related to dental sealants.
2. Identify sealant materials and classifications.
3. Describe how dental sealants work to penetrate and fill tooth pits and fissures.
4. Discuss indications for use, clinical procedures for application, and maintenance of dental sealants.

KNOWLEDGE EXERCISES

Write your answers for each question in the space provided.

1. In your own words, describe the purpose and action of a dental sealant.

_____

_____

_____

2. List the criteria for an ideal dental sealant.

_____

_____

_____

_____

_____

3. The many types of dental sealants have, to some extent, combined or overlapping characteristics. For example, autopolymerized dental sealants can be either clear or opaque in color. Identify all of the classifications and types of dental sealants.

_____

_____

_____

4. Study Table 36-1 in the textbook and review the section "Clinical Procedures" in Chapter 36 of the textbook to learn the basic procedures for application of dental sealants. List some general rules to follow during sealant application.

_____

_____

_____

_____

5. What is the purpose of debriding and cleaning the tooth surface before etching for sealant placement?

_____

_____

6. What materials can be used to isolate the area receiving a dental sealant?

_____

_____

7. After the tooth surface is etched, rinsed, and redried, what should you observe?

_____

8. What will prevent the dental sealant from penetrating to the bottom of the occlusal fissure?

_____

_____

9. Identify the factors that affect sealant retention.

_____

_____

COMPETENCY EXERCISES

Apply information from the chapter and use critical thinking skills to complete the competency exercises. Write responses on paper or create electronic documents to submit your answers.

1. You are collecting assessment data during an initial dental hygiene appointment for Dimitri Albergo, who is 12 years old. Dr. Donovan expects you to evaluate the need for dental sealants, record your findings on an assessment form, and then discuss your specific recommendations when he comes in to examine the patient. Together, you will make decisions for including sealants in Dimitri's dental hygiene care plan. What oral findings indicate a potential need for the placement of dental sealants?

2. Discuss why Dimitri's second molars are the most important teeth to evaluate for sealant placement.

3. During your oral examination of Dimitri, you find a pit-and-fissure area on tooth 30 that is questionable for the placement of a dental sealant. What next step will you take to determine whether that specific tooth surface is appropriate for sealant placement?

4. When you evaluate Dimitri's bitewing radiographs, no occlusal or proximal surface dental caries are present on tooth 14. What is the next step in deciding whether or not to select that tooth for placement of a dental sealant?

Everyday Ethics

Before completing the learning exercises below, reread and reflect on the Everyday Ethics scenario and Questions for Consideration in this chapter of the textbook. It may also be useful to review the Dental Hygiene Ethics discussion in Chapter 1, the Ethical Applications in the introduction pages for each section in the textbook, as well as the Codes of Ethics in Appendices I, II, and III.

Individual Learning Activity
Imagine that you are the dental hygienist in this scenario. Answer each of the questions for consideration at the end of the scenario.

Collaborative Learning Activity
Answer each of the questions for consideration at the end of the scenario in the textbook. Compare what you wrote with answers developed by another classmate and discuss differences/similarities.

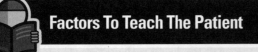

Factors To Teach The Patient

This scenario is related to the following factors listed in this chapter of the textbook:

- Sealants as part of a preventive program but not as a substitute for other preventive measures (e.g., limiting dietary sucrose, using fluorides, and controlling dental biofilm)
- What a sealant is and why such a meticulous application procedure is required
- What can be expected from a sealant, including how long it lasts and how it prevents dental caries
- Need for examination of the sealant at frequent, scheduled appointments and need for replacement when indicated

The dental hygiene care plan you develop for Dimitri (introduced in Competency Exercise question 1) recommends dental sealants for all four of his second permanent molars, plus teeth 14 and 3. Dimitri's mother has heard of dental sealants but does not understand why she should spend so much money to "fix" a tooth that has nothing wrong with it. To obtain consent from Dimitri's mother to apply the dental sealants, you must educate her.

Use the examples of patient conversations in Appendix D as a guide to develop a conversation to explain dental sealants to Mrs. Albergo.

CROSSWORD PUZZLE

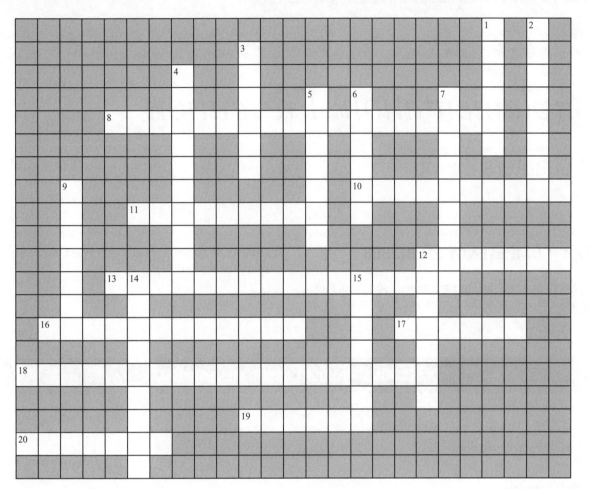

ACROSS

8. The self-curing, hardening process of pit-and-fissure sealants.
10. Tiny openings created during the acid etch step of sealant placement.
11. Refers to procedures that maintain a dry field during placement of dental sealants to keep saliva from contaminating the area to be etched.
12. Refers to the process of creating irregularities or micropores in the enamel.
13. The ability of things to exist together without harm.
16. A type of inked paper ribbon used to determine high spots by marking contacts between maxillary and mandibular teeth.
17. The appearance of the surface of a tooth after it is adequately etched and thoroughly dried during sealant application.
18. Polymerization with the use of an external light.
19. Within the living body (two words).
20. The physical adherence of a dental sealant to the microspaces between the enamel rods of the tooth structure.

DOWN

1. The process by which the plastic dental sealant becomes rigid.
2. Ingredient released by some dental sealants that enhances caries resistance.
3. The type of sealant that contains glass, quartz, silica, and other composite materials make the sealant more resistant to abrasion.
4. The type of acid used in a 15–50% solution to etch the tooth before placement of a dental sealant.
5. An organic polymer that flows into the pit or fissure of a tooth and bonds to the enamel surface by mechanical retention.
6. Bisphenol A-glycidyl methacrylate (abbreviation, without the hyphen).
7. Resistance to flow as a result of molecular cohesion.
9. A compound of high molecular weight formed by a combination of a chain of simpler molecules.
12. Refers to the phosphoric acid solution used to prepare the enamel surface of the tooth prior to placement of dental sealants.
14. Caries limited to the enamel.
15. Under laboratory conditions (two words).

Implementation: Prevention

■ Chapters 25–36

 COMPETENCY EXERCISES

Apply information from the chapter and use critical thinking skills to complete the Competency exercises. Write

responses on paper or create electronic documents to submit your answers.

SECTION V—PATIENT ASSESSMENT SUMMARY

Patient Name: Harold Wilmot	Age: 44	Gender: ☒ M ☐ F	☑ Initial Therapy
			☐ Maintenance
Provider Name: D.H. Student	Date: Today		☐ Re-evaluation

Chief Complaint:
Recently moved into this community—"I need my teeth cleaned."

ASSESSMENT FINDINGS

Health History

- Asthma; uses steroid inhaler
- Hypertension (148/82); controlled with beta-blocker medication
- Tobacco use: ½ to 1 pack per day for about 25 years
- ASA Classification—II
- ADL level—0

At Risk For:

Social and Dental History

- Has had regular dental visits (1 per year); last visit 1 year ago
- Has received tobacco cessation education and regular oral hygiene instructions at previous dental visits.
- Has tried twice to quit smoking, but relapsed because of withdrawal symptoms.

At Risk For:

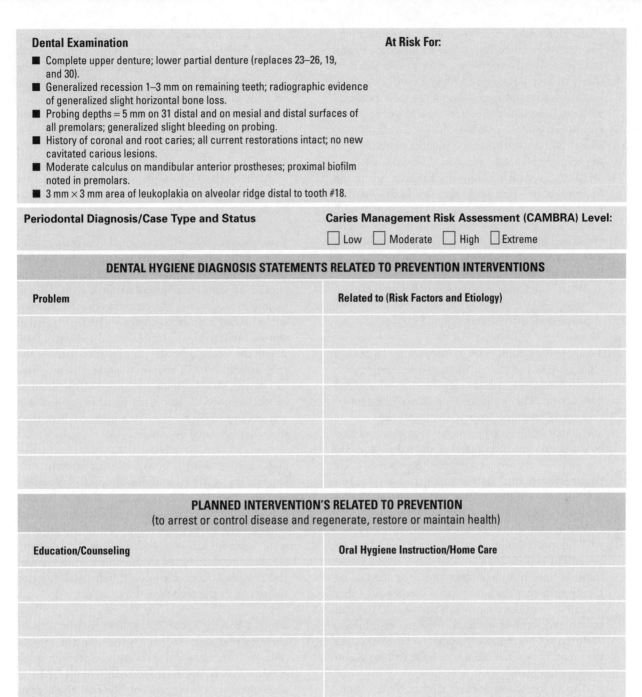

Dental Examination

- Complete upper denture; lower partial denture (replaces 23–26, 19, and 30).
- Generalized recession 1–3 mm on remaining teeth; radiographic evidence of generalized slight horizontal bone loss.
- Probing depths = 5 mm on 31 distal and on mesial and distal surfaces of all premolars; generalized slight bleeding on probing.
- History of coronal and root caries; all current restorations intact; no new cavitated carious lesions.
- Moderate calculus on mandibular anterior prostheses; proximal biofilm noted in premolars.
- 3 mm × 3 mm area of leukoplakia on alveolar ridge distal to tooth #18.

At Risk For:

Periodontal Diagnosis/Case Type and Status

Caries Management Risk Assessment (CAMBRA) Level:

☐ Low   ☐ Moderate   ☐ High   ☐ Extreme

DENTAL HYGIENE DIAGNOSIS STATEMENTS RELATED TO PREVENTION INTERVENTIONS

Problem	Related to (Risk Factors and Etiology)

PLANNED INTERVENTION'S RELATED TO PREVENTION
(to arrest or control disease and regenerate, restore or maintain health)

Education/Counseling	Oral Hygiene Instruction/Home Care

Review the Section V Patient Assessment Summary for Mr. Harold Wilmot to help you answer questions 1 through 3. The template included with his assessment summary will provide spaces for you to record your answers for these questions.

1. Complete the blank "At Risk For", Periodontal Diagnosis, and CAMBRA sections of the assessment form as best you can with the information in the patient assessment.

2. Write at least three dental hygiene diagnosis statements for Mr. Wilmot's dental hygiene care plan.

3. List the PREVENTION interventions you will plan to help Mr. Wilmot *arrest or control disease* and *regenerate, restore, or maintain* oral health.

4. Maria Hernandez is a 19-year-old single mother who has just received health insurance, including dental insurance. This is only her second visit ever to a dentist. The first was when she had a tooth extracted, because of dental caries, at age 14. She presents with swollen gingiva, multiple areas of severe dental caries, and extensive biofilm along the gingival margins of all her teeth. She is 5 months pregnant with her second child and has no other health issues.

Maria is nearly fluent in English, although Spanish is her first language; she lives with her mother and younger siblings. Maria's first child, who is 4 years old, has been receiving care in the clinic and has, within the last 6 months, had extensive dental work, including crowns and extractions because of dental caries.

What aspects of prevention will you focus on during a series of perhaps four dental hygiene appointments with Maria?

5. Today you examine Victor Azure, an 11-year-old child who lives on the nearby Navajo reservation with his mother, father, and two older brothers who attend high school. The results of Victor's dental examination reveal multiple restorations in primary molars and dental sealants on first molars that were provided by the dental practice located on the reservation. He has no currently active caries, but you observe a few demineralized areas on the maxillary incisors. You also observe swollen gingiva and extensive biofilm along the gingival margins of all of Victor's teeth.

Victor states that he brushes nearly every day with fluoridated toothpaste but really hates to do it because it is boring. Victor sometimes uses a home fluoride rinse but more often uses a strong-tasting mouthwash that his father likes. Victor states that his father uses the mouthwash because he has bad breath and some of his teeth wiggle. Victor knows that some of his remaining primary teeth are getting loose and hopes that the mouthwash will keep him from losing them.

The interview with Victor's mother, Skye, regarding his dental history indicates that Victor was exposed to fluoridated water for only the first 3 years of his life, before the family came back home from Chicago to live on the reservation, which does not have fluoridated water. Victor did not ever visit a dentist until last year, when all the restorative work was done, and his mother states that she plans to try to maintain the regular schedule of visits to the dentist that was recommended when Victor was there 6 months ago.

Skye states that the dentist told her that Victor's high rate of decay is linked to his diet, which is high in frequent carbohydrate intake, including large amounts of carbonated beverages, which he drinks all day long. But she also states that she isn't worried about the high rate of decay in the primary teeth because those are going to fall out soon anyway. She states proudly that she allowed the placement of the sealants to protect his adult teeth from decay.

When you go over Victor's medical history with his mother, you find that except for the fact that he is extremely overweight, there are no current health problems. There is, however, a family history of diabetes.

Identify the factors in this case scenario that you will address in your plan for preventive dental hygiene care for Victor.

6. Your patient, Mrs. Edmons, makes a frantic telephone call to the clinic this morning. Her normal, healthy, and very curious 2-year-old son, Nick, has sucked out and eaten most of a tube of fruit-flavored children's toothpaste. She estimates that he has consumed about 3 oz. of toothpaste. The first question you ask her is to identify the kind and amount of fluoride in the toothpaste. She states that the back of the tube indicates 0.15% sodium fluoride. Discover how to convert Mrs. Edmons's estimate of the amount of toothpaste Nick has eaten into the approximate amount in milliliters. Has Nick ingested more than the safely tolerated dose of fluoride?

7. Get together with a group of your student colleagues and gather examples/samples of a variety of adjunctive dental hygiene aids, such as flossing aids or holders, oral irrigators, and different types of interdental cleaners. Each one of you will then be responsible for learning how to use one oral hygiene aid, demonstrating it to all the others in the group, and providing feedback to each individual as he or she practices the technique for using the aid.

8. Explore patient records available in your school clinic to find cases for which the assessment data indicate the need for preventive interventions. A patient that you have personally collected the assessment data for is probably the best choice, but any patient record will do for this exercise. Use the assessment data to develop a patient-specific dental hygiene care plan for that patient that addresses all the relevant aspects of oral-disease prevention and oral-health promotion discussed in this section of the textbook.

DISCOVERY EXERCISES

1. Identify teaching materials currently available in your school clinic to use for patient education. Investigate sources for new or additional materials, and request samples. When you receive them, analyze them for

accuracy, readability, and appeal. Decide which ones are most appropriate and valuable for providing information for the patients you will see in your school clinic.

2. Create a product-comparison Infomap. This discovery exercise will help you compare chemotherapeutic agents used in dentistry and is best done by working together in small groups of three to six students.

   Step 1: Gather a variety of mouth rinses, dentifrices, or other dental products that contain chemotherapeutic ingredients recommended by dental hygienists for prevention of dental disease. Have each group member be responsible for finding particular products. You can gather over-the-counter products as well as those that are commonly dispensed only by prescription. You will need to make sure that you have the available packaging information for each product.

   Step 2: Assemble small plastic cups, long cotton swabs, and some paper towels so that you can do a taste test.

   Step 3: Develop an Infomap that will help you compare these products. There are examples of Infomaps throughout this workbook to give you ideas as you develop this one. Your Infomap should allow you to compare similar products in such areas as active chemotherapeutic ingredients, alcohol content, ADA Seal of Approval, cost, taste, efficacy of the product based on current research findings, and any other topic areas you think are important for your comparison.

   The Infomap you create can be used to help you compare products when you are making recommendations to your patients. After your student group develops the basic framework for the Infomap, you can continue to add products as you become aware of them to keep a currently updated review of products for recommending to your patients.

3. Use the information in the textbook to create an Infomap that compares various kinds of manual toothbrushes that you can recommend for your patients. How about an Infomap comparing the various brands and types of dental floss? What other prevention products could you compare in an Infomap format?

4. Being able to apply evidence-based prevention protocols as we make recommendations for patients requires practice in accessing, analyzing, and applying information from the dental and oral health literature. Select a prevention topic, and perform a review of the literature to obtain a list of current scientific research articles related to that topic. Obtain the full-text articles either online or at the library.

Write a short review of the literature to summarize what you learned from reading the articles. Be sure to include recommendations for patient care that are based on your analysis of the literature.

5. Work with your student colleagues to create an annotated list of Web sites that provide information on topics related to the prevention of oral disease. Each student should select a topic, and then perform an Internet search using the search engine of his or her choice. Make sure the Web sites you select provide valid, scientific, and reliable information.

   Write a brief summary of the information you learned from the Web site, and be sure to include the correct Internet address (URL) at the top of the page. Provide electronic copies of your brief description of the Web site to your instructor or to a student colleague who is willing to compile the information into one document that can be shared by all students.

6. Investigate prevention in the news. Collect articles from the current popular literature—such as newspapers, magazines, and television or radio announcements—that provide information on prevention of oral diseases. Also, look for dental product advertisements that appear in the popular press. This is the information that your patients see and will probably ask you about when you are providing patient education.

   ■ Is the information that you find presented in the popular media valid and scientifically accurate?
   ■ How can this information affect the way in which the dental profession is perceived?
   ■ Does the media information you find agree with the recommendations you make for dental preventive care?

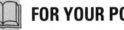 **FOR YOUR PORTFOLIO**

1. Include a copy of the original product comparison Infomap your student group created in the Discovery exercise above. As you update the Infomap with new product information, also include your most currently updated Infomap in your portfolio. Having both the original and the updated Infomaps will help you demonstrate your commitment to continued learning.

2. Provide written examples that describe dental hygiene education and counseling interventions you have provided for specific patients. Select examples that illustrate your ability to communicate, motivate, and educate particular patients so

that positive health outcomes result. Structure your examples so that each includes a discussion of the following:

- Significant assessment findings
- Prevention topics and methods presented
- Oral-health techniques demonstrated
- Method of patient practice used
- Methods for evaluating success of the patient's compliance, motivation levels, and learning styles (Discuss any factor/s that affected your ability to communicate with the patient and factors that affected compliance with your recommendations.)

3. Include copies of patient-specific care plans you have developed that illustrate your ability to plan individualized prevention for specific patient cases. Include some early attempts at developing care plans as well as some care plans that you have developed near the end of your student career. Provide a short written analysis of how the early examples compare with the later examples of care planning to demonstrate your growth toward competency in care planning for prevention.

4. Include the literature review you wrote in the Discovery exercise above. Later you can update your search to see if there is new information available that might change any recommendations you made in your first review.

5. Collect as many examples of prevention in the news as you can during the time you are a student and jot down notes analyzing each example. Later on, you can use your notes to write an analysis of all the examples you collected. Take time to identify trends in how preventive dentistry is presented in the popular media. How does the popular view of dentistry affect the way your patients perceive and are motivated by your prevention interventions and recommendations?

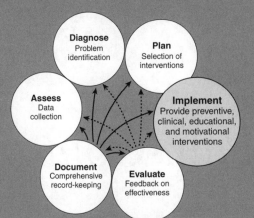

Implementation: Clinical Treatment

Chapters 37–45

■ LEARNING OBJECTIVES

Completing the exercises in this section of the workbook will prepare you to:

1. Manage patient anxiety and pain during dental hygiene treatment.
2. Provide a variety of dental hygiene treatment interventions.
3. Document all aspects of dental hygiene treatment.

■ COMPETENCIES FOR THE DENTAL HYGIENIST

Competencies supported by the learning in Section VI

Core Competencies: C3, C4, C5, C7, C9, C10, C11, C12, C13

Health Promotion and Disease Prevention: HP1, HP2, HP4, HP5, HP6

Patient/Client Care: PC4, PC10, PC11, PC13

Anxiety and Pain Control

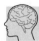 **KNOWLEDGE EXERCISES**

Write your answers for each question in the space provided.

1. In your own words, describe the interaction between the two components of pain.

   _____

   _____

   _____

2. Each individual person's reaction to pain is different. Individuals who react strongly or quickly to a painful stimulus are said to have a _____ pain threshold. Those who do not react strongly to the same painful stimulus are said to have a _____ pain threshold.

3. List the factors that can influence your patient's reaction to dental pain.

   _____

   _____

   _____

   _____

   _____

   _____

4. Which of the five pain-control mechanisms alter pain reaction?

   _____

   _____

   _____

5. Which of the pain-control mechanisms relies for success on your ability to communicate with and educate your patient?

   _____

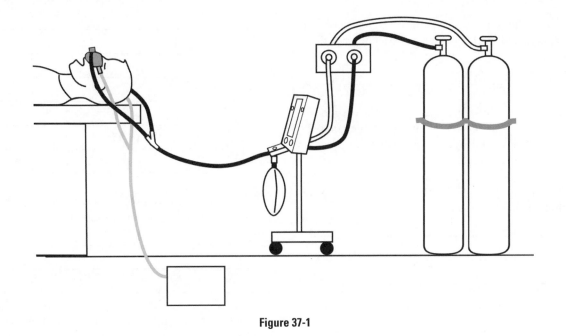

Figure 37-1

6. Figure 37-1 above shows a nitrous oxide delivery system. Label the following components on the figure. It might be useful to use colored pencil (use green for oxygen and blue for nitrous oxide, of course!). Note that some components may not be easy to identify or locate on the figure, but do your best; then investigate or ask your instructor to find out if your idea was correct.

- Oxygen tank (add a notation to identify the gas pressure)

- Nitrous oxide tank (add a notation to identify the gas pressure)

- Cylinder valves used to open and close each tank (*Hint:* There is one on each tank.)

- Hoses that carry only oxygen gas

- Hoses that carry only nitrous oxide gas

- Hoses that can carry both nitrous oxide gas and oxygen

- Regulator or reducing valve (location not discussed in the textbook)

- Flow meter (location not discussed in the textbook) (*Hint:* The clinician uses this to control the level of each gas administered to the patient.)

- On-demand valve (*Hint:* Probably located near the flow meter.)

- Reservoir bag

- Nasal hood, nose piece, or mask

- Scavenger system

- Areas where there are connectors (It is important to know where these are because you will regularly need to inspect and test them for potential leaks.)

7. Conscious sedation, produced by administration of a combination of nitrous oxide and oxygen, is frequently used to reduce patient anxiety and perception of pain during short dental procedures that are expected to cause a low level of pain. Identify the two properties of nitrous oxide that are useful for reducing pain.

_____

_____

8. Why is nitrous oxide sedation especially useful for control of soft tissue discomfort during dental hygiene procedures?

_____

_____

9. During dental hygiene procedures, a range of _____ % to _____ % nitrous oxide is administered in combination with oxygen to achieve optimum pain control for most patients, with the primary saturation of blood occurring in _____ min to _____ min.

10. What is the minimum amount of oxygen flow that is maintained by the gas delivery system for patient safety?

    _____

11. You will administer _____ % oxygen to your patient for several minutes after the completion of the dental hygiene procedure to prevent _____ _____.

12. List contraindications for the use of nitrous oxide during dental hygiene care.

    _____

    _____

    _____

    _____

    _____

    _____

13. Attention to the details of providing an effective scavenging system, rigorous equipment maintenance, and the initiation of other methods for preventing overexposure are imperative when nitrous oxide is used during patient care. What are the potential health hazards for clinicians who are exposed to excessive levels of nitrous oxide?

    _____

    _____

    _____

    _____

14. Without looking in the textbook, list the steps you will use to administer nitrous oxide–oxygen analgesic during patient care. For each step, when appropriate, indicate the time frame and the amount of oxygen or nitrous flow.

    _____

    _____

    _____

    _____

    _____

    _____

    _____

    _____

    _____

    _____

    _____

    _____

    _____

15. In your own words, explain how the nitrous oxide gas is titrated during administration.

    _____

    _____

    _____

16. Identify at least three advantages and three disadvantages of using conscious sedation anesthesia (such as nitrous oxide) to reduce patient pain and anxiety during dental hygiene treatment.

    ■ Advantages

    _____

    _____

    _____

    _____

    _____

    _____

    ■ Disadvantages

    _____

    _____

    _____

    _____

    _____

    _____

17. List three important components to include in your patient's progress notes after you administer nitrous oxide during dental hygiene treatment.

    _____

    _____

    _____

18. Which of the five basic pain-control mechanisms alter pain perception?

_____

_____

_____

19. A nonopioid analgesic is effective in altering pain perception by blocking what?

_____

_____

20. Pretreatment analgesics, if they are recommended, should be administered when?

_____

_____

21. List the indications for applying topical anesthetic to reduce your patient's perception of intraoral pain.

_____

_____

_____

_____

_____

22. Identify the active ingredients that are available as noninjectable or topical anesthetic preparations and the amount of time that each provides anesthesia to the tissues.

_____

_____

_____

_____

23. Match each description below with the correct amide type of local anesthesia. Each type of anesthesia is used more than once; some descriptions apply to more than one type of anesthesia.

TYPE OF AMIDE ANESTHETIC	DESCRIPTION
A. Articaine	_____ Long-acting amide drug
B. Bupivacaine	_____ Short- or medium-acting amide drug
C. Etidocaine	_____ Citanest plain and Citanest forte
D. Lidocaine	_____ Carbocaine, Polocaine, Isocaine
E. Mepivacaine	_____ Duranest
F. Prilocaine	_____ Marcaine
	_____ Septocaine, Septanest, and Ultracaine
	_____ Xylocaine, Octocaine, Lignospan
	_____ Available in 1.8 m/L of solution in cartridge
	_____ Most widely used amide; also available as a topical
	_____ Causes less vasodilation, so can be used without a vasoconstrictor
	_____ Diffuses best through soft and hard tissues
	_____ Provides extended period of analgesia to manage postcare pain
	_____ Metabolic by-products can temporarily reduce the oxygen-carrying capacity of blood
	_____ Potential drug interaction if patient is taking the drug cimetidine

24. Match each description below with the correct dental cartridge ingredient.

DENTAL CARTRIDGE INGREDIENT	DESCRIPTION
A. Amide anesthetic	_____ Creates isotonic match with the body
B. Antioxidant	_____ Blocks the transfer of ions across the nerve membrane
C. Sodium chloride	_____ Constricts blood vessels
D. Sterile water	_____ Preservative for the vasoconstrictor
E. Vasoconstrictor	_____ Diluent

25. Match each description below with the correct group of local anesthesia drugs. Each group is used more than once.

LOCAL ANESTHESIA DRUG GROUP	DESCRIPTION
A. Amide B. Ester	_____ Currently used only in topical anesthetics _____ Metabolized in blood plasma _____ Low incidence of allergic reactions _____ Less effective and shorter acting _____ Higher incidence of allergic reactions _____ Less effective and shorter acting _____ Metabolized by the liver _____ Causes vasodilation

26. Which ingredient in noninjectable topical anesthetic is most likely to cause an allergic reaction in your patient?

_____

27. Which ingredient in noninjectable topical anesthetic is the most likely to cause a toxic reaction in your patient?

_____

28. In your own words, describe the techniques and armamentarium used for administering noninjectable anesthesia.

_____

_____

_____

29. What techniques can be used to apply topical anesthesia to oral tissues?

_____

_____

30. Identify two vasoconstrictors that are commonly used in dental anesthetic and indicate the standard concentration of each one.

_____

_____

31. A vasoconstrictor offsets the vasodilating action of the local anesthetic. List the reasons for including a vasoconstrictor in local anesthetic solution.

_____

_____

_____

_____

32. What preservative for the vasoconstrictor can cause a potential allergic reaction?

_____

_____

_____

33. What potential drug interactions can cause an adverse reaction when dental anesthetics with vasoconstrictors are used?

_____

_____

_____

_____

34. What drug can be injected to reverse the effects of local anesthetic, and what is the action that reverses the effects?

_____

_____

35. You will consider your patient's medical history, the type of dental hygiene procedures that are planned, the potential for patient discomfort, and patient preference when you determine whether to include local anesthesia in your patient's plan for care. What are the sources of information that you will use to assess your patient before providing local anesthetic?

_____

_____

_____

_____

_____

36. What patient risk factors will you consider when selecting which local anesthetic solution to use during dental hygiene treatment?

_____

_____

_____

_____

37. What medical conditions indicate the need for patient-specific evaluation and very careful consideration when determining local anesthesia use during dental hygiene treatment?

_____

_____

_____

_____

_____

_____

_____

38. List the armamentarium you will assemble before providing local anesthesia.

_____

_____

_____

_____

_____

_____

_____

_____

_____

39. Why do you position the patient with the head lower than the heart during a local anesthesia injection?

_____

40. What is prevented from happening when you aspirate before injecting local anesthesia solution?

_____

_____

41. In your own words, describe the procedure for aspiration using a conventional anesthetic syringe.

_____

_____

_____

_____

42. The steps for syringe assembly are listed on the next page. Some of the structures are printed in boldface; label each one on Figure 37-2.

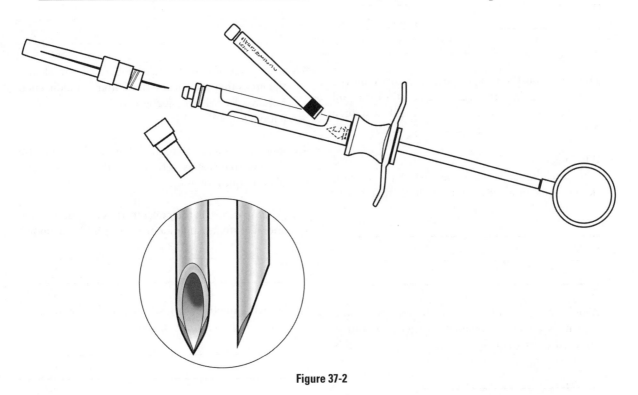

Figure 37-2

■ Step 1: Pull back on the **thumb ring.**

■ Step 2: Insert the **cartridge** that contains the selected type of anesthetic. Identify the **rubber stopper** and the **diaphragm end** of the cartridge. Identify the **volume** of solution in the cartridge. Identify the **window** openings in the syringe that will allow you to view the cartridge during aspiration.

■ Step 3: Set the **harpoon** into the appropriate end of the cartridge and test for lock.

■ Step 4: Discard the **safety cap** from the **cartridge end** of the needle.

■ Step 5: With your fingers holding the **needle hub,** screw the needle securely onto the end of the syringe. Identify the **needle** that is used for injection. Indicate the available **lengths** and **diameters** of the needles that are used for injecting dental anesthetic.

■ In the detail, identify the **bevel** of the needle and draw a line to indicate where the **bone** will be relative to the bevel when the needle is inserted for injection.

43. Describe what you will do if you see blood in the anesthetic cartridge when you aspirate while providing local anesthetic for your patient.

_____

_____

_____

44. The local anesthetic solution is deposited slowly, _____ min to _____ min for a full cartridge, to prevent _____ and to reduce potential for a _____ _____.

45. What injections will ensure complete soft and hard tissue anesthesia for your patient when you are providing periodontal treatment for all of the teeth in the mandibular left quadrant.

_____

_____

_____

46. Which injection will be needed to anesthetize the lingual tissue so that complete patient comfort is achieved during dental hygiene procedures in this area of the mouth?

_____

_____

_____

_____

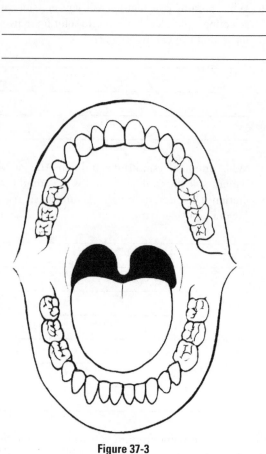

Figure 37-3

_____

_____

_____

47. Use a colored pencil to mark Figure 37-3 to identify the areas that are anesthetized after a middle superior alveolar (MSA) injection on the right side of the patient's mouth.

48. Use a colored pencil to mark Figure 37-3 to identify the area that is anesthetized after the injection identified in question 45.

49. What structure in the molar teeth is not anesthetized after a posterior superior alveolar (PSA) injection?

_____

_____

50. Which injections anesthetize only the terminal nerve endings for one individual tooth?

_____

_____

51. It is important that you are able to identify the type and the cause of any patient reaction quickly when you are providing local anesthesia. Match each description with the correct symptom. Some symptoms are used more than once; some descriptions apply to more than one type of symptom.

SYMPTOM	DESCRIPTION
A. Adequate anesthesia	_____ Anxiety reaction
B. Allergy	_____ Can be the result of too rapid absorption of a drug into bloodstream
C. Epithelial desquamation	_____ Can indicate that topical anesthetic was left in contact with the tissue for too long
D. Hematoma	_____ Can result from reduced ability to eliminate or metabolize the local anesthesia drug
E. Overdose	_____ Caused when a vein or artery is opened and leaks blood into the surrounding tissue
F. Paresthesia	_____ Experience of a profound effect for the duration of the procedure
G. Psychogenic reaction	_____ Extended duration of anesthesia effect
H. Trismus	_____ Hypersensitive state that can result in exaggerated response to a subsequent exposure to local anesthesia drug
	_____ Onset may range from a few seconds to many hours later
	_____ Patients will sometimes report this reaction as an allergy to local anesthesia
	_____ Response can range from mild to generalized life-threatening anaphylaxis
	_____ Spasm of jaw muscle that restricts opening after injection
	_____ Syncope and hyperventilation are the most common responses
	_____ Tissue sloughing
	_____ Toxic levels of local anesthesia drug are present in the bloodstream
	_____ Prevention of these complications relies on the use of excellent injection technique
	_____ This response can be made less likely if you use excellent patient communications skills and gentle administration techniques when you are injecting local anesthesia

COMPETENCY EXERCISES

Apply information from the chapter and use critical thinking skills to complete the competency exercises. Write responses on paper or create electronic documents to submit your answers.

1. Today you are presenting your dental hygiene care plan for four-quadrant, initial therapy scaling and root planing to Mr. Shizoka. You will ask the patient to sign an informed consent form before you begin your treatment. Mr. Shizoka does not have much previous dental experience. When you were collecting assessment data for the care plan, he appeared to be very nervous. He asked many questions about what you were doing and stopped you frequently when you were trying to probe because he was concerned about whether he would feel pain.

   Mr. Shizoka's medical history indicates that he has iron-deficiency anemia and takes a daily ferrous iron supplement. He has hypertension and takes an antihypertensive medication; but he tells you that whenever he is highly stressed, he gets a headache. Write a dental hygiene diagnosis statement related to Mr. Shizoka's anxiety about receiving dental hygiene treatment.

2. In the dental hygiene care plan you have developed, you plan to use nitrous oxide-oxygen for pain and anxiety control during Mr. Shizoka's four scaling and root planing appointments. You have already explained to Mr. Shizoka what nitrous oxide–oxygen sedation is and how it works. Explain the advantages and disadvantages so that he can be completely informed about the use of this pain and anxiety control measure.

3. Mr. Shizoka agrees to try the nitrous oxide–oxygen sedation for at least his first dental hygiene appointment to see if he is comfortable with it. Use your institution's guidelines for writing in patient records to document that you have fully informed Mr. Shizoka and that he has agreed to the use of nitrous oxide analgesia during his dental hygiene treatment.

4. At his next appointment, you carefully titrate the nitrous oxide–oxygen combination for Mr. Shizoka, and he shows all the signs of ideal sedation. When you begin the injection of local anesthesia into the area where you will be providing care, Mr. Shizoka becomes agitated and starts moving his arms and legs. His rate of respiration increases significantly, he starts to sweat, and his eyes tear up. You immediately stop injecting the local anesthesia. He says he feels sick to his stomach and wants to sit up. Discuss two possibilities for what is happening in this scenario?

5. What will you do next in the situation that is described in question 4?

6. Use your institution's guidelines for writing in patient records to document what happened today at Mr. Shizoka's dental hygiene appointment.

7. Explain, in patient-appropriate language, how the noninjectable local anesthesia patch is administered.

Everyday Ethics

Before completing the learning exercises below, reread and reflect on the Everyday Ethics scenario and Questions for Consideration in this chapter of the textbook. It may also be useful to review the Dental Hygiene Ethics discussion in Chapter 1, the Ethical Applications in the introduction pages for each section in the textbook, as well as the Codes of Ethics in Appendices I, II, and III.

Individual Learning Activity
Imagine that you are the dental hygienist in this scenario. Answer each of the questions for consideration at the end of the scenario.

Collaborative Learning Activity
Answer each of the questions for consideration at the end of the scenario in the textbook. Compare what you wrote with answers developed by another classmate and discuss differences/similarities.

Factors To Teach The Patient

This scenario is related to the following factors listed in this chapter of the textbook:

■ Be careful not to bite lip, cheek, or tongue while tissues are without normal sensations. Warn and watch children to prevent injury. Do not test anesthesia by biting the lip.
■ Avoid chewing hard foods and avoid hot food and drinks until normal sensation has returned.

Because a scheduled patient did not arrive and you have some time free, you are asked to spend the time speaking to Miriam's mother. Miriam Carroll is 9 years old. She has many dental problems but is always cooperative during treatment. At Miriam's appointment today, Dr. Steve will extract three primary molar root tips, and both the maxillary and mandibular arches on the left side of her mouth will be anesthetized for the extractions. This is the first time Miriam will experience the effects of local anesthesia.

Use the example of a patient conversation in Appendix D as a guide to prepare a conversation that you might use to provide postoperative follow-up information to Miriam's mother.

CHAPTER 38

Instruments and Principles for Instrumentation

Learning Objectives

Upon successful completion of these exercises, you will be able to:

1. Identify and define key terms and concepts related to dental instruments and instrumentation.
2. Identify the components of dental instruments.
3. Describe the purpose, characteristics, and principles for use of a variety of types of dental instruments.
4. Describe methods for developing dexterity and preventing cumulative trauma injuries during dental hygiene instrumentation.
5. Identify techniques for maintaining sharp dental instruments.

 KNOWLEDGE EXERCISES

Write your answers for each question in the space provided.

The following questions help you look at each type of instrument from several perspectives. If possible, have real instruments available to examine as you are doing these exercises so you can thoroughly understand the instruments' similarities and differences.

1. Locate and label each of the following parts on the instrument shown in Figure 38-1.

   ■ Blade

   ■ Shank

   ■ Lower shank

   ■ Handle

   ■ Serrated surface of the handle

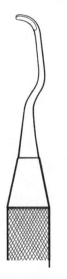

Figure 38-1

2. The instrument shown in Figure 38-1 has a relatively straight shank shape and is intended for use on _____ teeth.

3. Label the instruments shown in Figure 38-2.

   ■ Scaler

   ■ Curet

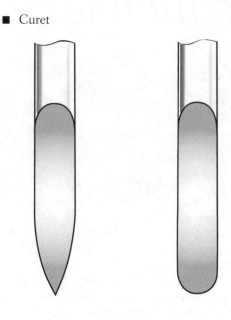

Figure 38-2

4. Label the following areas of both instruments shown in Figure 38-2.

   ■ *Pointed tip*

   ■ *Rounded toe (tip)*

   ■ *Cutting edges*

   ■ *Area of the cutting edge that is adapted to the tooth during scaling*

   ■ *Face of the blade*

   ■ *Terminal shank*

5. Match each description below to the letter that indicates the appropriate instrument shown in Figure 38-3 by writing the correct letter in the space provided.

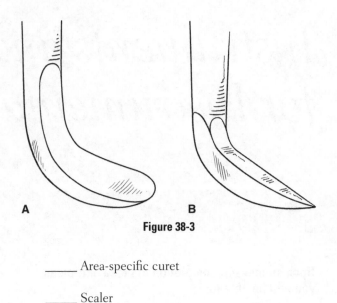

Figure 38-3

_____ Area-specific curet

_____ Scaler

6. Label the following areas on the working ends of each of the instruments shown in Figure 38-3.

   ■ Rounded toe (tip)

   ■ Pointed tip

   ■ Face of the blade

   ■ Cutting edges

   ■ Area of the cutting edge that is adapted to the tooth when scaling

   ■ Terminal shank

   ■ Lateral surface and back of the blade

7. Match each description below to the letter that indicates the appropriate instrument shown in Figure 38-4 by writing the correct letter in the space provided.

_____ Area-specific curet

_____ Universal curet

_____ Scaler

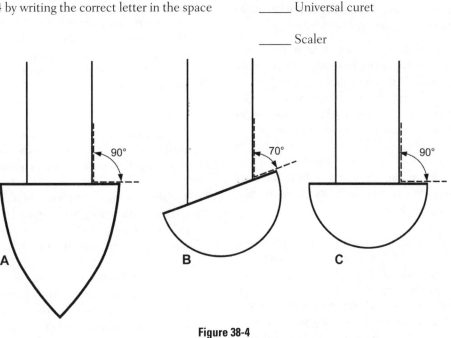

Figure 38-4

8. Label or mark the following areas on the working ends of each instrument shown in Figure 38-4.

   ■ Face of the blade

   ■ Cutting edges

   ■ Terminal shank

   ■ Lateral surface(s)

   ■ Back of the blade

9. Without looking at the figure in the textbook, draw a straight line on Figure 38-4 to indicate how the face of the sharpening stone would be placed (and angled) to sharpen *each* of the cutting edges of each instrument shown. After you draw your lines and label each angle, use a protractor to measure those angles. If your diagram is not correct, erase your lines and redraw them, using the protractor to help you place the angle of your sharpening stone correctly.

10. Imagine that you are using the moving-stone technique to sharpen the instruments shown in

Figure 38-4. Draw an arrow to indicate the direction of the stroke in which you would apply the most pressure as you move the stone. (*Hint:* This is also the direction you would finish each area as you are sharpening.)

11. When you are activating your instruments during dental hygiene treatment, the proper modified pen grasp is controlled and firm, but not tight and rigid. What are the effects of a grasp that is too tight and rigid?

_____

_____

_____

_____

12. What factors can influence your risk for cumulative trauma injury and pain from incorrect use of instruments during dental hygiene procedures?

_____

_____

_____

✓ COMPETENCY EXERCISES

Apply information from the chapter and use critical thinking skills to complete the competency exercises.

The only real way to become competent in the skills described in this chapter of the textbook is to practice. It is, of course, difficult to help you do that in a workbook format. However, here are some exercises you can do on your own to help you become competent in identifying instruments and practicing the principles of instrumentation. If you would like, work in small groups with two or three of your student colleagues. Using the information and descriptions in Chapter 38 in the textbook, group members can provide feedback about each person's instrument technique.

1. Gather a variety of instruments and lay them out on a table in front of you. Examine them carefully and thoroughly, identifying the instrument parts, the types, and the adaptation characteristics (such as the angle of the shank) of each instrument you have available. Then practice picking up the instrument in the modified pen grasp, placing a fulcrum on the tip of the thumb of your nondominant hand, and adapting the blade of the instrument on your fingernail in the correct position for activation.

2. Examine each instrument to determine its characteristics—such as balance, shank length, fabrication materials, and shape and rigidity of the shank. Discuss the purpose and uses of each instrument. Think about area of the mouth the instrument is appropriate for, the technique the instrument is intended for (e.g., heavy calculus or root planing), and any other indications/contraindications for use that pertain to the instrument's design.

3. Examine each instrument to determine whether the cutting edge is sharp. Practice the correct placement of a sharpening stone to sharpen each instrument.

4. To develop your dexterity, practice each of the strength, stretching, writing, and instrument exercises described in the "Dexterity Development" section of Chapter 38 in the textbook.

5. Sit comfortably in a chair that has no arms. Practice placing shoulders, arms, elbows, and wrists in a neutral position. While you are sitting there, practice each of the exercises in Figures 38-20 and 38-21 in the textbook.

Everyday Ethics

Before completing the learning exercises below, reread and reflect on the Everyday Ethics scenario and Questions for Consideration in this chapter of the textbook. It may also be useful to review the Dental Hygiene Ethics discussion in Chapter 1, the Ethical Applications in the introduction pages for each section in the textbook, as well as the Codes of Ethics in Appendices I, II, and III.

Individual Learning Activity

Imagine that you have observed what happened in the scenario, but are not one of the main characters involved in the situation. Write a reflective journal entry that:

■ describes how you might have reacted (as an observer-not as a participant),
■ expresses your personal feelings about what happened, or
■ identifies personal values that affect your reaction to the situation.

Discovery Activity

Ask a dental hygienist who has been practicing for a year or more to read the scenario. Provide them with a copy of one of the Codes of Ethics as well. Share the responses you have made to answer each question and ask that person to discuss the situation with you. What insights did you have or what did you learn during this discussion?

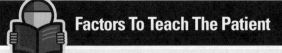

Factors To Teach The Patient

This scenario is related to the following factors listed in this chapter of the textbook:

- Why it is necessary to use a variety of instruments for scaling
- Benefits of using a finely sharpened instrument for calculus removal
- Harmful effects of using dull instruments

Today is your first scaling and root-planing appointment with Mr. Nicholas Diamond. When you open your sterilized instruments and line them up on the tray, Mr. Diamond expresses amazement at the number of them and comments on their different shapes. When you begin to check each instrument for sharpness before using them, he wants to know what you are looking for.

Use the examples of patient conversations in Appendix D as a guide to write a statement explaining to Mr. Diamond why you have so many instruments on your tray and why you need to make sure they are well sharpened before you begin his treatment. Use the conversation you create to educate a patient or friend who is not a student colleague.

CROSSWORD PUZZLE

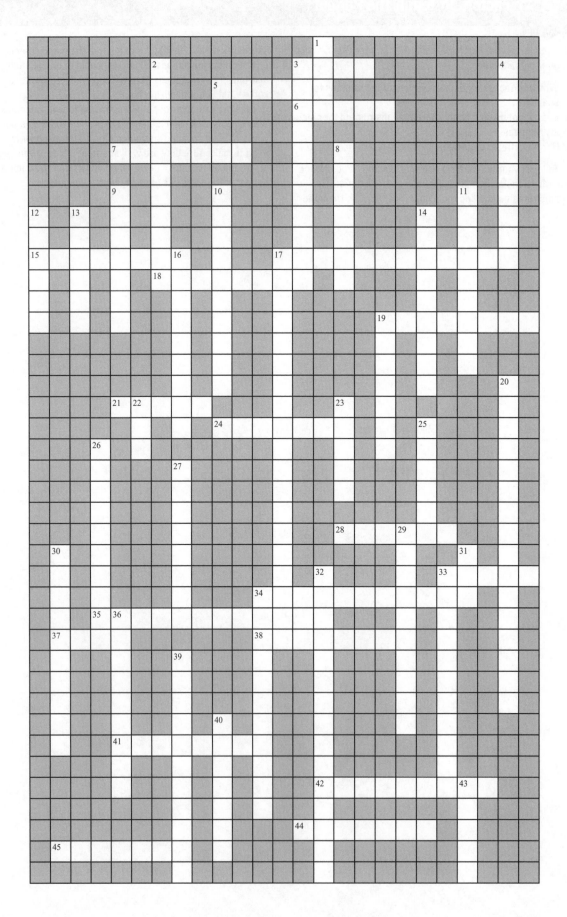

ACROSS

3. Refers to the cutting edge of an instrument that visually presents a rounded, shiny surface that reflects light.
5. This instrument is used to dislodge heavy calculus by pushing horizontally from facial to lingual on the proximal surface of teeth.
6. Another term for the sharpened working end of a dental instrument.
7. The combined push-and-pull stroke commonly used to activate a periodontal probe.
15. Refers to the size of the instrument handle; usually available in four sizes.
17. This type of lateral pressure when scaling contributes to burnishing of calculus.
18. Refers to the hand that is usually used for holding a scaling instrument during treatment.
19. This thinner type of instrument shank may provide more tactile sensitivity and is used to remove fine calculus or for maintenance root debridement.
21. Connects the handle and the working end of a dental instrument.
24. To smooth and polish the surface of calculus (usually with an instrument that is not sharp) instead of removing it completely with a well-sharpened instrument.
28. The position of the blade of an area-specific Gracey curet.
33. A scaling instrument with a rounded working end; there are two types: universal and area- specific.
34. Dental hygiene instrument that is usually held by the non-dominant hand using a modified pen grasp (two words).
35. Describes the relationship between the working end of the instrument and the tooth surface being treated.
37. A type of scaling instrument that has multiple cutting edges lined up on a round, oval, or rectangular base.
38. A working stroke that is parallel with the long axis of the tooth being treated.
41. Refers to the use of a mirror to view an area of the mouth.
42. This body part is relaxed and level when working in the neutral position.
44. Refers to the instrument stroke that is applied with an instrument to accomplish a task, such as removing calculus.
45. Stroke that applies definite, well-controlled pressure on the surface of a tooth; refers to instrumentation of a tooth to remove calculus.

DOWN

1. The type of stroke that is used when activating most scaling instruments.
2. This type of instrument has paired working ends that may be either mirror image or complementary (two words).
3. Refers to a light pressure stroke that disrupts dental biofilm from the root surface of a previously root-planed tooth surface.
4. Provides stabilization and control during instrumentation (two words).
8. One of three types of strokes that can be applied against the tooth surface with an instrument; a diagonal stroke.
9. The pressure that is required of an instrument to the tooth during a scaling procedure.
10. Refers to the unique area of each instrument that is used to carry out the purpose and function of that instrument (two words).
11. This type of lateral pressure can result in gouging of the root surface, patient discomfort, and clinician fatigue.
12. When you are using the modified pen grasp, the position of the instrument against this finger is extremely important to instrument control.
13. Refers to any scaling instrument with two cutting edges that meet in a point; can have a curved or straight blade.
14. A name for a type of scaler; refers to a straight scaler.
16. Refers to a stroke that is dependent on the surface texture of the area being instrumented; lighter pressure is applied progressively as strokes continue and the surface becomes smooth (two words).
17. Area of the tooth where treatment is indicated and the stroke of the dental instrument is applied (two words).
19. The support upon which your scaling hand finger rests so that force can be exerted during the scaling procedure in order to remove calculus.
20. The hand position that is used to hold a dental instrument (three words).
22. A type of scaling instrument that has a single straight cutting edge that is turned at a 99° angle to the shank.
23. Refers to the cutting edge of an instrument that is a fine line, has no width, and does not reflect light.
25. Single, unbroken movement of the instrument as it is applied against the tooth surface.
26. A working stroke that is applied parallel with the occlusal surface of the tooth being treated.
27. This type of instrument shank indicates the instrument is primarily used in anterior teeth.
29. Refers to the acceptable state for the sharpening stone and testing stick before use for sharpening dental instruments.
30. The finger that establishes a fulcrum when using a modified pen grasp during instrumentation (two words).
31. Metal particles removed during sharpening that remain attached to the edge of the instrument.
32. A sharpening method in which the flat stone is placed on a steady surface and the instrument is moved across the surface of the stone (two words).
33. The type of instrument shank that is designed to help adapt the instrument to difficult-to-reach areas, such as the distal surfaces of molars (two words).
34. Refers to a sharpening technique in which the dental instrument is stabilized against the edge of an immovable work area with the nondominant hand and the stone is applied at the appropriate angle (two words).
36. Refers to development of the control, coordination, and strength needed to become proficient in the efficient and effective use of dental instruments.
39. Refers to the fine line where the face and the lateral surfaces of a well-sharpened dental instrument meet (two words).
40. The position of wrist, forearm, elbow, and shoulder that prevents occupational pain risk for dental hygienists.
43. The thick, stronger, less flexible instrument shank needed for the removal of heavy calculus deposits.

Nonsurgical Periodontal Instrumentation

Learning Objectives

Upon successful completion of these exercises, you will be able to:

1. Identify and define key terms and concepts related to nonsurgical periodontal treatment.
2. Define the scope, purpose, and effect of nonsurgical periodontal therapy.
3. Describe appointment preparation and follow-up procedures for nonsurgical periodontal treatment.
4. Identify and describe techniques used for nonsurgical periodontal instrumentation.
5. Identify the types and components of power-driven scalers.
6. Describe techniques for using and maintaining power-driven scalers and manual instruments.

 KNOWLEDGE EXERCISES

Write your answers for each question in the space provided.

1. What is the aim of periodontal debridement interventions you provide for your patients?

   _____

   _____

2. List procedures that can be included when you plan periodontal debridement for your patient.

   _____

   _____

   _____

3. Nonsurgical interventions for periodontal disease can provide the definitive treatment for many of your patients with periodontal infections. Some patients with more advanced disease will require additional treatment after the initial debridement therapy that you provide for them. Describe the aims and expected outcomes of providing complete and carefully performed nonsurgical periodontal therapy.

   _____

   _____

   _____

   _____

4. What are the clinical end points that indicate successful nonsurgical instrumentation?

   _____

   _____

   _____

5. What changes occur in the subgingival microflora after instrumentation procedures during periodontal debridement.

_____

_____

_____

_____

6. List situations that indicate the need to plan multiple appointments for completion of periodontal debridement procedures.

_____

_____

_____

7. In your own words, describe tissue conditioning.

_____

_____

_____

8. If multiple dental hygiene appointments are planned for nonsurgical periodontal therapy, when should you evaluate the success of your initial periodontal debridement?

_____

_____

_____

9. Identify the components of an immediate evaluation.

_____

_____

10. What postcare instructions will you provide your patient with after scaling and root planing procedures?

_____

_____

_____

_____

11. What factors are taken into account when determining a maintenance interval after completion of nonsurgical periodontal treatment?

_____

_____

_____

_____

_____

12. In your own words, explain full-mouth disinfection.

_____

_____

_____

13. A recommended plan for dental hygiene care includes complete and thorough scaling of each segment of the mouth. List the problems associated with providing a full-mouth incomplete or preliminary partial scaling at the first appointment and then planning to have your patient schedule additional appointments for more definitive treatment.

_____

_____

_____

_____

14. What assessment strategies will you use to assess your patient in order to formulate a plan for instrumentation?

_____

_____

_____

15. What will you look for during a visual examination of your patient's gingival tissues that will help you formulate your strategy for instrumentation?

_____

_____

16. Why will you perform a tactile subgingival examination, using a periodontal probe and explorer, before beginning periodontal instrumentation to remove calculus?

_____

_____

_____

17. Why is it important to have your patient's radiographs available for review during scaling and root planing procedures?

_____

_____

18. List the factors that affect which instruments you will select for calculus removal during an individual patient's nonsurgical care.

_____

_____

_____

_____

19. Removal of subgingival calculus is more difficult than removal of supragingival calculus and is complicated by several significant factors. List the factors and variables that make instrumentation of subgingival surfaces more complex.

_____

_____

_____

_____

_____

20. The steps for providing manual scaling are listed below. Put the list in the correct order (1 = first step; 10 = last step).

STEP NUMBER	DESCRIPTION
_____	Select the correct cutting edge of the instrument.
_____	Stabilize your hand in your patient's mouth, using a finger rest.
_____	Adapt the toe of the cutting edge of the instrument against the tooth surface.
_____	Use smooth, overlapping, light-pressured finishing strokes that provide maximum sensitivity to minute irregularities of the tooth surface.
_____	Apply sufficient (moderate to heavy) lateral pressure for calculus removal.
_____	Angle the instrument blade for insertion to the base of the periodontal pocket.
_____	Apply light lateral pressure for instrument insertion and confirmation of soft tissue attachment.
_____	Activate the instrument, maintaining the angulation and adaptation of the cutting edge evenly during the stroke.
_____	Pick up the instrument using a light modified pen grasp.
_____	Repeat in overlapping, channeled strokes to remove all calculus.

21. Explain how a well-sharpened instrument reduces the amount of lateral pressure necessary for complete calculus removal.

_____

_____

22. Describe the clinician's hand motion that helps maintain adaptation of the toe of the cutting edge of the instrument to the tooth surface during scaling procedures.

_____

23. Your dental hygiene care plan for a patient may include a blended approach that uses both manual and power-driven dental hygiene instrumentation techniques. List general clinical preparation measures that you will follow before using a power-driven scaler during patient care.

_____

_____

_____

_____

_____

24. List the steps used to prepare an ultrasonic unit.

_____

_____

_____

_____

_____

25. List the steps for preparing your patient before you use a power-driven scaler.

_____

_____

_____

_____

_____

_____

_____

26. Complete Infomap 39-1 with information from the textbook to help you compare the different types of power-driven scaling devices.

INFOMAP 39-1						
TYPE	**FREQUENCY**	**MODE OF ACTION**	**TIP TYPE AND MOVEMENT**	**WATER USE**	**CONTRAINDICATIONS, PRECAUTIONS, AND RISK FACTORS FOR USE**	**PRINCIPLES OF INSTRUMENTATION AND TECHNIQUE FOR USE**
Sonic scaler						
Ultrasonic magnetostrictive						
Ultrasonic piezoelectric						

27. Figure 39-1 shows three ultrasonic tips. Identify the following components for each one. One way to do this is to use a different-colored pencil to fill in or identify each area on the drawing.

   ■ The point of the tip

   ■ The tip

   ■ The grip

   ■ The area in which you would likely find the O-ring on a magnetostrictive insert

   ■ The area in which the metal stack would be located on a magnetostrictive insert

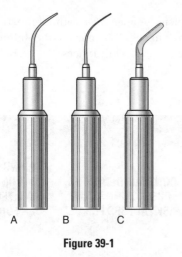

A   B   C

Figure 39-1

28. Match each description to the appropriate tip shown in Figure 39-1 by writing the correct letter in the space provided next to each statement. Each letter may be used more than once; some descriptions apply to more than one tip.

_____	Designed for removal of heavy supragingival calculus
_____	Thinner tip designed for subgingival instrumentation
_____	Universal tip generally used for removal of moderate to heavy deposits from supragingival or relatively shallow pockets
_____	Tip that is intended for use on only low or medium power if it is attached to a magnetostrictive insert
_____	Tip that can be useful for removing orthodontic cement

✓ COMPETENCY EXERCISES

Apply information from the chapter and use critical thinking skills to complete the competency exercises. Write responses on paper or create electronic documents to submit your answers.

The only real way to become competent in the skills described in this chapter of the textbook is to practice. It is, of course, difficult to help you do that in a workbook format. One way to enhance your competency in instrumentation skills is to work with a partner to provide feedback for each other during clinical exercises. Exercise 1, below provides one scenario for you to consider. As you work with student colleagues, you will find many more opportunities to explain and provide feedback on each other's instrumentation skills.

1. You are watching your student colleague, Mary Neely, while she is scaling. You have been designated as her mentor colleague, and your task for today is to give her verbal feedback about all areas of her clinical performance while she is providing patient care. Tomorrow she will observe you providing patient care and will have feedback for you.

   While you are observing Mary, you notice that as she is scaling in the maxillary posterior areas, she is having some trouble placing a comfortable fulcrum during her activation stroke. You also observe that as she activates the instrument her wrist motion seems to move the instrument handle from side to side and her hand pivots back and forth on her finger rest.

   Explain what this type of hand motion might indicate about the angle of the blade of the instrument against the surface of the tooth down inside the periodontal pocket. Explain what Mary is doing incorrectly and how she might change the motion of her hand to increase her ability to remove calculus. (*Hint:* You can practice moving your instrument on a typodont or model to help you visualize what you are trying to describe.)

2. In your own words, explain why the interrelationship among dental biofilm, endotoxins, cementum, and calculus is important to consider when you plan dental hygiene treatment to eliminate the cause of periodontal infection.

Everyday Ethics

Before completing the learning exercises below, reread and reflect on the Everyday Ethics scenario and Questions for Consideration in this chapter of the textbook. It may also be useful to review the Dental Hygiene Ethics discussion in Chapter 1, the Ethical Applications in the introduction pages for each section in the textbook, as well as the Codes of Ethics in Appendices I, II, and III.

Collaborative Learning Activity

Work with another student colleague to role-play the scenario. The goal of this exercise is for you and your colleague to work though the alternative actions in order to come to consensus on a solution or response that is acceptable to both of you.

Discovery Activity

Ask a dental hygienist who has been practicing for a year or more to read the scenario. Provide them with a copy of the Code of Ethics as well. Share the responses you have made to answer each question and ask that person to discuss the situation with you. What insights did you have or what did you learn during this discussion?

Factors To Teach The Patient

This scenario is related to the following factors listed in this chapter of the textbook:

- The rationale for follow-up evaluation following the completion of scaling and root planing

At the last appointment in a multiple appointment series, during which you have provided quadrant by quadrant scaling and rootplaning for Mr. Davis, you remind him to schedule a treatment evaluation appointment in 3 to 4 weeks with the front desk manager on his way out. He complains that he really does not want to come to see you one more time this year and he feels that a recall visit 6 months from now will be sufficient.

Use the example of patient conversations in Appendix D as a guide to prepare a conversation that you will use to explain the need for final evaluation before determining an appropriate recall interval. Use the conversation you create to educate a patient or friend. Then modify your conversation based on what you learned from their feedback.

CROSSWORD PUZZLE

ACROSS

1. Refers to scaling techniques that uses overlapping strokes to ensure complete removal of calculus from a tooth or root surface.
2. Lateral pressure used during assessment procedures and instrument insertion.
5. Therapeutic washing.
8. Another name for the magnetostrictive insert in the handpiece of a power-driven scaler.
9. Refers to the action or stroke that applies pressure and maintains the cutting edge of the instrument on the tooth in order to remove calculus.
10. A device that converts energy or power from one form to another.
12. Formation and collapsing of bubbles in the water surrounding an ultrasonic tip.
14. Refers to an area of calculus on a tooth.
15. A term that refers to instrumentation of the crown or root surfaces of a tooth.
16. The type of power-driven scaler that is driven by compressed air.
17. Type of metal rod used in magnetostrictive ultrasonic unit inserts.
19. The type of power-driven scaler that produces tip vibrations by dimensional changes in crystals housed in the handpiece.
20. Instrumentation to remove dental biofilm and calculus.
22. Can be used for coolant and lavage in some ultrasonic units to help reduce levels of pathogens in aerosols when using a power- driven scaler; can also be used as a preprocedural rinse to reduce microorganisms.
23. Refers to the direction of the pressure of the cutting edge of a scaling instrument against the surface of the tooth; if the force is not sufficient, calculus may not be totally removed.
24. Refers to the use of an antimicrobial mouthrinse to reduce aspiration of contaminated materials by both the patient and the clinician during the use of a power-driven scaler.

DOWN

1. Ultrasonic tip shape that has curvatures designed to adapt to posterior surfaces of teeth.
2. Pressure that is applied during instrumentation, depending on the nature of the calculus deposit and the type of therapy being performed.
3. The type of power-driven scaler that produces tip vibrations by expansion and contraction of a metal stack or rod.
4. Can be produced if a power-driven scaler is not used appropriately; can cause damage to the pulp tissue of a patient's tooth.
6. Lipopolysaccharide (LPS) complex found in the cell wall of many gram-negative microorganisms; toxic to human tissue.
7. Refers to the area between the roots of a multirooted tooth.
11. The last step of calculus removal in which the clinician uses an explorer to determine the end point of the treatment.
13. Refers to the outermost third of the instrument cutting edge that is kept in contact with the tooth surface during instrumentation.
18. Resolving inflammation, shrinking spongy tissue, and converting a pocket to a sulcus brings your patient s gingival tissue to _____.
21. Refers to an instrument blade that is likely to burnish calculus instead of removing it.

CHAPTER 40

Nonsurgical Periodontal Therapy: Supplemental Care Procedures

Learning Objectives

Upon successful completion of these exercises, you will be able to:

1. Intify and define key terms and concepts related to nonsurgical, supplemental periodontal therapy.

2. Describe and compare delivery methods and types of supplemental antimicrobial therapies for periodontal disease.
3. Document supplemental periodontal therapy procedures.

 KNOWLEDGE EXERCISES

Write your answers for each question in the space provided.

1. Antimicrobial therapy is only one supplemental care procedure that you will plan for your patients. List additional supplemental procedures carried out by dental hygienists.

   _____

   _____

   _____

   _____

   _____

   _____

2. What is the objective of antimicrobial therapy?

   _____

   _____

3. Identify three situations where professional subgingival irrigation can help reduce microorganisms.

   _____

   _____

   _____

4. What conditions may indicate a recommendation of antimicrobial therapy for your patient who is in the maintenance phase of periodontal treatment?

   _____

   _____

   _____

5. What factors increase the likelihood of success of local delivery methods for antimicrobial therapy?

   _____

   _____

   _____

6. What are the products that can be used as antimicrobial agents for subgingival irrigation?

_____

_____

_____

_____

7. How is definitive assessment of instrumentation of a furcation achieved?

_____

_____

8. At reevaluation of adjunctive treatment, what is the indication that the pocket lining is ulcerated and still infected?

_____

9. A biodegradable doxycycline polymer is delivered in a syringe containing liquid _____
_____ and using a _____, narrow-diameter cannula.

10. Describe the method for preparing the cannula to make it easier to insert into the periodontal pocket.

_____

_____

11. What steps follow the irrigation of a pocket with doxycycline polymer liquid?

_____

12. How is minocycline hydrochloride delivered?

_____

_____

13. What is the dose in a chlorhexidine gluconate chip?

_____

14. How large is the chlorhexidine chip? Use a periodontal probe to measure it, and make a full-sized drawing of a chip.

_____

_____

15. What factors do you consider when placing chlorhexidine chips if more than one pocket is to be treated?

_____

_____

16. Why doesn't the chlorhexidine chip have to be removed after it is placed?

_____

17. What does the acronym PARQ stand for?

_____

✓ COMPETENCY EXERCISES

Apply information from the chapter and use critical thinking skills to complete the competency exercises. Write responses on paper or create electronic documents to submit your answers.

1. Describe how the supplemental therapy strategies described in Chapter 40 can enhance outcomes of treatment for patients with advanced periodontal disease.

2. Explain why it is important to be extremely careful to control the pressure with which you express the liquid when using a cannula to provide irrigation into a periodontal pocket.

3. Develop an Infomap to help you compare information about the type and amount of active ingredient or agent that is delivered to the sulcus, delivery methods, placement procedures, and care and storage of each of the different types of local delivery antimicrobials.

   ■ To make this a Discovery Exercise, gather samples of each of the products that are described in the book and use the packaging information to complete the Infomap.

   ■ To enhance your ability to make evidence-based decisions for planning patient care, consult Chapter 2 in the textbook to help you complete a review of the current literature about one or more of the local delivery systems described in this chapter.

4. You are filling out the patient record for Bruce McDonald after his appointment. Today you placed one cartridge of minocycline in a 6-mm pocket on the mesiolingual surface of tooth 3 and another one in a 7-mm pocket on the mesial surface of tooth 5. You educated Mr. McDonald about the self-care regimens he will follow for the next few days, and you scheduled an appointment for follow-up procedures. Using your institution's guidelines for writing in patient records, document Mr. McDonald's appointment procedures.

Everyday Ethics

Before completing the learning exercises below, reread and reflect on the Everyday Ethics scenario and Questions for Consideration in this chapter of the textbook. It may also be useful to review the Dental Hygiene Ethics discussion in Chapter 1, the Ethical Applications in the introduction pages for each section in the textbook, as well as the Codes of Ethics in Appendices I, II, and III.

Individual Learning Activity

Imagine that you are the dental hygienist in this scenario. Answer each of the questions for consideration at the end of the scenario.

Discovery Activity

Ask a friend or relative who is not involved in healthcare to read the scenario and discuss it with you from the perspective of a "patient" who receives services within the healthcare system. Discuss what you learned from the concerns, insights, or difference in perspective that person expressed.

Factors To Teach The Patient

This scenario is related to the following factors listed in this chapter of the textbook:

■ What a periodontal pocket is and why it needs to be treated
■ How the treatment using minocycline hydrochloride, chlorhexidine chip, or doxycycline polymer affects the infection in the pocket
■ The success of all periodontal therapy depends on the daily personal dental biofilm control by the patient.

Your care plan for Ms. Johnetta Sullivan outlines a series of four quadrant scaling and root planing appointments plus a variety of educational and counseling interventions, with the goal of arresting her significant periodontal disease, which is characterized by generalized deep probing depths and attachment loss. When you are explaining the care plan to Johnetta to obtain informed consent, she asks many, many questions. She has heard about the concept of putting

antibiotics "right into the gums" from her friend, who has recently received this treatment in one area of her mouth. Johnetta wants to know why she cannot receive this procedure instead of having to undergo all the "scraping and hurting" that is outlined in your care plan. You know that it is important for the interventions you have planned to be completed before antibiotic therapy is considered.

Use the examples of patient conversations in Appendix D as a guide to prepare a conversation that you might use to educate Johnetta about why and how local delivery supplemental care procedures are used in the treatment of periodontal disease and about why they are not appropriate for her at this time.

Use the conversation you create to role-play this situation with a fellow student. If you are the patient in the role-play, be sure to ask questions. If you are the dental hygienist, try to anticipate questions and answer them in your explanation.

WORD SEARCH

```
C  J  I  Z  P  S  Y  R  I  N  G  E  B  I  K  G  J  M  B  S
E  O  I  M  G  C  A  R  T  R  I  D  G  E  R  E  K  V  I  Y
W  A  N  U  O  O  M  W  A  N  U  K  G  X  S  N  K  E  O  S
O  W  L  T  V  P  F  Y  M  X  L  M  V  Y  S  I  J  N  D  T
E  P  O  C  R  S  P  Q  T  N  A  R  Q  V  C  T  X  D  E  E
X  D  A  U  Q  O  T  O  A  D  U  H  X  Y  M  B  N  O  G  M
O  M  G  Y  U  M  L  V  R  V  A  Z  J  Z  J  O  K  G  R  I
G  Q  S  J  N  I  G  L  R  T  T  N  P  O  I  N  X  E  A  C
E  M  M  Y  G  C  E  D  E  F  U  W  T  T  H  P  G  N  D  L
N  N  T  N  G  R  L  B  X  D  B  N  A  I  S  R  V  O  A  N
O  I  U  Q  X  O  A  E  P  H  R  G  I  F  B  S  N  U  B  Y
U  B  R  T  Z  M  T  K  O  G  I  E  D  S  J  I  I  S  L  G
S  Z  E  H  B  I  I  Q  S  R  E  N  L  T  T  A  O  A  E  I
N  L  J  J  Q  N  N  O  R  F  T  K  W  E  F  I  P  T  K  S
L  T  N  Y  J  I  C  I  M  F  L  J  Y  G  A  B  C  Y  I  B
Z  S  B  H  V  I  H  Z  Y  Z  O  M  H  U  W  S  C  G  Y  C
F  X  X  A  X  Y  I  X  N  P  D  C  W  G  D  A  E  D  F  Z
U  G  I  X  L  N  P  X  C  A  N  N  U  L  A  U  G  N  R  N
A  N  T  I  M  I  C  R  O  B  I  A  L  L  Z  N  L  Q  J  B
A  C  H  E  M  O  T  H  E  R  A  P  Y  G  M  X  V  U  W  B
```

WORD SEARCH CLUES

1. An agent produced by or obtained from microorganisms that can kill other microorganisms or inhibit their growth
2. Can be broken down by a biological process, such as by bacterial or enzymatic reaction
3. Method of delivering antibiotics to the infected area through blood circulation
4. Method of delivering any liquid substance directly into subgingival spaces
5. Method of delivering chlorhexidine directly into subgingival spaces (two words)
6. Method of delivering doxycycline directly into subgingival spaces
7. Method of delivering minocycline directly into subgingival spaces
8. Refers to therapy that uses chemical or pharmaceutical agents for the control or destruction of microorganisms
9. Refers to the placement of antimicrobials directly into the subgingival pocket, directly at the site where they are needed (two words)
10. Treatment by means of a chemical or pharmaceutical agent
11. Tubular end of an instrument placed in a cavity that is used to introduce or withdraw fluid
12. Type of infection caused by normal flora from the skin, nose, mouth, intestinal, or urogenital tracts
13. Type of infection that is caused by acquired organisms that are not normal flora
14. Type of infection that can occur from organisms that are not usually harmful if an individual's immune system is impaired or altered
15. A type of area-specific instrument or Gracey curet that is useful for fitting into confined areas of furcations during root planing

Acute Periodontal Conditions

Upon successful completion of these exercises, you will be able to:

1. Identify and define key terms and concepts related to acute periodontal conditions.
2. Identify the causes, clinical signs and symptoms, and risk factors for acute periodontal infections.
3. Identify the causes, clinical signs and symptoms of primary herpetic gingivostomatitis (PHG).
4. Plan dental hygiene care for a patient with acute periodontal or primary herpetic infections.

 KNOWLEDGE EXERCISES

Write your answers for each question in the space provided.

1. In your own words, explain the difference between an acute and a chronic condition.

2. Describe what you would observe during the examination of a patient diagnosed with necrotizing ulcerative gingivitis.

3. What is a pseudomembrane?

4. Identify and describe the four microscopic layers of the gingival tissue that contain spirochetes in necrotizing lesions.

5. What types of microorganisms are found in greater numbers in necrotizing lesions?

6. What health-related factors can predispose your patient to necrotizing oral conditions?

_____

_____

_____

_____

_____

7. What personal factors predispose an individual to necrotizing oral conditions?

_____

_____

_____

_____

8. What is NUP?

_____

_____

9. Briefly describe necrotizing stomatitis.

_____

_____

10. What is malaise, and what additional health-related symptoms may accompany a diagnosis of necrotizing oral conditions?

_____

_____

_____

11. When you are taking the medical history of a patient who presents with signs of necrotizing ulcerative oral lesions, what additional questions will you ask to aid in the diagnosis?

_____

_____

_____

12. In your own words, describe an abscess.

_____

_____

13. What is a fistula?

_____

_____

14. In your own words, define the term "gum boil."

_____

_____

15. Identify the factors that can cause the formation of a gingival or periodontal abscess.

_____

_____

_____

_____

16. List the classic signs of a periodontal abscess.

_____

_____

_____

_____

17. What are the objectives for immediate treatment if your patient presents with a periodontal abscess?

_____

_____

_____

_____

18. What methods are used to establish drainage of a periodontal abscess?

_____

_____

_____

_____

19. What post-treatment instructions will you give your patient after you have provided dental hygiene care for a periodontal abscess?

_____

_____

_____

_____

20. What is pericoronitis?

_____

_____

21. What is the usual causative agent for primary herpetic gingivostomatitis (PHG) and how is it spread?

_____

_____

22. What are the clinical manifestations of PHG?

_____

_____

_____

23. What are the implications of PHG for dental or dental hygiene treatment?

_____

_____

24. What are the oral hygiene concerns during the acute phase of PHG?

_____

_____

COMPETENCY EXERCISES

Apply information from the chapter and use critical thinking skills to complete the competency exercises. Write responses on paper or create electronic documents to submit your answers.

1. Mr. Rufus is introduced in the Everyday Ethics box in Chapter 41 of the textbook. Read about the details of his health history and oral inspection. Then use the Patient-Specific Dental Hygiene Care Plan Template (Appendix B) and the outline for appointments to provide care for acute stage necrotizing infection in Chapter 41 of the textbook to develop a complete care plan for the dental hygiene treatment of Mr. Rufus's condition. Include a plan for follow-up procedures.

2. Develop an Infomap or table that will help you to compare primary gingovstomatitis (PGS) and necrotizing ulcerative periodontitis (NUP). Include information related to signs, symptoms, etiology, oral manifestations, resolution, diagnosis, management, and treatment considerations for each condition.

3. Develop an Infomap to compare the development, etiology, clinical signs and symptoms, tooth vitality, and radiographic appearances between a periodontal abscess and a pulpal abscess.

Everyday Ethics

Before completing the learning exercises below, reread and reflect on the Everyday Ethics scenario and Questions for Consideration in this chapter of the textbook. It may also be useful to review the Dental Hygiene Ethics discussion in Chapter 1, the Ethical Applications in the introduction pages for each section in the textbook, as well as the Codes of Ethics in Appendices I, II, and III.

Collaborative Learning Activity
Answer each of the questions for consideration at the end of the scenario in the textbook. Compare what you wrote with answers developed by another classmate and discuss differences/similarities.

Discovery Activity
Ask a dental hygienist who has been practicing for a year or more to read the scenario. Provide them with a copy of the _Code of Ethics_ as well. Share the responses you have made to answer each question and ask that person to discuss the situation with you. What insights did you have or what did you learn during this discussion?

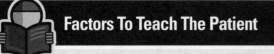

Factors To Teach The Patient

This scenario is related to the following factors listed in this chapter of the textbook:

- Premature discontinuation of treatment for NUG because acute signs have subsided and can lead to recurrence of the infection
- The role of diet, rest, and dental biofilm control in the prevention of NUG
- The avoidance of an oral irrigating device in the presence of acute inflammatory conditions (Microorganisms may be forced into the tissues beneath a pocket, and bacteremia can be produced.)

After you complete the care plan for Mr. Rufus in Competency Exercise question 1, use the details of your plan and the examples of patient conversations in Appendix D as guides to prepare a conversation educating Mr. Rufus about the condition in his mouth. Explain the dental hygiene interventions you have planned so that Mr. Rufus can give his informed consent for treatment.

CHAPTER 42

Sutures and Dressings

Upon successful completion of these exercises, you will be able to:

1. Identify and define key terms and concepts related to sutures and periodontal dressings.
2. Identify components/materials used for sutures and periodontal dressings.
3. Explain procedures for placement and removal of sutures and periodontal dressings.
4. Discuss rationale for and provide post-treatment instructions to patients with periodontal dressings.
5. Identify the components of appropriate documentation for surgical treatment, and suture and dressing placement and removal.
6. Document suture removal procedures in the patient record.

 KNOWLEDGE EXERCISES

Write your answers for each question in the space provided.

1. List three functions of postsurgical suture placement.

   _____

   _____

   _____

2. Which type of suture is capable of causing adverse tissue reaction?

   _____

3. What type of intraoral sutures must be removed by a dentist or dental hygienist within a specific period of time?

   _____

4. Many types of suturing needles are available. What three factors influence selection of a specific type?

   _____

   _____

   _____

5. Which part of the needle is grasped by a needle holder during the suturing procedure?

   _____

6. List at least three requirements of an acceptable surgical suture needle.

   _____

   _____

   _____

7. Suture knots tied on the _____ surface of the alveolar ridge and tied with a _____-mm suture tail left in place are easy to remove later.

8. Removable sutures should not be left in place longer than _____ days.

9. When removing a suture, it is necessary to raise the knot and hold it with a slight tension, slightly depress the tissue with the back of the scissors blade, and cut the suture in the part that was previously buried in the tissue. In your own words, describe why this procedure is followed.

    _____

    _____

10. Describe the characteristics of an acceptable dressing material.

    _____

    _____

    _____

11. List three disadvantages of zinc oxide with eugenol dressing material.

    _____

    _____

    _____

12. List three advantages of chemical-cured dressings.

    _____

    _____

    _____

13. An absorbable dressing that can be placed directly on clean, moist, or bleeding wounds to promote wound healing is a _____ dressing.

14. A surgical dressing is typically left in place for _____ days.

15. Identify a necessary component of the patient dismissal process following the placement of a periodontal dressing.

    _____

16. List the components of the detailed documentation required following suture removal.

    _____

    _____

    _____

    _____

    _____

17. Following the removal of sutures or dressing, when should the return appointment to observe the surgical area be scheduled?

    _____

COMPETENCY EXERCISES

Apply information from the chapter and use critical thinking skills to complete the competency exercises. Write responses on paper or create electronic documents to submit your answers.

1. Mrs. Belinda Hawkins had periodontal surgery about 10 days ago. She is scheduled with you this afternoon for suture removal. List and explain the purpose of all the items and instruments you will need to set up in your treatment room to prepare for her postsurgical dressing and suture removal appointment.

2. After you seat Mrs. Hawkins and update her medical history, you examine the surgical areas and find out that the dressing is completely intact on the maxillary arch but that on the mandibular arch has partly broken off and the sutures are uncovered. One suture appears as though it may be partially embedded in the dressing material. You note that all areas are fairly free of debris, and the surrounding mucosal tissue looks healthy. Describe the procedure you will use for removing the periodontal dressings.

3. Explain why you need to place each suture on a gauze sponge for postprocedural counting.

4. You gently rinse and examine Mrs. Hawkins' mouth. All areas appear to be healing well, with only slight redness in the area of tooth 30 where the suture had been embedded in the dressing. Explain follow-up bacterial biofilm control procedures to Mrs. Hawkins.

5. Write a progress note to document Mrs. Hawkins' suture removal procedure. Follow your institution's guidelines for writing in patient records.

? QUESTIONS PATIENTS ASK

What sources of information can you identify that will help you answer your patient's questions in this scenario?

When you greet Mrs. Hawkins in the reception room and walk with her back to your treatment room for her suture removal appointment, she is clearly nervous about the impending procedure. She asks, "Will it hurt? Will there be any bleeding?"

Everyday Ethics

Before completing the learning exercises below, reread and reflect on the Everyday Ethics scenario and Questions for Consideration in this chapter of the textbook. It may also be useful to review the Dental Hygiene Ethics discussion in Chapter 1, the Ethical Applications in the introduction pages for each section in the textbook, as well as the Codes of Ethics in Appendices I, II, and III.

Individual Learning Activity
Imagine that you are the dental hygienist in this scenario. Answer each of the questions for consideration at the end of the scenario.

Discovery Activity
Ask a friend or relative who is not involved in healthcare to read the scenario and discuss it with you from the perspective of a "patient" who receives services within the healthcare system. Discuss what you learned from the concerns, insights, or difference in perspective that person expressed.

Factors To Teach The Patient

This scenario is related to the following factors listed in this chapter of the textbook:

■ Explanations for the items in Table 42-1 in the textbook
■ Care of the mouth during the period after surgical treatment while wearing a periodontal dressing
■ That tobacco use is detrimental and delays healing

Because you provided initial therapy care for Mr. Bruce Barrimundi, you are very interested in observing when he is scheduled for periodontal surgery. After the surgical procedure is complete and the sutures and dressings are placed, you are asked to give him the printed instructions for post-treatment care that you have developed based on the information in Table 42-1 in the textbook.

You know that compliance with recommendations is always better if you provide verbal instructions as well as written. Besides, there are several factors that you think

are important to emphasize. You know that Mr. Barramundi still smokes (although you have told him how bad it is for his periodontal health). You also know that he has a very vigorous tooth brushing style and is always working very hard to make sure every tiny area of dental biofilm is completely removed.

Use the patient instructions for posttreatment care (Table 42-1 in the textbook) and the example of a patient conversation in Appendix D as a guide to prepare an outline for a verbal reinforcement of posttreatment instructions for Mr. Barramundi.

Use the conversation you create to role-play this situation with a fellow student. If you are the patient in the role-play, be sure to ask questions. If you are the dental hygienist, try to anticipate questions and answer them in your explanation.

WORD SEARCH

```
I  Q  T  S  M  O  N  O  F  I  L  A  M  E  N  T  C
Q  N  H  Y  D  R  O  L  Y  S  I  S  S  N  L  T  E
B  S  T  P  R  O  T  E  C  T  I  V  E  M  Z  L  T
H  B  E  E  H  E  M  O  S  T  A  S  I  S  L  U  A
F  Y  L  Y  R  D  D  R  E  S  S  I  N  G  B  A  B
J  Q  X  A  P  D  D  L  F  V  J  M  O  R  K  P  S
I  M  C  I  N  T  E  R  R  U  P  T  E  D  T  P  O
M  J  M  O  B  K  Q  N  S  O  Z  W  Y  T  Y  O  R
I  Z  B  Y  N  O  E  O  F  T  E  D  O  W  S  B
E  C  K  U  G  T  R  T  Z  A  E  Q  S  K  Y  I  A
S  L  I  N  G  O  I  V  V  M  L  A  B  L  A  T  B
W  A  R  D  S  W  O  N  D  R  P  A  C  K  S  I  L
W  Z  V  Y  B  R  A  Q  U  C  O  A  P  T  W  O  E
M  Q  M  M  U  P  E  R  I  O  C  A  R  E  A  N  Q
P  R  E  S  S  U  R  E  M  Q  U  Q  G  M  G  Y  O
S  T  E  R  I  L  I  T  Y  C  Y  S  X  Y  E  F  J
Y  O  A  O  V  B  O  R  D  E  R  M  O  L  D  A  X
```

WORD SEARCH CLUES

1. Suture that is broken down by body enzymes or by water
2. Suturing procedure that forms loops on one side of an incision and a series of stitches directly over the incision; also called a continuous lock
3. Shaping of the peripheries of a dressing by manual manipulation of the tissue adjacent to the borders to duplicate the contour and size of the vestibule. (two words)
4. Approximate the edges of a wound with no overlap
5. Suture that is an uninterrupted series of stitches tied at one or both ends
6. Material used to cover or protect a wound; also called a pack
7. Termination of bleeding by mechanical or chemical means
8. Process in which water penetrates and causes breakdown of a suture
9. Suture that joins flaps on both the lingual and the facial sides of the dental arch
10. Application of a suture to hold or constrict tissue
11. Single-strand suture
12. Paste–gel type of chemical-cured dressing; a brand name
13. Type of dressing used to control bleeding
14. Type of dressing that shields an area from injury or trauma
15. Suture used when the flap is only one side; also called a suspension suture
16. Important characteristic of a suture or needle for preventing infection
17. Stitch or series of stitches made to secure apposition of the edges of a surgical or traumatic wound
18. Eyeless end of a needle that allows suture material and needle to act as one unit
19. Sounds like the name of a superhero but is really a well-known brand name of a zinc oxide with eugenol dressing

CHAPTER 43

Dentin Hypersensitivity

Learning Objectives

Upon successful completion of these exercises, you will be able to:

1. Identify and define key terms and concepts related to dentin hypersensitivity.
2. Discuss the etiology of hypersensitivity and the hydrodynamic theory of pain transmission.
3. Identify factors that influence desensitization.
4. Identify pain characteristics and determine and document potential differential diagnoses.
5. Plan dental hygiene interventions to manage dentin hypersensitivity.

KNOWLEDGE EXERCISES

Write your answers for each question in the space provided.

1. In your own words, define *hypersensitivity*.

   _____

   _____

2. List at least three *patient* behaviors that can trigger a hypersensitivity pain response.

   _____

   _____

   _____

   _____

   _____

3. What condition precedes the development of dentinal hypersensitivity?

   _____

   _____

4. Describe the role of dentinal tubules in the development of hypersensitivity.

   _____

   _____

   _____

   _____

   _____

5. How are odontoblasts related to the transmission of pain as explained by the hydrodynamic theory?

   _____

   _____

6. There are many, many factors that contribute to gingival recession, subsequent root exposure, and potential dentin hypersensitivity. Name as many as you can before looking in the textbook to check your answer.

   _____

   _____

7. In about _____ % of teeth, the enamel and the cementum do not meet, leaving an area of exposed dentin.

8. What factors contribute to erosion on an exposed root surface?

_____

_____

_____

9. In your own words, describe *abfraction*.

_____

_____

10. Which natural desensitization mechanism is related to narrowing of the inside wall of the dentin tubules?

_____

11. A smear layer can reduce dentin sensitivity by blocking the dentin tubules. What causes a smear layer?

_____

_____

_____

12. What is the *negative* effect of a smear layer?

_____

_____

13. Two different patients can experience pain from hypersensitivity in different ways—in other words, pain perception is subjective. What does that mean?

_____

_____

14. List the components to document in your patient's dental history of hypersensitivity.

_____

_____

_____

_____

_____

15. Identify two patient response–related diagnostic tests that can be used to determine location and severity of tooth pain.

_____

_____

16. Without looking at the textbook (you won't always have it with you when you are interviewing a patient), identify at least three trigger questions you can ask your patient about tooth pain.

_____

_____

_____

_____

_____

17. You can use a VRS to rate the level of pain your patient is feeling. If your patient describes her tooth-related pain as a "level 3," what does she mean?

_____

_____

18. Identify the clinical examination techniques used to differentiate among the variety of potential causes for dental pain.

_____

_____

_____

_____

_____

19. No one best method has been identified for the treatment of hypersensitivity. Treatment options offered to the patient should begin with the most _____ and least _____ measures.

20. List at least five factors that you will take into consideration when selecting a desensitizing agent.

_____

_____

_____

_____

_____

21. What patient actions can help reduce dental hypersensitivity?

_____

_____

22. Identify the ingredients in over-the-counter (OTC) desensitizing dentifrices.

_____

_____

23. Identify _therapeutic ingredients_ that chemically block the pain response by occluding the dentinal tubules.

_____

_____

_____

_____

24. List the types of calcium phosphate used to improve dental hypersensitivity

_____

_____

_____

_____

25. List two means of physically covering exposed dentinal tubules at the CEJ.

_____

_____

26. How is a laser used to treat hypersensitivity?

_____

_____

_____

27. What dental hygiene procedures can increase potential pain related to hypersensitivity?

_____

_____

28. Define iontophoresis.

_____

_____

29. The highest prevalence of hypersensitivity is found in _____. Prevalence and severity usually _____ in older folks due to the occurrence of natural mechanisms of desensitization.

COMPETENCY EXERCISES

Apply information from the chapter and use critical thinking skills to complete the competency exercises. Write responses on paper or create electronic documents to submit your answers.

1. Explain how abfraction differs from abrasion.

2. Using patient-appropriate language, describe the hydrodynamic theory.

3. Compare and contrast the two different subjective pain assessment scales (the VAS and the VRS) identified in Box 43-3 in the textbook. Why would you use both of them together for patient assessment?

4. Mr. Mustafa's chief complaint is a frequently occurring, sharply painful sensation on the right side of his mouth. The pain often occurs when he grinds his teeth together during stressful moments at work. He says sometimes that area of his mouth causes pain when he drinks very cold water or chews on cold or hard, crunchy foods.

   Dr. Bedron, who is busy with another patient and cannot take time to examine Mr. Mustafa today, asks you to assess Mr. Mustafa's complaint and document your findings and differential diagnosis in the patient record for him to read at the appointment Mr. Mustafa has scheduled with him next week. Your intraoral examination discovers many areas of deep recession along the facial cervical margins, toothbrush abrasion along the facial surfaces of all his molar teeth, and numerous large MOD restorations that were placed a very long time ago. Several of the restorations are beginning to break down, but you do not find any current large carious lesions.

   You know that Dr. Bedron will need to do a very thorough clinical examination and question your patient carefully before he can diagnose the problem. But, using the information you have here and your school's guidelines for writing progress notes, document your differential diagnosis for conditions may potentially be causing Mr. Mustafa's tooth pain? Support your selections using the information in Table 43-1 in the textbook.

❓ QUESTIONS PATIENTS ASK

What sources of information can you identify that will help you answer your patient's questions in this scenario?

Some patients express concerns related to a friend's experiences. "My friend bleached her teeth and said that it caused sensitivity. Should I avoid bleaching my teeth?"

A patient may express concern over the diagnosis of hypersensitivity for a specific area. "How do you know that I have sensitivity and not a cavity?"

Many patients will want to understand more completely how the desensitizing agents will work to help their problem. "How soon after I start using sensitivity toothpaste will I notice an improvement in my hypersensitivity? Will I need to use a desensitizing product forever? Will I ever be able to have ice in my summer drinks again? Should I drink my morning orange juice before or after I brush my teeth?"

Everyday Ethics

Before completing the learning exercises below, reread and reflect on the Everyday Ethics scenario and Questions for Consideration in this chapter of the textbook. It may also be useful to review the Dental Hygiene Ethics discussion in Chapter 1, the Ethical Applications in the introduction pages for each section in the textbook, as well as the Codes of Ethics in Appendices I, II, and III.

Individual Learning Activities
■ Imagine that you are the dental hygienist in this scenario. Answer each of the questions for consideration at the end of the scenario.

■ Imagine the scenario from the patient's perspective. How might the patient's response to the questions following the scenario be different from those of the dental hygienist involved?

Factors To Teach The Patient

This scenario is related to the following factors listed in this chapter of the textbook:

■ Activities and habits that may contribute to dentin hypersensitivity
■ Importance of appropriate oral hygiene self-care techniques, such as using a soft toothbrush and avoiding vigorous brushing, which may contribute to gingival recession and subsequent abrasion of root surface
■ That toothbrushing should not immediately follow consumption of acidic foods or beverages or use of acidic mouthwashes

You are at your desk writing out a dental hygiene care plan for Mrs. Jernigan. Her chief symptom of tooth pain has been diagnosed by Dr. Hockwater as dentin hypersensitivity. Mrs. Jernigan is scheduled with you later this week for education and counseling. This is the first patient you have counseled regarding the management of dentin hypersensitivity, and you want to be thorough.

Use the examples of patient conversations in Appendix D of this workbook as a guide to create a conversation and to role-play this situation with a fellow student.

CHAPTER 44

Extrinsic Stain Removal

Learning Objectives

Upon successful completion of these exercises, you will be able to:

1. Identify and define key terms and concepts related to removal of extrinsic dental stain.
2. Identify the science, effects, indications, contraindications, precautions, and procedures for selective dental polishing.
3. Describe polishing agents, instruments, and techniques used for removal of extrinsic stains.
4. Document removal of tooth stain in patient record.

KNOWLEDGE EXERCISES

Write your answers for each question in the space provided.

1. Coronal polishing can remove _____ _____ (two words) and _____, but does not remove _____.

2. The use of polishing agents for stain removal is a selective procedure that not every patient needs, especially on a routine basis. List the potential negative effects of polishing.

_____

_____

_____

_____

_____

_____

_____

3. Identify actions you can take and polishing techniques you can use to minimize the negative effects of polishing.

_____

_____

_____

_____

4. Which abrasives commonly used in dental cleaning and polishing agents have a Mohs hardness value that indicates that they are less likely to scratch your patient's exposed tooth surfaces?

_____

_____

_____

_____

5. What characteristics and application principles affect the abrasive action of polishing agents?

■ Characteristics of abrasive particles

_____

_____

_____

_____

■ Application principles

_____

_____

_____

6. In your own words, explain the difference between cleaning and polishing agents.

_____

_____

7. Ultra- or high-speed handpieces rotate between _____ and _____ revolutions per minute. Low-speed handpieces, typically used for polishing extrinsic stains, rotate between _____ and _____ revolutions per minute.

8. Describe the kinds of prophylaxis angle attachments (polishing cups) that are available for you to use when polishing stain in different areas of the tooth.

_____

_____

_____

9. In your own words, describe the procedure used for applying the polishing agent to an area of stained enamel.

_____

_____

_____

_____

10. How is a bristle brush used?

_____

_____

11. How can stain be removed from proximal surfaces of teeth?

_____

_____

12. What special care is required when using finishing strips to remove stain from proximal surfaces of anterior teeth?

_____

_____

13. How does an air-powder polisher work and when is it used?

_____

_____

_____

14. In your own words, describe the techniques you will use for reducing your exposure to aerosolized spray and for protecting both your patient and yourself when polishing, especially when using an air-powder polisher.

_____

_____

_____

_____

15. What are the indications for polishing?

_____

_____

16. List the clinical findings that indicate you should NOT polish your patient's teeth during the dental hygiene appointment.

_____

_____

_____

_____

_____

_____

17. What is tribiology?

    _____

    _____

18. What is a three-body abrasive polishing agent?

    _____

    _____

19. What is the most common cause of aerosol production when using air-powder polishing?

    _____

    _____

20. Describe potentially negative effects and sequellae of incorrectly directing the handpiece nozzle during air-powder polishing.

    _____

    _____

21. How can the clinician prevent potential injury while using the air-powder polisher?

    _____

    _____

✓ COMPETENCY EXERCISES

Apply information from the chapter and use critical thinking skills to complete the competency exercises. Write responses on paper or create electronic documents to submit your answers.

1. What is the difference between polishing and abrasion? In what ways can you produce one but not the other when you remove stain from your patient's teeth?

2. Winston Nottingham always brings you a small packet of tea from England when he comes in for his regular periodontal maintenance appointment. He drinks tea every day, and you usually notice staining on the lingual surfaces of his maxillary and mandibular anterior teeth and on a few lingual proximal surfaces of the lower premolars. He has significant recession, especially on the facial surfaces on his lower molars and the facial and lingual surfaces of his maxillary molars owing to previous history of periodontal infection.

   Write a dental hygiene diagnosis statement identifying Mr. Nottingham's condition in relation to the stain and the recession.

3. What dental hygiene intervention is appropriate for addressing Mr. Nottingham's problem?

4. Using your institution's guidelines for writing in patient records, document the procedure you used to remove the tea stain from Mr. Nottingham's teeth.

5. Mr. Nottingham's son, Will, who is 12 years old, is also your patient. He is in the office for a regularly scheduled 6-month prophylaxis appointment. You are glad he has returned as scheduled, because there are several areas of demineralization that you are monitoring. Will also has significant areas of dental stain because he drinks tea every morning with his parents. You point out the areas of stain to him and you mention that you must polish quite a few areas in his mouth.

   While you are preparing to polish his teeth, Will picks up the container of polishing paste and notices that it contains fluoride. He points that out to you and wants to know why he must also undergo the "icky" fluoride treatment after you finish polishing. He wants to know why you can't just polish all of the areas of his teeth and then skip the regular fluoride treatment completely. Discuss why the use of a fluoride-containing polishing paste is not a replacement for a conventional topical application of fluoride.

Everyday Ethics

Before completing the learning exercises below, reread and reflect on the Everyday Ethics scenario and Questions for Consideration in this chapter of the textbook. It may also be useful to review the Dental Hygiene Ethics discussion in Chapter 1, the Ethical Applications in the introduction pages for each section in the textbook, as well as the Codes of Ethics in Appendices I, II, and III.

Individual Learning Activity
Identify a situation you have experienced that presents a similar ethical dilemma. Write about what you would do dif-

ferently now than you did at the time the incident happened—support your discussion with concepts from the dental hygiene codes of ethics.

Discovery Activity
Ask a friend or relative who is not involved in healthcare to read the scenario and discuss it with you from the perspective of a "patient" who receives services within the healthcare system. Discuss what you learned from the concerns, insights, or difference in perspective that person expressed.

Factors To Teach The Patient

This scenario is related to the following factors listed in this chapter of the textbook:

■ How dental biofilm and stains form on the teeth and their replacements

As noted in the Everyday Ethics case for this chapter in the textbook, Carol explained to Mr. Jackson that colorings from food and drink could stain both natural teeth and the cosmetic restorations he had placed a year ago. Carol

encouraged him to cut back on drinking tea, reinforced his role in stain prevention, and stressed the benefits to his appearance of compliance.

Use the examples of patient conversations in Appendix D as a guide to prepare an outline for a conversation for discussing the concept of stain formation with Mr. Jackson. Use the outline you create as the starting point to educate a patient or friend (not a student colleague) about stain formation.

CHAPTER 45

Tooth Bleaching

Upon successful completion of these exercises, you will be able to:

1. Identify and define key terms and concepts related to tooth bleaching.
2. Compare types of procedures, and discuss the processes of tooth bleaching systems.
3. Discuss the risks and potential side effects of bleaching.
4. Identify indications and contraindications for dental bleaching treatment.

KNOWLEDGE EXERCISES

Write your answers for each question in the space provided.

1. What is the difference between bleaching and whitening?

   _____

   _____

   _____

2. External tooth bleaching/whitening procedures can be used for both _____ and _____ teeth.

3. Describe the process for bleaching non-vital teeth.

   _____

   _____

4. What ingredients are used for bleaching non-vital teeth?

   _____

   _____

5. Describe the mechanism of bleaching vital teeth.

   _____

   _____

   _____

6. Explain the action of each of the two active ingredients that are used in bleaching systems for vital teeth.

   _____

   _____

   _____

7. Explain the difference in working time for each of the two active ingredients used in bleaching systems for vital teeth.

   _____

   _____

   _____

8. How long does hydrogen peroxide continue to work on the vital tooth after placement?

_____

_____

9. How long does carbamide peroxide continue to work on the vital tooth after placement?

_____

_____

10. List and describe the purpose of additional ingredients used in bleaching systems.

INGREDIENT(S)	PURPOSE

11. Identify the safety concerns or effects of bleaching that are associated with each of the following factors.

FACTOR	SAFETY CONCERNS/EFFECTS OF BLEACHING
Tooth Structure	
Oral Soft Tissue	
Restorative Materials	
Systemic Effects	

12. Which vital tooth conditions would respond favorably to tooth bleaching?

_____

_____

13. Which vital tooth conditions would not respond favorably to tooth bleaching?

_____

_____

14. What tooth conditions indicate need for a dental care intervention prior to tooth bleaching?

_____

_____

15. Describe effective methods for reducing sensitivity related to bleaching.

_____

_____

_____

_____

16. What factors can influence the final outcome of tooth bleaching treatment?

_____

_____

_____

_____

17. Explain why vital teeth appear whiter immediately after completion of a tooth bleaching procedure.

_____

_____

18. What are the potential *reversible* side effects of bleaching?

_____

_____

_____

19. Identify potential *irreversible* effects of bleaching on tooth structure.

_____

_____

_____

_____

20. List methods used for vital tooth bleaching.

_____

_____

_____

 COMPETENCY EXERCISES

Apply information from the chapter and use critical thinking skills to complete the competency exercises. Write responses on paper or create electronic documents to submit your answers.

1. Although many of your patients will desire to have their teeth whitened, each must be assessed carefully to determine the safety and appropriateness of this dental procedure. Identify contraindications for tooth bleaching. As you answer this question, take into consideration all of the factors you will assess in relation to each of the various types of tooth bleaching systems that are available.

2. Maria Kennedy is a new patient. Right after you seat her in the dental chair, she points to a darkened front tooth and tells you that the tooth had a root canal

about 5 years ago. She wants to know why the over-the-counter tooth-whitening product she has applied almost made it look worse. How will you answer her question?

3. As you continue to talk with Maria, you mention that there is a procedure to whiten a nonvital tooth. She gets excited about that possibility and wants to know how the procedure is done. Even though you would like to get started with her complete history assessment and oral exam first, you know that it is important to provide at least a brief answer to her question. How will you explain the procedure to her?

4. During your assessment, you determine that there are numerous demineralized areas on the surfaces of Maria's teeth, and you suspect that these are probably due to overuse of the whitening products. What interventions will you include in her care plan to address the issue?

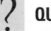 **QUESTIONS PATIENTS ASK**

What sources of information can you identify that will help you answer your patient's questions in this scenario?

"Which bleaching/whitening method is best?" "How white will my teeth actually get?" "Should I whiten my teeth before or after you place those new fillings in my front teeth?" "Can I have my teeth bleached in the office now and then use an over-the-counter product to keep them white?"

 DISCOVERY EXERCISES

1. Go to the American Dental Association Web site at http://www.ada.org/ and type the word "whitening" into the search box to find the latest ADA information about whitening products.

2. Systematic reviews offer the clinician the most reliable research and information. Do a literature search by using the following link to PubMed: http://www.ncbi.nlm.nih.gov/pubmed/ Choose clinical queries; then type "tooth whitening" in the search box. Learn about the most recent systematic reviews of tooth whitening products.

Everyday Ethics

Before completing the learning exercises below, reread and reflect on the Everyday Ethics scenario and Questions for Consideration in this chapter of the textbook. It may also be useful to review the Dental Hygiene Ethics discussion in Chapter 1, the Ethical Applications in the introduction pages for each section in the textbook, as well as the Codes of Ethics in Appendices I, II, and III.

Individual Learning Activity
Imagine that you are the dental hygienist in this scenario. Answer each of the questions for consideration at the end of the scenario.

Discovery Activity
Ask a friend or relative who is not involved in healthcare to read the scenario and discuss it with you from the perspective of a "patient" who receives services within the healthcare system. Discuss what you learned from the concerns, insights, or difference in perspective that person expressed.

Factors To Teach The Patient

This scenario is related to the following factors listed in this chapter of the textbook:

- In-office whitening may produce more sensitivity than over-the-counter and at-home products.
- In most cases, whitening must be periodically repeated to maintain desired tooth color.
- Existing tooth-colored restorations will not change color, therefore may not match and may need to be replaced after whitening.

Using the examples of patient conversations in Appendix D as a guide, write a conversation you could use to obtain informed consent for a light-activated, in-office tooth bleaching procedure. Use your conversation to educate a patient or a friend, and then modify it on the basis of what you learned from the interaction.

Implementation: Clinical Treatment

■ Chapters 37–45

 COMPETENCY EXERCISES

Apply information from the chapter and use critical think-ing skills to complete the competency exercises. Write *responses on paper or create electronic documents to submit your answers.*

SECTION VI—PATIENT ASSESSMENT SUMMARY

Patient Name: Aidan O'Connor	Age: 21	Gender: ☒ M F	☑ Initial Therapy
			☐ Maintenance
Provider Name: D.H. Student	Date: Today		☐ Re-evaluation

Chief Complaint:
"I came home from college this weekend and my mother made this appointment for me. I can't believe how much my teeth and gums are hurting. This upper right tooth—I think it is one of the molars—has just been throbbing for the past two weeks. And my mouth tastes terrible, but I can't even brush my teeth because my gums hurt so much!"

ASSESSMENT FINDINGS

Health History

■ No medical visits for two years—no current medications
■ High stress levels related to upcoming end-of-term exams
■ Tobacco use: 1 pack per day for 1 year—mostly while studying
■ Alcohol use: usually only 1 alcoholic drink daily; however, on questioning, he admits to occasional excess in alcohol use as a stress reduction measure.
■ ASA Classification—I
■ ADL level—0

At Risk for:

Social and Dental History

■ Had regular dental care as a child; Most recent visit was 2 years ago
■ Denies neglect of regular daily oral hygiene measures except for the past week or so when mouth has been hurting
■ Sips high sucrose, carbonated beverage while studying

At Risk for:

Dental Examination

- Generalized visible oral biofilm and debris in all areas of mouth
- Generalized visible calculus
- Generalized erythematic and sloughing gingival tissue; craterlike defects in lower anterior and lower left premolar area.
- No visible decay; No restorations; intact dental sealants detectable on #14 and #19. Broken sealant remnants on #3 and #30.

At Risk for:

Periodontal Diagnosis/Case Type and Status

Caries Management Risk Assessment (CAMBRA) Level:

Low   Moderate   High   Extreme

DENTAL HYGIENE DIAGNOSIS STATEMENTS RELATED TO TREATMENT INTERVENTIONS

Problem	Related to (Risk Factors and Etiology)

PLANNED INTERVENTIONS
(to arrest or control disease and regenerate, restore or maintain health)

Clinical Treatment Interventions

Review the Section VI Patient Assessment Summary for Aidan O'Connor to help you answer questions 1 through 3. The template included with his assessment summary will provide spaces for you to record your answers for these questions.

1. Complete the blank "At Risk for", Periodontal Diagnosis, and CAMBRA sections of the assessment form as best you can with the information in the patient assessment.

2. Write at least three dental hygiene diagnosis statements for Aidan's dental hygiene care plan that are related to clinical TREATMENT interventions that are within the scope of dental hygiene practice.

3. List the clinical TREATMENT interventions you will plan to help *arrest or control disease* and *regenerate, restore, or maintain* oral health in Aidan's mouth.

4. Describe the dental hygiene instruments and procedures you will select and use when you are providing dental hygiene care for each of the following patients. Discuss the rationale for your selections.

- Mrs. Louise Gaiter presents with heavy, tenacious ledges of subgingival calculus in all areas of her mouth. In most areas of her mouth, you have recorded 3- to 5-mm pocket probing depths, but in several molar areas, there is calculus to the base of 7- to 9-mm pocket probing depths. Her gingival tissues are keratinized from long-term tobacco use.

- Mr. Randall Forbes presents with spiny or nodular areas of calculus on surfaces just beneath the proximal contact areas of almost all of his teeth. His gingival tissues were bleeding heavily as you recorded 3 to 4 mm probing depths.

- Mrs. Amelia Pritchert, who has had previous periodontal surgery, presents for her maintenance appointment with some areas of slight calculus and no probing depths deeper than 3 mm. But you have recorded 3 to 4 mm of gingival recession in most of the areas of her mouth.

- Ms. Claudia Exeter drinks tea. She has very slight supragingival calculus in a few areas of her mouth but has a generalized moderate extrinsic stain on most of her tooth surfaces.

- Amal, who is 8 years old, presents with slight lower anterior calculus, generalized dental biofilm, and moderate gingivitis with bleeding on probing in all areas of his mouth.

- Mr. Robert Galen presents with slight generalized supragingival and subgingival calculus. He has a dental implant to replace tooth 38.

 ## DISCOVERY EXERCISES

1. Spend time searching the Internet to find manufacturer and/or product Web sites that provide information about instruments and local anesthesia–related products, such as syringes, cartridges, and needle-safety devices. Create a "Webliography" (similar to an annotated bibliography) that contains a list of Web addresses (URLs) for sites providing information about specific dental hygiene–related products; include a brief description of the information that each Web site contains.

2. Use the product information you find to compare current dental hygiene instruments in terms of availability, handle size, design, and price.

3. Search the literature to locate the most current evidence to support the use of a specific dental hygiene therapy, such as root planing, selective polishing, ultrasonic scaling, tooth whitening, or placement of local-delivery antibiotics during the treatment of periodontal disease. Write a brief report on your findings.

4. Search the American Dental Hygienists' Association Web site (www.adha.org) to find information about which states in the United States allow provision of local anesthesia within the scope of dental hygiene practice. Describe how the ability to provide pain control during dental hygiene procedures can affect the success of the patient's treatment.

5. Research to find out which treatment interventions described in this section of the textbook are legal dental hygiene scope of practice in your state.

6. Conduct a review of literature to determine:

- types of topical anesthesia that can be applied to an abraded or incompletely healed area.

- types of water based gel that can be used to soften crusted sutures.

FOR YOUR PORTFOLIO

1. Include a Webliography you create about any topic related to dental hygiene care (see Discovery Exercise 1).

2. A brief written report (make sure to cite your references accurately) summarizing the information you gathered during your literature search for Discovery Exercise 3 would provide excellent documentation of your ability to use outside sources to find current information about dental hygiene care.

3. Include a variety of patient care plans you have developed to highlight your expertise at planning patient-specific clinical interventions for your patients.

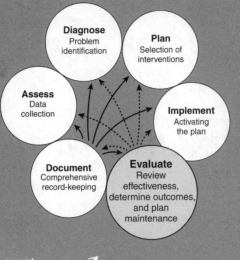

Diagnose
Problem
identification

Plan
Selection of
interventions

Assess
Data
collection

Implement
Activating
the plan

Document
Comprehensive
record-keeping

Evaluate
Review
effectiveness,
determine outcomes,
and plan
maintenance

Evaluation

Chapters 46–47

■ LEARNING OBJECTIVES

Completing the exercises in this section of the workbook will prepare you to:

1. Identify key concepts in evaluating the outcomes of dental hygiene interventions.
2. Apply outcomes assessment findings to plan maintenance care.
3. Document patient care outcomes and recommendations for follow-up care.

■ COMPETENCIES FOR THE DENTAL HYGIENIST (APPENDIX A)

Competencies supported by the learning in Section VII:

Core Competencies: C3, C4,C5, C6, C7, C9, C10, C11, C12, C13.

Health Promotion and Disease Prevention: HP2, HP4, HP5, HP6.

Patient Care: PC1, PC2, PC3, PC4, PC11, PC12, PC13.

Principles of Evaluation

Upon successful completion of these exercises, you will be able to:

1. Identify and define key terms and concepts related to evaluation of dental hygiene interventions.

2. Discuss standards for dental hygiene practice.
3. Identify skills related to self-assessment and reflective dental hygiene practice

 KNOWLEDGE EXERCISES

Write your answers for each question in the space provided.

1. State the purpose of evaluating treatment outcomes at the end of a sequence of dental hygiene interventions.

_____

_____

2. State the purpose of ongoing evaluation during each appointment of a multiappointment treatment sequence.

_____

_____

_____

3. What steps will you take to evaluate the dental hygiene care you provide for each patient?

_____

_____

_____

_____

4. List three ways to evaluate posttreatment outcomes.

_____

_____

_____

5. What is interview evaluation?

_____

_____

6. What is the reason for comparison of pre and posttreatment assessment findings?

_____

_____

7. List the six categories that provide guidance for adhering to the ADHA standards for clinical dental hygiene practice.

_____

_____

_____

_____

_____

8. List three sources for determining standard of care during a legal dispute.

_____

_____

_____

9. What is the purpose for ongoing self-assessment and personal reflection regarding professional skills and knowledge in dental hygiene practice?

_____

_____

10. Unscramble the following words help you learn about the skills you can develop for reflective dental hygiene practice.

■ kcabdeef _____

■ notiflecer _____

■ awaresself-nes _____

■ yanslais _____

■ notleavuai _____

11. Define the three steps that can be used to direct reflective thinking and self-assessment about everyday occurrences related to dental hygiene practice.

_____

_____

_____

 COMPETENCY EXERCISES

Apply information from the chapter and use critical thinking skills to complete the competency exercises. Write responses on paper or create electronic documents to submit your answers.

1. Explain the concept of professional Standards of Care. Discuss the role that dental hygiene standards of care can play in ongoing self-assessment and reflective dental hygiene practice.

2. Ms. Olivia Qaba has just moved into your town and is scheduled today as a new patient in your clinic. Dr. Kish briefly examines her, and then you spend the rest of the appointment collecting thorough assessment data and providing the dental hygiene clinical interventions and education that are required to meet her needs.

    When dental hygiene care is complete, you evaluate treatment outcomes. When you are planning maintenance care for Ms. Qaba (or for any patient), Dr. Kish requires that you consult with him to decide the appropriate maintenance interval for each case. Because Dr. Kish has only briefly examined Ms. Qaba before your treatment, he is unlikely to know as much about her as you do after your interaction with her during the series of dental hygiene appointments. What important knowledge do you bring to recommending a maintenance interval for your patient that Dr. Kish may not know after his brief examination? (*Hint*: Think about this question particularly in terms of the indicators you will use to measure the success of your dental hygiene interventions related to health behaviors).

 DISCOVERY EXERCISE

Initiate the practice of reflective self-assessment in your dental hygiene practice by starting a "Critical Incident" journal. Plan to write in the journal at least once every week until you graduate. Each week, select a situation related to your dental hygiene education that poses a question for you, causes you confusion, or is in some way meaningful for your professional development. Follow the three steps and use example questions from Table 46-2 in the textbook to write a brief (no more than 1 to 2 pages) journal entry that describes what happened, analyzes why it was important for your learning or professional practice, and outlines additional learning or next steps that will help you enhance your professionalism, clinical skills, or knowledge.

Everyday Ethics

Before completing the learning exercises below, reread and reflect on the Everyday Ethics scenario and Questions for Consideration in this chapter of the textbook. It may also be useful to review the Dental Hygiene Ethics discussion in Chapter 1, the Ethical Applications in the introduction pages for each section in the textbook, as well as the Codes of Ethics in Appendices I, II, and III.

Collaborative Learning Activity

Answer each of the questions for consideration at the end of the scenario in the textbook. Compare what you wrote with answers developed by another classmate and discuss differences/similarities.

Discovery Activity

Ask a dental hygienist who has been practicing for a year or more to read the scenario. Provide them with a copy of one of the Codes of Ethics as well. Share the responses you have made to answer each question and ask that person to discuss the situation with you. What insights did you have, or, what did you learn during this discussion?

Factors To Teach The Patient

This scenario is related to the following factors listed in this chapter of the textbook:

- The need for evaluation to establish the basis for "next step" treatment and maintenance decisions
- How outcomes from dental hygiene interventions are used to determine further treatment needs and maintenance interval

Salima, the dental hygienist in the Everyday Ethics scenario for this chapter, knows that she must educate her patient, Mrs. Midoun, during this appointment about the need to evaluate the outcomes of dental hygiene treatment. Use the examples of patient conversations in Appendix D to outline an approach that Salima can use as she provides information about the need for outcomes assessment for her patient.

CHAPTER 47

Maintenance

Upon successful completion of these exercises, you will be able to:

1. Identify the purposes, procedures, and methods for planning dental hygiene maintenance care.

2. Discuss factors that contribute to recurrence of periodontal infection.

3. Document maintenance interval recommendations.

 KNOWLEDGE EXERCISES

Write your answers for each question in the space provided.

1. If a disease does not respond to routine therapy, the disease is considered to be resistant, or _____.

2. The term _____ refers to the abatement of the symptoms of a disease.

3. The concept of continuing dental hygiene care is introduced to the patient in the initial dental hygiene care plan. Identify the purposes of a maintenance program for patients who successfully complete initial therapy.

_____

_____

_____

_____

_____

_____

4. List the factors you will consider when deciding upon a maintenance appointment interval that meets your patient's needs.

_____

_____

_____

_____

_____

_____

_____

_____

_____

5. After evaluating the success of your dental hygiene interventions, you will establish your patient's periodontal maintenance interval in consultation with your patient, the attending dentist, and sometimes even the patient's physician. What does the term *consultation* mean?

_____

_____

6. In your own words, define the types or categories of periodontal maintenance therapy.

_____

_____

_____

_____

_____

_____

7. Identify assessment procedures and dental hygiene interventions that are commonly provided during a dental hygiene maintenance appointment.

■ Assessment procedures

_____

_____

_____

_____

_____

_____

_____

_____

■ Dental hygiene interventions

_____

_____

_____

_____

_____

8. What factors contribute to the recurrence of periodontal disease?

_____

_____

_____

_____

_____

_____

9. You and the attending general dentist will decide together if there is a need to refer your patient to a periodontist for specialized periodontal therapy.

■ Under what conditions might you refer a new patient directly to a periodontist?

_____

_____

■ What criteria are used to determine referral when you evaluate treatment outcomes during a maintenance appointment after you have provided the initial therapy?

_____

_____

_____

_____

10. A dental clinic maintenance plan can be set up using a card-file system or a computer-assisted approach. Identify two administrative methods for implementing the maintenance plan and scheduling patient appointments.

_____

_____

✓ COMPETENCY EXERCISES

Apply information from the chapter and use critical thinking skills to complete the competency exercises. Write responses on paper or create electronic documents to submit your answers.

1. Many factors contribute to the success of periodontal therapy and the remission or recurrence of periodontal disease.

■ For which factors are the dental hygienist's actions particularly important in arresting disease?

■ How does patient compliance affect the recurrence of periodontal disease?

■ What risk factors for recurrence of periodontal disease are not easily modifiable by dental hygiene interventions?

■ How do all of these factors interplay when making decisions regarding the frequency of individualized patient maintenance appointments?

2. Follow your school guidelines to write a progress note documenting maintenance interval recommendations for Mrs. Qaba. (See the Factors to Teach the Patient exercise for this chapter for more information.)

DISCOVERY EXERCISE

Before you do this exercise, take a moment to read Chapter 2 in the textbook. Then read a bit about Ms. Qaba, in the Factors to Teach the Patient exercise below. Develop a PICO question related to determining an appropriate periodontal maintenance interval for Ms. Qaba. Use the PICO question you develop to find evidence in the dental literature to support your maintenance-interval recommendations.

Everyday Ethics

Before completing the learning exercises below, reread and reflect on the Everyday Ethics scenario and Questions for Consideration in this chapter of the textbook. It may also be useful to review the Dental Hygiene Ethics discussion in Chapter 1, the Ethical Applications in the introduction pages for each section in the textbook, as well as the Codes of Ethics in Appendices I, II, and III.

Individual Learning Activity
Imagine that you are the dental hygienist in this scenario. Answer each of the questions for consideration at the end of the scenario.

Collaborative Learning Activity
Work with another student colleague to role-play the scenario. The goal of this exercise is for you and your colleague to work though the alternative actions in order to come to consensus on a solution or response that is acceptable to both of you.

Factors To Teach The Patient

This scenario is related to the following factors listed in this chapter of the textbook:

- Purposes of follow-up and maintenance appointments
- Importance of keeping all maintenance appointments

Together, you and Dr. Kish decide that a 3-month maintenance interval is appropriate for Ms. Qaba (first introduced in the Competency Exercise in Chapter 46). One reason for this decision is that even though her tissues are healthy right now, she is HIV positive and has a history of significant bone loss from past periodontal infection. You know from her dental history that she has been scheduled previously for 3-month periodontal maintenance, but Ms. Qaba states that she is not sure there is much point to having her teeth cleaned so often. She says that she was really hoping to stretch the interval to 6 months because she no longer has dental insurance.

Use the example patient conversations in Appendix D as a guide to write a statement explaining your maintenance-interval recommendation to Ms. Qaba. Make sure to include a discussion of the literature articles you located when you did the discovery exercise above.

Evaluation

■ Chapters 46–47

COMPETENCY EXERCISES

Apply information from the chapter and use critical think-
ing skills to complete the Competency exercises. Write
responses on paper or create electronic documents to
submit your answers.

SECTION VII—PATIENT ASSESSMENT SUMMARY

Patient Name: Charen Woodmacher	Age: 15	Gender: M ☐ F ☒	☐ Initial Therapy
			☐ Maintenance
Provider Name: D.H. Student	Date: Today		☒ Re-evaluation

Chief Complaint:

Patient presents for re-evaluation following the completion of a series of quadrant scaling and root planing appointments with signifi-cant oral health educational interventions provided at each appointment.

RE-EVALUATION FINDINGS

Retreat ☐   **Refer** ☒   **Continuing care interval:** 6 months recall appointment
(in general practice office)

Description of posttreatment outcomes:

Resolution of carious lesion on tooth #30 (root canal completed, appointment for crown scheduled within 1 month). Patient appears to be more motivated in self-care practices and biofilm levels are significantly reduced. Generalized probing depths are reduced to 3 mm and tissue health improved: reduction in erythema, bulbous appearance and generalized bleeding. However, 6- to 8-mm pockets, with bleeding on probing, has not resolved in lower anterior sextant and in molar areas.

Referral to physician for complete medical work-up.

Referral to periodontist for assessment of specialized periodontal treatment needs.

**ASSESSMENT FINDINGS FROM CHAREN WOODMACHER'S
PRE-TREATMENT ASSESSMENT**
PROVIDED HERE FOR ADDITIONAL INFORMATION

Health History

- Recent diagnosis of bulimia—currently undergoing psychological assessment and treatment
- Iron-deficiency anemia
- Contraceptive pills
- Daily iron supplement
- ASA classification: II
- ADL level: 0

At Risk for:

- Enamel erosion
- Increased susceptibility to dental caries
- Increased gingival response to oral biofilm

Social and Dental History

- Regular dental care until 2 years ago when she started refusing to come to the dentist
- Good general knowledge, but admits to recent general neglect of oral hygiene
- Had orthodontic bands until 6 months ago, but all appliances were removed and treatment discontinued

At Risk for:

- Increased susceptibility to dental caries
- Demineralization
- Periodontal infection

Dental Examination

- Deep caries #30 with abscess visible on radiograph
- Evidence of lingual erosion on maxillary incisors
- General biofilm accumulation
- Heavy calculus in all areas
- Generalized erythema, bulbous papilla, and bleeding on probing
- Generalized 4 mm with 6- to 8-mm pockets in mandibular anterior sextant and on #3 mesial, #14 mesial and distal, and #18 mesial.

At Risk for:

- Oral pain
- Dental caries
- Gingival or periodontal infection/abscess

Read the Section I Patient Assessment Summary to help you answer questions #1 and #2.

1. According to the documentation in her re-evaluation section of her care plan, Charen Woodmacher has been referred to the periodontist for specialized care, even though her tissue health has improved because of the dental hygiene treatment she received. Explain why.

2. Even though Charen has been referred to the periodontist, the care plan recommends that a 6-month recall appointment is scheduled with the general practice dentist. Explain why. (*Hint:* It may be helpful to look at the pretreatment assessment data as you think about this question.)

 DISCOVERY EXERCISES

1. Investigate and describe the recall system that is used in your school clinic. What is your role as a student in making the system work and for making sure that complete oral health maintenance care is scheduled and delivered as needed for the patients you provide care for in your clinic?

2. As an exercise in self-evaluation, imagine that you are a clinical instructor assigned to evaluate your patient care and provide feedback at the end of a patient appointment. Before you call the instructor over at the end of one or more patient appointments, complete the same evaluation form your instructor will be using. Compare your own self-evaluation score with the score and feedback that is actually provided by your instructor for the same patient. How will differences you discover between the two evaluations redirect future self-evaluation of your clinical skills?

 FOR YOUR PORTFOLIO

Maintain a reflective journal by writing "critical incident" entries related to patient care experiences over several weeks or months during your education. Organize the individual journal entries by broad topic areas; for example ethical issues, healthcare knowledge, clinical skills, motivating patient behavior chance, etc. When you have collected several journal entries related to one topic, you can "reflect on your reflection." This action can enhance your understanding of your professional self and your ability to self-evaluate by analyzing and reflecting about what you have learned over time.

WORD SEARCH

```
E V A L U A T I O N R X Y C P R O F
F A M C X E Q F U G J N J P B E Z V
R H N T G N P Y C G M I V P N F J P
R Y Y R R E F R A C T O R Y H L K K
D G O K D P G J H X X Z L K I E P O
Z R E W B Y M F P L C M G X U C S M
Q Q D Y R C A S S E S S M E N T K Q
B D B A N A L Y S I S Y G F J I D S
U Y Y U O U T C O M E S P V M V Y O
B A C R I T I C A L I N C I D E N T
C C O M P L I A N C E G H U M P L V
E P F E E D B A C K F U A E R R Y X
R X M A F E Z P I K S Z J P D A P C
H C T T P G X X T H S O E Q A C K M
Q A S D P R E B O O K I M B G T S U
D C R I S K F A C T O R M X Z I P E
U J X M Q E D P R E C A L L Q C T N
S O X C O M P R O M I S E D M E I D
```

WORD SEARCH CLUES

1. Standard #5 in the ADHA Standards for Clinical Dental Hygiene Practice.
2. A reflective-practice journaling approach that is useful in guiding clinicians to assess and to document learning from their actions and responses during clinical situations. (two words).
3. A characteristic, habit, or predisposing condition taken into consideration when planning for the patient's maintenance interval following the evaluation of initial treatment outcomes (two words).
4. Information collected during the evaluation procedure.
5. Also called preventive maintenance and supportive periodontal therapy (an acronym).
6. Evaluated following the completion of dental hygiene treatment and patient education.
7. Refers to providing communication about the outcomes of dental hygiene treatment.
8. The "So what" component of reflection and self-assessment.
9. Perceptive self-awareness, judgment, critical analysis and synthesis of information, and application of new knowledge are key skills practitioners need for (two words).
10. This step in the dental hygiene process of care has many of the same components as the evaluation step.
11. One category of periodontal maintenance therapy (PMT).
12. The method of administering a patient's a maintenance plan by scheduling the next appointment before a patient leaves the current appointment.
13. Refers to the patient's health behavior actions that are in accordance with the clinician's recommendations.
14. A system of making appointments for the long-term maintenance needs of the patient.
15. Not responding to therapy.

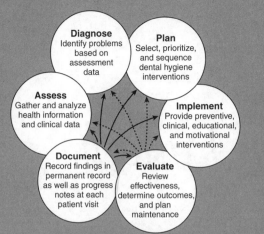

Diagnose
Identify problems based on assessment data

Plan
Select, prioritize, and sequence dental hygiene interventions

Assess
Gather and analyze health information and clinical data

Implement
Provide preventive, clinical, educational, and motivational interventions

Document
Record findings in permanent record as well as progress notes at each patient visit

Evaluate
Review effectiveness, determine outcomes, and plan maintenance

Patients With Special Needs

Chapters 48–69

■ LEARNING OBJECTIVES

Completing the exercises in this section of the workbook will prepare you to:

1. Identify treatment and education modifications necessary to meet the needs of individuals with physical, mental, and medical conditions or limitations.

2. Plan and provide dental hygiene care for individuals with special needs in both traditional and nontraditional practice settings.

3. Document all aspects of dental hygiene care.

■ COMPETENCIES FOR THE DENTAL HYGIENIST

All competencies listed in the *ADEA Competencies For Entry into the Profession of Dental Hygiene* (Appendix A) are supported by the learning in Section VIII.

The Pregnant Patient

Upon successful completion of these exercises, you will be able to:

1. Identify and define key terms and concepts related to the pregnant patient.
2. Identify the oral/facial development timetable in relationship to overall fetal development.

3. Describe oral findings common in pregnancy.
4. Plan and document dental hygiene care that addresses the unique physical, oral, and emotional considerations of the pregnant patient.

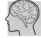 **KNOWLEDGE EXERCISES**

Write your answers for each question in the space provided.

1. The term applied to teaching ahead of time so that untoward conditions can be prevented.

   _____

2. One third of a pregnancy; a 3-month period.

   _____

3. A factor that can cause disease or malformation during fetal development.

   _____

4. An antibiotic that has the well-known effect of staining the infant's teeth if taken by the pregnant mother after 4 months of gestation.

   _____

5. A class of drug that, if taken by the mother, can cause low muscle tone and poor sucking reflex in the infant.

   _____

6. List three oral findings that are common during pregnancy.

   _____

   _____

   _____

7. In your own words, describe the clinical appearance and symptoms of a "pregnancy tumor."

   _____

   _____

8. List three signs you might observe in your pregnant patient that would make you suspect depression.

   _____

   _____

   _____

9. Is the following statement true or false? To ensure that the developing teeth of their unborn children will be protected, all pregnant women should

receive prenatal vitamins containing fluoride. Provide a rationale for your answer.

_____

_____

10. Visualizing a timeline can often help put information into perspective. Use the timeline (in Figure 48-1 below) to identify the oral/facial feature that is developing in the fetus during the approximate time indicated by each of the lettered segments.

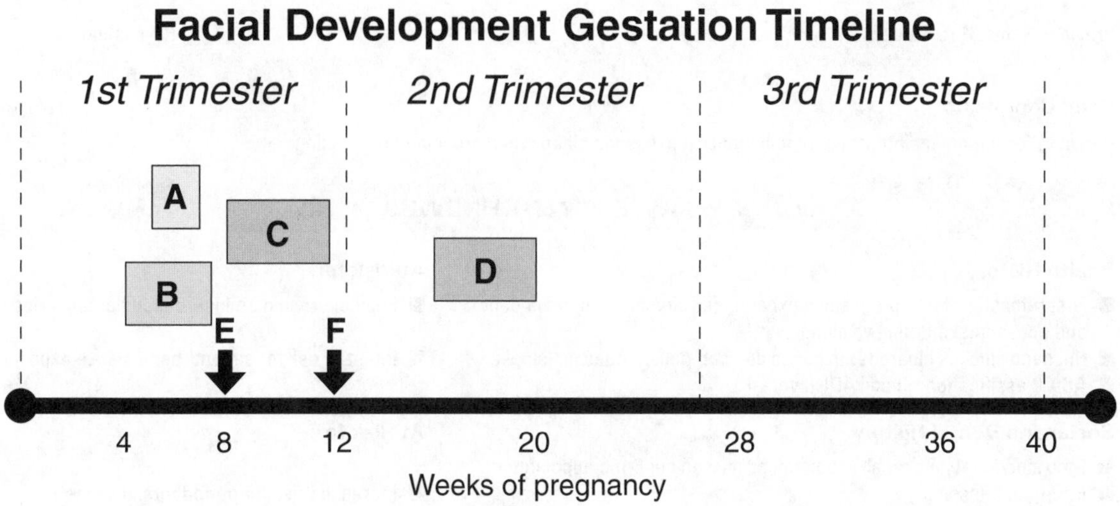

Facial Development Gestation Timeline

Figure 48-1

A. _____

B. _____

C. _____

D. _____

E. By this time (8th week) a _____ _____ is apparent in the developing fetus.

F. By this time (12th week) a _____ _____ is apparent in the developing fetus.

11. What are the possible adverse effects on the fetus when a woman smokes during pregnancy?

_____

_____

12. Identify reasons why some women have more problems with gingivitis during pregnancy.

_____

_____

13. What is the supine hypertensive syndrome?

_____

_____

_____

14. List the symptoms of supine hypertensive syndrome.

_____

_____

_____

✔ COMPETENCY EXERCISES

Apply information from the chapter and use critical thinking skills to complete the competency exercises. Write responses on paper or create electronic documents to submit your answers.

1. Mrs. Jill Mason, who is late in the second trimester of a healthy pregnancy, presents for her dental hygiene appointment with a toothache and a swelling on the right side of her mandible. The dentist orders a single periapical radiograph of the area. Mrs. Mason is concerned about the effect of the radiation on her developing baby. Using all the information available to you in Chapter 48, describe the educational approach, protective measures, and radiographic techniques you will use to relieve her fears and maximize safety for her and the baby.

2. Using the format for writing progress notes that is used in your school, document the patient position adaption that was used during Mrs. Mason's treatment.

CHAPTER 48—PATIENT ASSESSMENT SUMMARY

Patient Name: Mrs. Diane White   Age: 27   Gender: M [F]   ☐ Initial Therapy

☑ Maintenance

Provider Name: D.H. Student   Date: Today   ☐ Re-evaluation

Chief Complaint:

Presents for routine maintenance appointment. Gum tissues bleed when brushing and flossing.

ASSESSMENT FINDINGS

Health History

- First trimester of first pregnancy; experiences significant nausea daily and occasional morning vomiting
- Husband smokes cigarettes in house and car; patient does not smoke.
- ASA Classification - II and ADL level - 0

At Risk for:

- Enamel erosion and increased dental caries risk
- Infant at risk for second-hand smoke exposure

Social and Dental History

- 9 mo since previous recall appointment; missed her 6-mo appointment.
- Infrequent flossing
- Uses bottled water with no fluoride content; smell of fluoridated toothpaste makes her feel nauseated.
- Frequent high-carbohydrate snacks (graham crackers) to help control nausea

At Risk for:

- Increased risk for periodontal disease
- Increased caries risk and risk for enamel erosion
- Increased caries risk

Dental Examination

- No current cavitated lesions; a small number of occlusal surface restorations are all in good repair.
- Moderate biofilm along cervical margins and on proximal surfaces
- Generalized 4-mm probing depths; no radiographic indication of bone loss
- Generalized red, bulbous tissue and generalized bleeding on probing

At Risk for:

- Increased risk for caries and periodontal infection
- Oral infection, increased risk for periodontal/gingival infection
- Increased risk for periodontal/gingival infection and pyogenic granuloma

Periodontal Diagnosis/Case Type and Status

Gingivitis

Caries Management Risk Assessment (CAMBRA) Level:

☐ Low ☑ Moderate ☐ High ☐ Extreme

Read the Chapter 48 Patient Assessment Summary for Mrs. White to help you answer questions the following questions.

3. Mrs. White mentions that she frequently experiences nausea, gagging, and vomiting followed by an unpleasant taste. You realize from looking at the patient assessment data collected during her previous appointment that she is at risk for several additional oral problems. Identify the possible oral problems, and provide three self-care measures that will minimize their oral effects.

4. Using the dental hygiene diagnosis format, identify a cause or factor that could result in increased risk for dental caries during the course of Mrs. White's pregnancy.

5. Write a goal for the problem that you identified in your dental hygiene diagnosis in question 4. Include a time frame for meeting the goal. How will you measure whether your patient met the goal?

Everyday Ethics

Before completing the learning exercises below, reread and reflect on the Everyday Ethics scenario and Questions for Consideration in this chapter of the textbook. It may also be useful to review the Dental Hygiene Ethics discussion in Chapter 1, the Ethical Applications in the introduction pages for each section in the textbook, as well as the Codes of Ethics in Appendices I, II, and III.

Collaborative Learning Activity
Answer each of the questions for consideration at the end of the scenario in the textbook. Compare what you wrote

with answers developed by another classmate and discuss differences/similarities.

Discovery Activity
Ask a friend or relative who is not involved in healthcare to read the scenario and discuss it with you from the perspective of a "patient" who receives services within the healthcare system. Discuss what you learned from the concerns, insights, or difference in perspective that person expressed.

? QUESTIONS PATIENTS ASK

What sources of information can you identify that will help you answer your patient's questions in this scenario?

"Because of my nausea, I have to eat frequent small snacks. I usually nibble on granola bars—those are

healthy snacks, aren't they?" "I heard that pregnancy takes calcium away from my teeth, so is that why I seem to be getting more cavities?" "Should I just wait until after the baby is born to have my fillings done?" "Is it safe to use a mouthwash while I am pregnant?"

 ## Factors To Teach The Patient

This scenario is related to the following factors listed in this chapter of the textbook:

■ Why control measures are learned before and in conjunction with scaling
■ Facts of oral disease prevention and oral health promotion relevant to the patient's current level of health care knowledge and individual risk factors

Using the example Patient Assessment Summary for Mrs. White, your answers to the questions about her in the

Competency exercises for this chapter, and the example conversations provided in Appendix D as a guide, prepare an outline for a conversation that you might use to educate Mrs. White regarding one of the problems identified in the dental hygiene diagnosis. Use the conversation to educate a patient or friend, and then modify it based on what you learned by using the outline.

Pediatric Oral Health Care: Infancy Through Age 5

Upon successful completion of these exercises, you will be able to:

1. Identify and define key terms and concepts related to pediatric oral health care.
2. Identify risk factors for oral disease in children.
3. Discuss the role of the dental hygienist in providing early oral care intervention.
4. Discuss anticipatory guidance for parents of infants and toddlers.
5. Explain tooth development and eruption patterns.
6. Use knowledge of specific oral health issues, child management techniques, caries management by risk assessment and clinical procedures to plan dental hygiene care and oral health education for infants/toddlers and their parents.

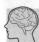 **KNOWLEDGE EXERCISES**

Write your answers for each question in the space provided.

1. Match the following term or concept with the most appropriate age-related phrase.

TERM/CONCEPT	AGE
_____ Weaning to a sippy cup	A. At 2 y of age
_____ Preschool child	B. Before 12 mo of age
_____ First dental visit	C. At approximately 6 mo of age
_____ Tiny "smear" of toothpaste	D. Tiny infant
_____ Toddler	E. 3–5 y of age
_____ Neonate	F. 1–3 y of age

2. List three indications for making a radiograph of a 3-year-old child's dentition.

_____

_____

_____

3. List the four principles of Caries Management by Risk Assessment (CAMBRA).

_____

_____

_____

_____

4. List at least three important factors to address when interviewing parents or guardians regarding their child's risk factors for oral disease.

_____

_____

_____

_____

_____

5. When the oral healthcare provider performs a knee-to-knee examination, who stabilizes the infant's legs and hands? For what purpose would this position be reversed?

_____

_____

6. How much toothpaste is appropriate for parents to place on the toothbrush of a 4-year-old?

_____

_____

7. List two common causes of halitosis (bad breath) in children.

_____

_____

8. List three indications that suggest need for orthodontic evaluation of a child patient.

_____

_____

_____

9. Identify at least three areas that are appropriate to address when you are providing anticipatory guidance for the parents of a 4-year-old.

_____

_____

_____

10. Provide anticipatory guidance and age-related guidelines for parents regarding the following oral health care milestones.

   a. Begin using fluoride toothpaste _____

   _____

   b. Find a dental home _____

   _____

   c. Eliminate thumb and finger sucking _____

   _____

   d. Wean from the bottle _____

   _____

   e. Clean the oral cavity _____

   _____

   f. Avoid feeding/grazing at will _____

   _____

   g. Examine the mouth for oral health problems _____

   _____

11. List the advantages of weaning a baby from the bottle to a regular cup.

_____

_____

12. Identify ways a mother could provide comfort to a child who is in pain from teething.

_____

_____

COMPETENCY EXERCISES

Apply information from the chapter and use critical thinking skills to complete the competency exercises. Write responses on paper or create electronic documents to submit your answers.

1. In your own words, define _early childhood caries_ as if you were explaining the concept to a parent.

2. Explain why knowledge of expected developmental milestones and the child's actual developmental level are necessary when providing dental care for that child.

3. Make up three terms/names for dental equipment or instruments (different from those mentioned in the textbook) that you might use to explain what is happening during a dental visit to an anxious preschooler. For extra fun, share your names with those of your student colleagues.

4. Angela Flores, 3 years old, sits quietly in the dental chair for several minutes while you speak with her mother. She allows you to tilt the chair into a supine position but begins to cry as soon as you approach her mouth with your mirror and explorer. She continues to cry and reach for her mother even after you explain all the fun games you will play together while you examine her teeth. Outline an appropriate response to this situation.

5. You are conducting an oral health education class for a mother's group at the community center near your house as part of a community service project. The mother of a darling 3-month-old girl asks you when

she can expect her baby's teeth to start coming in. Explain the development and eruption patterns of primary teeth.

6. Explain to this young mother why healthy primary teeth are important for the growth and development of a healthy permanent dentition.

7. Explain how a parent can transfer *Streptococcus mutans* from her mouth to the infant's mouth.

DISCOVERY EXERCISES

Go to your local pharmacy, grocery store, or department store and find different brands and types of pacifiers available for parents to select for their baby. Use the criteria listed in Chapter 49 of the textbook to determine which brand and type of pacifier you will recommend for your patients.

Everyday Ethics

Before completing the learning exercises below, reread and reflect on the Everyday Ethics scenario and Questions for Consideration in this chapter of the textbook. It may also be useful to review the Dental Hygiene Ethics discussion in Chapter 1, the Ethical Applications in the introduction pages for each section in the textbook, as well as the Codes of Ethics in Appendices I, II, and III.

Individual Learning Activity

Imagine that you have observed what happened in the scenario, but are not one of the main characters involved in the situation. Write a reflective journal entry that:

- describes how you might have reacted (as an observer- not as a participant),

- expresses your personal feelings about what happened, or
- identifies personal values that affect your reaction to the situation.

Discovery Activity

Ask a dental hygienist who has been practicing for a year or more to read the scenario. Provide them with a copy of one of the Codes of Ethics as well. Share the responses you have made to answer each question and ask that person to discuss the situation with you. What insights did you have or what did you learn during this discussion?

Factors To Teach The Patient

This scenario is related to the following factors:

- How the bacteria that cause dental caries can be transferred to a baby's mouth
- How fluoride makes enamel stronger and more resistant to the bacteria that cause dental caries
- Methods to prevent dental caries from developing in a young child's mouth
- How feeding methods and snacking patterns can contribute to dental caries
- How the parent can examine the infant/child's mouth and what to look for during the examination

Mr. and Mrs. Jacobson are in your treatment room with their son, Eric, who is 2.5 years old. The dentist has diagnosed incipient early childhood caries based on observations made during her examination. You have been asked to educate these very concerned parents about how and why this is happening to their son and what can be done to arrest the decay process and prevent further problems.

Use the example of a patient conversation in Appendix D as a guide to outline a conversation you might have with the Jacobsons. Compare your conversation with a student colleague's to identify any missing information.

CHAPTER 50

The Patient With a Cleft Lip and/or Palate

Learning Objectives

Upon successful completion of these exercises, you will be able to:

1. Identify and define key terms and concepts related to oral/facial clefts.
2. Identify prenatal risk factors and developmental time frame for oral/facial clefts.
3. Describe treatment for oral/facial clefts.
4. Use knowledge of the oral, physical, and personal characteristics of the patient to plan and document dental hygiene care and oral hygiene instructions.

 KNOWLEDGE EXERCISES

Write your answers for each question in the space provided.

1. Describe the direction of the formation/fusion of the lip and palatal structures during development.

   _____
   _____

2. During which embryonic weeks does the palate develop?

   _____

3. How is a class 3 craniofacial cleft defined?

   _____

4. Which classes of facial cleft involve lack of fusion in the premaxilla?

   _____

5. Which class of cleft is identified as a submucous, imperfect muscle union cleft across the soft palate, producing an incomplete closure of the pharynx?

6. List three environmental risk factors for craniofacial clefts.

   _____
   _____
   _____

7. List three common characteristics that can affect the *teeth* of a patient with a craniofacial cleft.

   _____
   _____
   _____

8. List the three categories of professionals who contribute members to an interdisciplinary team for treatment of an individual with cleft lip and/or palate.

   _____
   _____
   _____

9. Identify one of the dental specialties in which clinicians may provide care for a patient with a cleft and describe that practitioner's role in the treatment of the patient.

_____

_____

10. Ideally, treatment of a craniofacial cleft is begun before the infant is 6 months old. What is the purpose for such early intervention?

_____

_____

_____

_____

11. What are the goals of surgical treatment for cleft lip and palate?

_____

_____

_____

_____

_____

12. In your own words, describe the benefits a dental prosthesis can provide for a patient with a cleft lip and palate.

_____

_____

_____

_____

✓ COMPETENCY EXERCISES

Apply information from the chapter and use critical thinking skills to complete the competency exercises. Write responses on paper or create electronic documents to submit your answers.

1. Discuss why lack of prenatal care is considered a risk factor for cleft lip and/or palate.

2. Describe characteristics that may make it difficult to communicate with an individual who has an incomplete palatal closure.

3. Adam Horconcitos, a 12-year-old, has recently come to America from Honduras to live with Mr. and Mrs. Mehlisch, his American adoptive parents. Adam has a class 5 unilateral (left side) facial cleft that was not treated when he was an infant. He is scheduled for his first surgical procedure in about 3 weeks. You are a member of Adam's care team, and you are seeing him today for the first time to evaluate his oral status.

The only dental visits Adam has had previously were about 2 years ago with a prosthodontist in Honduras. The doctor fabricated an appliance to provide for some closure of the palatal opening to enhance Adam's ability to swallow and speak.

When you talk with Adam and the Mehlisches before the boy's examination, you find that Adam speaks fairly good English, because he went to an American school in his own country. He is a handsome, personable, and likable young man; but he is really very shy and frequently hides his mouth and nose behind his hand as he speaks to you. His voice has a kind of nasal sound, but his hearing is normal, and with a bit of concentration, you can understand him fairly well. Adam does not have any major health problems, except for a susceptibility to frequent sore throats and ear infections.

Adam did not enjoy a good dental experience during the fabrication of his prosthesis or during his recent visits with the oral surgeon to plan his surgical care. He is extremely fearful of anyone or anything that comes near his mouth. In spite of that, he is wearing the prosthetic appliance every day, and it seems to be working well for him.

You are successful in using all of your most comforting patient management techniques, and you convince Adam to allow his mouth to be examined. During your examination, you discover that he has a mixed dentition with five primary molars still being retained, significant malocclusions, and two missing anterior teeth in the area of the cleft. His level of dental caries is fortunately quite low—only one small cavity in a deciduous molar that is already loose. You conclude, from a discussion with Mrs. Mehlisch, that Adam's snacking habits are not highly cariogenic.

His gingival health, however, is another matter. He won't usually let anyone touch his mouth, and he doesn't like to have a toothbrush near his mouth even when he does it himself. You find extensive biofilm accumulation on his teeth, gums, and tongue as well as on the prosthodontic appliance he wears. His mother complains that his breath is often very bad. His gums bleed extremely easily when they are touched.

Using the information in the case description above and a copy of the Dental Hygiene Care Plan template in Appendix B of the workbook, write an individualized dental hygiene care plan for Adam.

4. Using your school's format for writing progress notes, document the assessment visit for Adam's permanent record.

Everyday Ethics

Before completing the learning exercises below, reread and reflect on the Everyday Ethics scenario and Questions for Consideration in this chapter of the textbook. It may also be useful to review the Dental Hygiene Ethics discussion in Chapter 1, the Ethical Applications in the introduction pages for each section in the textbook, as well as the Codes of Ethics in Appendices I, II, and III.

Individual Learning Activities

■ Imagine that you are the dental hygienist in this scenario. Answer each of the questions for consideration at the end of the scenario.

■ Identify a situation you have experienced that presents a similar ethical dilemma. Write about you would do differently now than you did at the time the incident happened—support your discussion with concepts from the dental hygiene codes of ethics.

Factors To Teach The Patient

This scenario is related to the following factors listed in this chapter of the textbook:

■ Parental anticipatory guidance (Tables 49-1 and 49-2 in Chapter 49 of the textbook)

Today your patient is Mrs. Diane White, who you first met in the Chapter 48 Competency Exercises. You have been providing dental hygiene care for her since she was in her first trimester of pregnancy. About 3 months ago, her little girl was born with a class 3 cleft palate. Although the child is well cared for by an interdisciplinary team of healthcare

workers at the local hospital, Mrs. White notes that there is no dental hygienist on the team. She asks you for advice in providing oral care for her child as she grows.

Use information about cleft palate (Chapter 50 in the textbook) and what you have learned about parental anticipatory guidance (in Chapter 49 in the textbook) to role-play this situation with a fellow student. If you are Mrs. White in the role-play, be sure to ask questions. If you are the dental hygienist, try to anticipate questions and answer them in your explanation.

CROSSWORD PUZZLE

ACROSS

1. A prosthesis designed to cover the cleft of a hard palate.
4. Pertaining to the part of the skull that encloses the brain and the face.
8. This insufficiency affects closure of the opening between the mouth and nose in speech, resulting in a nasal-sounding voice.
11. Genetic transmission of traits from parents to offspring.
13. A term describing a cleft of the uvula.
15. Tissue transplanted and expected to become a part of the host tissue.
16. Plastic surgery of nose and lip.
17. Pertaining to or arising through the action of many factors.
20. Replaces or improves function of any absent part of the human body.
21. Combination of symptoms commonly occurring together.
22. Pertaining to the function of the skeletal system and its associated functions.
23. Type of surgical procedure that repositions parts of the maxilla or mandible.
24. Bilateral cleft lip separates this from its normal fusion with the entire maxilla.
25. Plastic reconstruction of the palate.

DOWN

2. Insertion of an indwelling tube to facilitate passage of air or evacuation of secretions.
3. One source of the bone used for an autogenous bone graft.
5. Present at and existing from the time of birth.
6. The process of restoring a person's abilities to the maximum possible fitness.
7. A surgical repair of a lip defect.
9. The process of acquiring fitness for the first time; associated with persons who have acquired disabilities.
10. A graft transferred from one part of the patient's body to another part.
12. One important member of the interdisciplinary team who will treat the patient with a cleft lip and/or palate (two words).
14. An agent, such as drugs of abuse during the first trimester of a pregnancy, that can increase risk for cleft lip and palate.
18. When this normal process does not happen during development, a facial cleft can result.
19. A type of graft placed before the eruption of maxillary teeth at a cleft site to create a normal architecture through which the teeth can erupt.

CHAPTER 51

The Patient With an Endocrine Disorder or Hormonal Change

Upon successful completion of these exercises, you will be able to:

1. Identify and define key terms and concepts related to hormonal function and hormone disorders.
2. Identify the major endocrine glands and describe the function of each.

3. Identify and describe physical, mental, emotional, and oral health factors commonly associated with adolescence and puberty.
4. Identify and describe physical, mental, emotional, and oral health factors commonly associated with menses and menopause.

 KNOWLEDGE EXERCISES

Write your answers for each question in the space provided.

1. Hormones that, together with the nervous system, maintain body homeostasis are excreted by _____ _____ and transported to body cells or other glands by _____ or _____.

2. List the major endocrine glands and briefly describe the function of each.

_____
_____
_____
_____
_____
_____
_____

_____
_____
_____
_____

3. Both _____ _____ and _____ _____ of a hormone can affect a patient's physical and mental status.

4. Identify the term defined or described by each of the following statements relating to hormones, puberty, and the female menstrual cycle.

a. A chemical produced by the human body that has a specific regulatory function on other body cells or organs

_____

b. A collective name for the hormones produced by the ovaries; responsible for development of female characteristics

_____

c. A hormone that, along with estrogen, is present at various levels during the female menstrual cycle

_____

d. A collective name for the hormones produced by the testes; responsible for the development of male characteristics

_____

e. A synthetic hormone contained, either as a combination with estrogen or as a single preparation, in oral contraceptives

_____

f. The period of time from the beginning of one menstrual flow to the beginning of the next menstrual flow

_____

g. A term referring to menstruation

_____

h. Menstrual intervals >45 days

_____

i. Absence of spontaneous menstrual cycles during the reproductive years

_____

j. Difficult and painful menstruation

_____

k. A condition of the endometrium that causes pelvic pain

_____

l. The lining of the uterus

_____

m. A cluster of behavioral, somatic, affective, and cognitive disorders that appear in the luteal phase of the menstrual cycle and resolve rapidly with the onset of menses

_____

n. A feeling of fullness, soreness, or pain in the breast

_____

o. Feeling unwell, unhappy, or depressed

_____

p. Pertaining to secretion of a substance directly into blood or lymph rather than into a duct; the opposite of exocrine

_____

q. Enlargement of the thyroid gland, may indicate Grave's disease or Hashimoto's thyroiditis

_____

r. Thickening of the skin, blunting of the senses and intellect, labored speech associated with hypothyroidism

_____

5. Cyclic menstruation is regulated by fluctuations in estrogen and progesterone and, with some variations and irregularities, is usually about 28 days in length. In your own words, explain how the levels of each of these two hormones vary relative to menstruation and ovulation during the menstrual cycle. (*Hint:* Describe Figure 51-2 in the textbook.)

_____

_____

_____

_____

_____

_____

6. Some women experience discomfort for several days preceding the beginning of their menstrual flow. If your patient mentions that she is feeling the effects of premenstrual symptoms, what is she likely to be experiencing?

_____

_____

_____

_____

_____

7. Define the two types of dysmenorrhea.

   _____

   _____

   _____

   _____

8. If your patient is experiencing irregularity or other problems with her menstrual cycle, a careful assessment and review of her health history is imperative, because she can also be experiencing other _____ _____ problems.

9. List the side effects of oral contraceptives that will be of concern when you are providing dental hygiene care for your patient.

   _____

   _____

   _____

10. Identify the term defined or described by each of following statements relating to adolescents.

    a. Chronic skin disorder associated with hormone fluctuation in adolescents

       _____

    b. Early is 10 to 13 years of age, middle is 14 to 17 years of age, and late is 18 to 21 years of age

       _____

    c. The period during which the gonads mature and begin to function

       _____

    d. Referring to someone around the age of puberty

       _____

    e. Coming to the age of sexual maturity

       _____

    f. Identifies the onset of menstruation

       _____

    g. The process of male sperm production

       _____

11. Summarize the effects of puberty-linked hormone increases have on the physical development of both males and females.

    _____

    _____

    _____

    _____

12. List the three health basics that teens need for general well-being.

    _____

    _____

    _____

13. What dental disease related to eating habits has a higher incidence during adolescence than any other age group?

    _____

14. A healthy diet is important at any age. Identify two eating disorders that are especially associated with teens who have a distorted body image.

    _____

    _____

15. What nutritional deficiency is related to the onset of menstruation in teenage girls?

    _____

16. Hormonal changes during puberty can cause an _____ response to bacterial biofilm and increase your adolescent patient's risk for _____.

17. List factors that increase your adolescent patient's risk for periodontitis.

    _____

    _____

    _____

    _____

    _____

    _____

    _____

18. Between 5% and 47% of adolescents around the world demonstrate evidence of periodontal loss of attachment. Which two periodontal diseases are most likely implicated?

_____

_____

19. List examples of oral problems you may observe when you perform an oral assessment of a teenage patient.

_____

_____

_____

_____

_____

20. The dental hygienist who understands the psychosocial development that adolescents are undergoing as they mature can communicate more successfully while teaching them about their oral health. List common emotional and behavioral changes that can affect teaching/learning of oral health measures during _early_ adolescence.

_____

_____

_____

_____

21. List educational approaches you can take that will have the most impact on motivation and compliance of your teenage patients and thus the most significant influence on their oral health status.

_____

_____

_____

_____

_____

22. Identify the term defined or described by each of the following statements relating to menopause.

a. A normal condition of aging in which there is complete and permanent cessation of menstrual flow

_____

b. Physiologic reaction that causes the hot flashes and night sweats characteristic of menopause

_____

c. A prescription of purified or synthetic hormone to correct or prevent undesirable symptoms of menopause

_____

23. Most adverse oral changes related to menopause can be prevented or diminished with adequate nutrition and thorough daily oral hygiene care. List the oral changes that can be associated with menopause.

_____

_____

_____

_____

_____

_____

✓ COMPETENCY EXERCISES

Apply information from the chapter and use critical thinking skills to complete the competency exercises. Write responses on paper or create electronic documents to submit your answers.

Charen Woodmacher, 15 years of age, and her mother both arrive for Charen's scheduled dental hygiene appointment. You haven't seen Charen in almost 2 years because, as her mother told you on the telephone, Charen has simply refused to come for dental appointments. Mrs. Woodmacher told you also that Charen's braces were finally removed about 6 months ago and the treatment was never completed because of Charen's attitude.

You greet Charen in the reception room, and she just rolls her eyes. She continues to slouch in the comfortable chair and keeps her book open. Mrs. Woodmacher sighs and pulls Charen upright; they both follow you down to the treatment room.

When you update the teen's medical history, her mother informs you that Charen has recently been diagnosed with bulimia and is currently under medical and psychological treatment for the disorder. Charen has iron-deficiency anemia and is taking a daily supplement; she also takes a combination estrogen/progestin oral contraceptive.

Mrs. Woodmacher finally goes back to the waiting room, and you direct your next few questions to Charen. She states, "That tooth on the lower left side has been bothering me, and my mother says that I need my teeth cleaned." Your intraoral assessment findings include deep occlusal decay on tooth 30, with evidence of an abscess on the periapical radiograph of that area.

You document evidence of enamel erosion on the maxillary anterior teeth, generalized biofilm accumulation and heavy calculus in all areas, and generalized erythematous and bleeding tissues. Probing depths in the anterior teeth are generally 4 mm, and there are numerous areas of 6- to 7-mm depth in the posterior teeth.

Make a copy of the Patient Specific Care Plan in Appendix B, or use the format for care planning used in your school to write a care plan for Charen.

1. What are Charen's oral and general health risks based on the significant findings from her assessment data?

2. Dr. Hillcrest, the dentist where you practice, prescribes antibiotics for the abscess on Charen's lower right molar. What specific counseling/patient education topic will you need to address with Charen because of this prescription?

3. Write at least two dental hygiene diagnosis statements for Charen's dental hygiene care plan.

4. What dental hygiene interventions will you plan to address in each of the dental hygiene diagnosis statements written in question 3?

5. Write one goal for each problem identified in the dental hygiene diagnoses in question 3. Include a time frame for meeting the goals. How will you measure whether or not your patient met the goals?

Everyday Ethics

Before completing the learning exercises below, reread and reflect on the Everyday Ethics scenario and Questions for Consideration in this chapter of the textbook. It may also be useful to review the Dental Hygiene Ethics discussion in Chapter 1, the Ethical Applications in the introduction pages for each section in the textbook, as well as the Codes of Ethics in Appendices I, II, and III.

Individual Learning Activity
Imagine that you are the dental hygienist in this scenario. Answer each of the questions for consideration at the end of the scenario.

Collaborative Learning Activity
Work with another student colleague to role-play the scenario. The goal of this exercise is for you and your colleague to work though the alternative actions in order to come to consensus on a solution or response that is acceptable to both of you.

Factors To Teach The Patient

This scenario is related to the following factors listed in this chapter of the textbook:

- The benefits of fluoride throughout life
- The importance of nutrition, exercise, and sleep for good health

Today is the first time you are providing dental hygiene care for Rosalee Ayers, age 55 years. She arrives late and mentions that because she is under high stress these days and hasn't been eating or sleeping very well; she overslept this morning. Rosalee is a high-powered businesswoman who takes great pride in her youthful appearance and her healthy lifestyle. As you update her health history, you note that she has received regular dental hygiene care for the last 15 years. Her general health status is very good, and she takes no medications. A notation in her record states that she is in menopause; her menses ceased 1 year ago.

When you begin your oral examination, Rosalee mentions that because of the oral hygiene instruction she has received at this clinic, she has always brushed and flossed every day. Lately, however, she has noticed that her mouth frequently feels really dry, and sometimes she feels a burning sensation on her tongue, palate, and inside her lips.

Your assessment findings indicate that her biofilm levels are very low, there are very few dental restorations, and there are no current carious lesions.

Her oral tissues are generally very healthy looking. Periodontal pocket depths are all <3 mm. Past periodontal charts have recorded generalized 2- to 3-mm recession in all premolar and molar areas, but there are no changes in the level of recession when you do your periodontal charting today.

After your assessment is complete, you write a brief care plan and, because of your patient's increased risk for root caries, you include a recommendation for fluoride treatment.

When you discuss your care plan with Rosalee, she chuckles and says, "Look, I'm not a kid any more. What on earth do I need a fluoride treatment for?"

Use the examples of patient conversations in Appendix D as a guide to write a conversation explaining your recommendations to Rosalee.

CHAPTER 52

The Older Adult Patient

Upon successful completion of these exercises, you will be able to:

1. Identify and define key terms and concepts related to aging.
2. Identify physical, general health, and oral health changes that are characteristic of aging.
3. Describe the effects of osteoporosis and Alzheimer disease on oral health status.
4. Plan and document dental hygiene interventions and health education approaches that enhance the oral health of the elderly patient.

KNOWLEDGE EXERCISES

Write your answers for each question in the space provided.

1. In your own words, define the following terms related to aging.

   a. Aging

   _____
   _____

   b. Senescence

   _____
   _____

   c. Gerontology

   _____
   _____

   d. Geriatrics

   _____
   _____

   e. Biologic age

   _____
   _____

   f. Chronologic age

   _____
   _____

   g. Psychological age

   _____
   _____

   h. Life expectancy

   _____
   _____

2. There are two common classifications used to define individuals from elderly populations: age related and function related. These two systems used together can help provide an accurate description of your aging patients. List the categories for each of these classifications.

a. Age-related classifications

_____

_____

_____

_____

b. Function-related classifications

_____

_____

_____

3. Differentiate between the terms *primary aging* and *secondary aging*.

_____

_____

_____

_____

4. For each of the following body systems, describe at least two changes that occur because of primary aging.

a. Musculoskeletal

_____

_____

_____

b. Skin

_____

_____

_____

c. Cardiovascular

_____

_____

_____

d. Respiratory

_____

_____

_____

e. Gastrointestinal

_____

_____

f. Central and Peripheral Nervous

_____

_____

_____

g. Senses

_____

_____

_____

h. Endocrine

_____

_____

_____

i. Immune

_____

_____

_____

5. The elderly may react differently to disease than your younger patients. Identify the differences mentioned in the textbook.

_____

_____

_____

_____

6. List four of the most common chronic health conditions of the elderly.

_____

_____

_____

_____

7. What risk factor related to chronic diseases is associated with increased risk for dental caries in older adult patients?

_____

_____

8. List the risk factors for osteoporosis.

_____

_____

_____

_____

_____

_____

_____

9. Your older patient with osteoporosis is considered to be at greater risk for periodontal bone loss. List the factors that relate osteoporosis to periodontal disease.

_____

_____

10. What medication, sometimes used in treatment for osteoporosis is a contraindication for dental surgery?

_____

11. Briefly describe each of the five progressive stages of Alzheimer's disease and indicate the patient care modifications or dental hygiene management considerations appropriate for each stage.

STAGE	DESCRIPTION	DENTAL HYGIENE CARE CONSIDERATIONS
1		
2		
3		
4		
5		
6		
7		

12. Identify the age-associated oral conditions described by each of the following statements:

    a. Difficulty swallowing

    _____

    b. Oral lesion that appears as skinfolds with fissuring at the corner of the mouth; not specifically an age-related lesion but is frequently seen among elderly persons

    _____

    c. Burning, smooth, shiny, bald tongue with atrophied papillae; related to nutritional deficiencies

    _____

    d. Deep red or bluish nodular masses commonly found during an intraoral examination of older individuals on either side of the midline on the ventral surface of the tongue

    _____

    e. Oral condition often noted in the elderly that is related to pathologic states, drug-induced changes, or radiation-induced degeneration of salivary glands

    _____

    f. Dental disease occurring in older folks that is related to cementum exposed by periodontal infections and often to xerostomia

    _____

13. A dry, purse-string opening of your elderly patient's lips may make wide opening difficult during dental hygiene treatment. What causes this condition?

    _____

    _____

14. In your own words, describe common age-related degenerative changes to oral mucosa.

    _____

    _____

15. Identify the risk factors for oral candidiasis that may be present in your elderly patient.

    _____

    _____

    _____

16. Identify risk factors that may contribute to root caries in the elderly.

    _____

    _____

    _____

    _____

    _____

17. Periodontal findings reflect the patterns of health and disease over the years of your older patient's life. Describe the range of tissue changes that may be noted when examining an older patient.

    _____

    _____

    _____

    _____

    _____

18. Identify the barriers that can negatively impact access to dental hygiene care for an elderly individual.

    _____

    _____

    _____

    _____

19. Older patients often use more prescription drugs and more over-the-counter medications than other age groups. List the ways you can be sure that you know what drugs your patient is taking and that you make appropriate decisions when you plan dental hygiene care.

    _____

    _____

    _____

    _____

20. List factors likely to occur in your elderly patient that can contribute to accumulation and retention of dental biofilm and increased difficulty in removal.

    _____

    _____

    _____

    _____

21. Describe specific biofilm removal methods and techniques that you can recommend for an elderly patient.

_____

_____

_____

22. Caloric intake must decrease to control weight as elderly individuals become less physically active. However, nutritional needs of older individuals are not different from those of younger adults. What factors can contribute to dietary and nutritional deficiencies in your older patients?

_____

_____

_____

_____

_____

_____

_____

_____

_____

_____

_____

_____

_____

_____

Everyday Ethics

Before completing the learning exercises below, reread and reflect on the Everyday Ethics scenario and Questions for Consideration in this chapter of the textbook. It may also be useful to review the Dental Hygiene Ethics discussion in Chapter 1, the Ethical Applications in the introduction pages for each section in the textbook, as well as the Codes of Ethics in Appendices I, II, and III.

Collaborative Learning Activity
Work with another student colleague to role-play the scenario. The goal of this exercise is for you and your colleague to work though the alternative actions in order to come to consensus on a solution or response that is acceptable to both of you.

Discovery Activity
Ask a friend or relative who is not involved in healthcare to read the scenario and discuss it with you from the perspective of a "patient" who receives services within the healthcare system. Discuss what you learned from the concerns, insights, or difference in perspective that person expressed.

Factors To Teach The Patient

This scenario is related to the following factors listed in this chapter of the textbook:

■ That dentition can last a lifetime
■ The value of a well-balanced diet
■ Importance of drinking fluoridated water

You have recently learned that Marie Tonawonda (introduced in the competency exercises) has been moved to an extended-care facility. Her nephew, Stan, comes in for his regular appointment and thanks you again for all the information you provided when Ms. Tonawonda was in for her appointment. He reaffirms his commitment to maintaining his aunt's oral health.

He mentions his concern about your instructions to limit Ms. Tonawonda's exposure to high-sucrose foods. In order to increase nutritional intake, the residents at the Sunshine Residence Home, where she is now residing, seem to have access to food at any time they desire and, unfortunately, that includes availability of cookies all the time. Stan has encouraged the staff to provide support for his aunt's efforts at limiting sweets and conducting daily brushing and flossing, but he isn't sure his wishes are being met.

You decide that you will investigate the possibility of volunteering to provide staff in-service presentations about oral health to the caregivers at the extended-care facility. Develop an outline of the topics you would cover in these presentations.

COMPETENCY EXERCISES

Apply information from the chapter and use critical thinking skills to complete the competency exercises. Write responses on paper or create electronic documents to submit your answers.

1. Explain why an older patient's slowness to learn new oral hygiene techniques does not necessarily mean an inability to learn.

2. Discuss why it is important to develop an aggressive preventive care plan for a patient in the early stages of Alzheimer's disease.

CHAPTER 52—PATIENT ASSESSMENT SUMMARY

Patient Name: Marie Tonawonda	Age: 89	Gender: M [F]	☐ Initial Therapy
			☑ Maintenance
Provider Name: D.H. Student	Date: Today		☐ Re-evaluation

Chief Complaint:
Her nephew states: "I brought her in today for her regular cleaning appointment."

ASSESSMENT FINDINGS

Health History

- Taking calcium-channel blocker for hypertension and sublingual nitroglycerine tablet as needed for occasional angina
- Recent antidepressant prescription
- Osteoporosis – exhibits curvature of upper back
- Increasing mental confusion and cognitive disability
- Decreased visual acuity even when corrected with glasses
- Wears a hearing aid
- ASA Classification – II and ADL level – 2

At Risk for:

Social and Dental History

- History of dental visits every 4 months
- Recent increase in sucrose intake (described by nephew)
- High dental literacy—but recent cognitive decrease
- Assisted with daily care by her nephew who has little dental knowledge

At Risk for:

Dental Examination

- Xerostomia
- Generalized recession: 3–5 mm.
- Generalized 3–4 mm probing depths; generalized slight bleeding at gingival margins
- Several class 1 and class II furcations in molar areas
- Very few restorations—all in good condition

At Risk for:

Periodontal Diagnosis/Case Type and Status
History of generalized, controlled chronic periodontitis with recent increase in marginal gingivitis

Caries Management Risk Assessment (CAMBRA) Level:
☐ Low ☑ Moderate ☐ High ☐ Extreme

3. Today your patient is Marie Tonawonda, age 89 years. Refer to her Patient Assessment summary as you complete the following exercises.

Ms. Tonawonda has been a patient in your clinic for many, many years, and she comes in every 4 months, like clockwork, for her periodontal maintenance appointments. Her father was a dentist, and she was his dental assistant when she was a young girl, so she loves to talk about the changes she has observed in dentistry.

As her nephew, Stan, escorts her slowly into your treatment room, you notice that, although she greets you cheerfully as usual, she is becoming increasingly frail. As Stan helps with a health history update, he mentions that his aunt has recently been placed on an antidepressant by her physician. Stan visits his aunt in her home nearly daily and recently noticed that she hasn't been eating regular meals. There has been other evidence that Ms. Tonawonda has been decreasingly able to provide her own daily self-care, and Stan says that, even when he reminds her, she does not always remember to brush her teeth or comb her hair every day.

Stan states that he will continue to bring her in for her regular dental care and that Ms. Tonawonda's insurance will continue to cover the cost of any dental needs she has.

While your dental assistant is taking radiographs of Ms. Tonawonda's teeth, you begin to jot down notes for her dental hygiene care plan. You suddenly remember the OSCAR assessment approach to identifying the needs of older individuals (see Table 23-2 in the textbook). Complete an OSCAR Assessment to identify factors of concern for Ms. Tonawonda.

4. Using the assessment data from Ms. Tonawonda's Patient Assessment Summary, your OSCAR assessment notes, and the information in Chapter 52 of the textbook, write three dental hygiene diagnosis statements for Ms. Tonawonda's care plan.

5. Because Ms. Tonawonda's cognitive abilities are declining, her need for education and oral hygiene instruction are very different from that of most of your other patients. Ms. Tonawonda will need ways to receive reminders for daily oral care. Using your school's format for writing progress notes, document the education and home care instructions you will provide during today's appointment.

? QUESTIONS PATIENTS ASK

What sources of information can you identify that will help you answer your patient's question in this scenario?

A healthy, functionally independent 70-year-old patient asks you if, at her age, she should consider dental implants for the molar teeth that were recently extracted. How will you respond?

The Edentulous Patient

Upon successful completion of these exercises, you will be able to:

1. Identify and define key terms and concepts related to an edentulous patient.
2. Identify potential adverse effects of dental prostheses on oral tissues.
3. Plan and document dental hygiene interventions that address patient needs before and after insertion of a denture.
4. Identify criteria and procedures for marking dentures.

 KNOWLEDGE EXERCISES

Write your answers for each question in the space provided.

1. Identify reasons for wearing a denture to replace the missing teeth in an edentulous arch.

   _____

   _____

   _____

2. List three reasons why a denture may be constructed to replace primary dentition for a child patient.

   _____

   _____

   _____

3. What is the purpose of a provisional or interim dental prosthesis?

   _____

   _____

4. Why is it often necessary to reline or remake an immediate denture approximately 6 months after initial placement?

   _____

   _____

5. As a dental hygienist, you may provide counseling and education for your patient both before and after he or she receives a new denture. Explain the purpose of predelivery patient counseling.

   _____

   _____

6. When a denture is placed immediately after extractions, you instruct your patient to leave the denture in place for _____ to _____ hours without removing it, to aid in control of bleeding and swelling.

7. Because adjustments can be expected when a new denture is placed over healed ridges, you instruct your patient to return within _____ hours; you then make reappointments as needed.

8. What is the purpose of a postinsertion appointment with the dental hygienist after a new denture is placed? (*Hint:* The dentist, not the dental hygienist, will adjust the new denture, if needed.)

_____

_____

9. List the potential effects of alveolar ridge remodeling after placement of a complete denture.

_____

_____

_____

_____

_____

10. Your patient may resort to _____ remedies to relieve the effects of alveolar remodeling or poor denture fit, but you will counsel him or her to seek dental care if there are any problems, because these kinds of remedies are _____ if used improperly or over time.

11. List factors that contribute to the varying tissue reactions experienced by patients who wear dentures.

_____

_____

_____

_____

_____

12. Xerostomia can adversely affect denture _____ and tissue _____.

13. List two negative oral effects related to the sensory changes that may be experienced by your patient who wears complete dentures.

_____

_____

14. For most of your patients who wear complete dentures, how often should they come back for a maintenance appointment (unless they are experiencing problems)?

_____

15. At dental hygiene appointments, it is important to thoroughly examine the oral tissues of a patient who wears complete dentures. In your own words, describe the tension test for examining the mouth of your edentulous patient.

_____

_____

16. List the three *most common* causes of oral lesions under a dental prosthesis.

_____

_____

_____

17. What is the effect of xerostomia for your patient who wears dentures?

_____

_____

18. What is an epulis fissuratum?

_____

_____

19. Name the common fungal infection that can result in denture stomatitis.

_____

20. List three factors that can contribute to angular cheilitis in your patient who wears dentures.

_____

_____

_____

21. If you observe a localized ulcerated lesion related to an overextended denture border that persists longer than normal healing times, you should bring the situation to the attention of the dentist so that the lesion can be _____.

22. List the topics to include when you are educating your patient about ways to prevent damage to oral tissues related to wearing dentures.

_____

_____

_____

23. List three reasons to mark your patient's denture with identifying information.

    _____

    _____

    _____

24. In your own words, briefly summarize the criteria for an adequate denture-marking system relative to the following issues.

    a. The denture

    _____

    _____

    b. The material used

    _____

    _____

    c. The procedure used

    _____

    _____

25. List two areas in which identification information can be incorporated as a denture is fabricated.

    _____

    _____

26. Where should an inclusion identification marker be placed on an existing denture that was not previously labeled?

    a. Maxillary denture

    _____

    b. Mandibular denture

    _____

27. Identify two methods for marking identification information on the surface of a denture.

    _____

    _____

28. What information is included when marking the denture of a patient who is in a long-term care nursing home?

    _____

    _____

✓ COMPETENCY EXERCISES

Apply information from the chapter and use critical thinking skills to complete the competency exercises. Write responses on paper or create electronic documents to submit your answers.

1. Explain why regular dental hygiene maintenance care is important for edentulous patients, whether or not they are wearing complete dentures.

2. Explain why caries-control methods are important to teach your patient who wears an overdenture.

3. After discussing several alternate treatment plans with the dentist, Mr. Bruehner has decided to have all of his remaining natural teeth extracted and immediate maxillary and mandibular dentures placed. He is very concerned, because his mother wore dentures and had many problems with them over the years. He has confided to Dr. Joseph that his mother's dentures didn't look like they belonged to her face and mouth, that she couldn't eat what she wanted to, that the dentures were not comfortable, and—worst of all—that his mother always had what he calls "dragon breath."

   Mr. Bruehner has an appointment with you today to begin preinsertion patient counseling before he schedules the extraction appointment. You are developing a dental hygiene care plan before he arrives.

   When you read the assessment data in his patient record, you learn that Mr. Bruehner has been receiving his dental treatment in this practice for a bit longer than 1 year. His general health status is relatively good, and he is currently taking one medication for hypertension that contributes to xerostomia. He has a history of periodontal disease for which the original prognosis was rated as poor. He has a fairly high dental IQ because of education provided by the previous dental hygienist, but the counseling he received was focused on his periodontal status and the attempt to arrest the progress of oral disease.

   Use a copy of the Patient-Specific Dental Hygiene Care Plan Template in Appendix B and the information in Table 53-1 in the textbook to develop a dental hygiene care plan for a series of preinsertion and postinsertion appointments for Mr. Bruehner. Be sure to include at least one preinsertion appointment (more if you think he might need them), an appointment for instructions the day of his extractions, and a postinsertion appointment for instructions after he receives his dentures in the care plan you write.

4. Use your school's format for writing progress notes to document the dental hygiene education you provided during a preinsertion appointment for Mr. Bruehner.

Everyday Ethics

Before completing the learning exercises below, reread and reflect on the Everyday Ethics scenario and Questions for Consideration in this chapter of the textbook. It may also be useful to review the Dental Hygiene Ethics discussion in Chapter 1, the Ethical Applications in the introduction pages for each section in the textbook, as well as the Codes of Ethics in Appendices I, II, and III.

Individual Learning Activity

Identify a situation you have experienced that presents a similar ethical dilemma. Write about what you would do differently now than you did at the time the incident happened—support your discussion with concepts from the dental hygiene codes of ethics.

Collaborative Learning Activity

Identify a situation in which you have resolved a similar ethical dilemma and share the story with a classmate. Discuss how that person might have acted differently to resolve the situation.

Factors To Teach The Patient

This scenario is related to the following factors listed in this chapter of the textbook:

■ Dentures and tissues must be examined at least once a year for care of the tissue-supported removable prosthesis; implant-supported dentures require more frequent examination. The frequency of maintenance appointments is geared to the individual, depending in part on that patient's ability to clean the dentures and to keep them free from biofilm, stain, and calculus.

■ Dentures may need periodic replacement. Tissues under the dentures change.

■ Avoid the use of drugstore remedies, reliners, and other home-applied materials unless the dentist has provided specific instructions.

■ There are specific methods of care for dentures.

■ Leave the dentures out of the mouth overnight in accord with the dentist's directions.

Mr. Bruehner (introduced in the competency exercises in this chapter) received his immediate denture 2 days ago. This morning, he is scheduled with Dr. Joseph for a postinsertion appointment to check healing at the extraction sites; then he has an appointment with you for postinsertion education and counseling.

Use the patient-specific dental-hygiene care plan you created for Mr. Bruehner and the examples of patient conversations in Appendix D as guides to prepare an outline for a conversation that you will have with Mr. Bruehner during this appointment.

WORD SEARCH

```
I  W  J  G  L  E  B  W  B  X  U  C  P  T  B  N  E  G  U  Y
M  D  Q  M  L  I  X  C  O  V  E  R  D  E  N  T  U  R  E  W
M  E  J  H  V  L  N  O  Q  H  A  A  G  K  D  W  D  W  J  P
E  N  C  M  M  I  V  I  S  U  T  S  D  N  X  I  L  X  X  A
D  T  X  R  L  I  T  D  N  T  G  B  N  H  A  T  C  A  Z  L
I  U  V  O  E  H  O  N  D  G  O  B  V  F  E  P  V  L  J  A
A  R  E  S  O  R  P  T  I  O  N  S  A  C  K  S  R  O  K  T
T  E  C  Z  Y  S  P  E  C  I  A  L  I  Z  E  D  I  Q  J  I
E  V  X  O  H  K  P  I  M  R  Q  H  V  S  O  O  M  V  A  N
K  Y  A  O  M  X  B  N  P  R  O  S  T  H  E  S  I  S  E  U
U  U  N  M  M  A  N  D  I  B  U  L  A  R  I  S  W  N  U  S
P  A  P  I  L  L  A  R  Y  H  Y  P  E  R  P  L  A  S  I  A
X  P  E  S  K  O  J  K  T  I  R  R  E  S  E  C  T  I  O  N
P  U  C  H  A  R  A  C  T  E  R  I  Z  A  T  I  O  N  U  G
B  V  S  H  Z  P  Y  Z  J  M  A  S  T  I  C  A  T  O  R  Y
Y  C  E  B  A  N  G  U  L  A  R  C  H  E  I  L  I  T  I  S
F  K  S  W  Q  L  X  S  X  K  P  S  U  B  M  U  C  O  S  A
B  D  I  H  V  Y  V  X  B  L  B  A  N  O  D  O  N  T  I  A
E  V  F  P  X  S  W  U  F  O  R  F  Y  N  O  P  Z  D  O  L
Y  C  H  D  C  A  N  D  I  D  A  A  L  B  I  C  A  N  S  E
```

WORD SEARCH CLUES

1. Term for an artificial replacement of one or more teeth and associated oral structures.
2. Term for an artificial substitute for missing natural teeth.
3. Type of complete denture fabricated for placement directly after the removal of natural teeth or surgical preparation of dental arches.
4. Removable prosthesis that covers remaining teeth, roots, or implants.
5. Modification of the form and color of the denture base and teeth to produce a more lifelike appearance.
6. The mucosa that covers the floor of the mouth, vestibules, and cheeks.
7. Type of mucosa that covers the edentulous ridge and hard palate.
8. The cushion of connective tissue, vessels, nerves, adipose tissue, and glands between mucosa and bone on the edentulous ridge.
9. Excision of a segment of any part (e.g., of the jawbone) or removal of articular ends of bones forming a joint.
10. The tori usually removed from the lingual premolar area before fabrication of a denture.
11. Bony enlargement (torus) that is surgically removed before fabrication of a maxillary denture.
12. Bony changes in the alveolar ridge over time that can lead to loss of denture support, changes in facial structure, and changes in oral functioning.
13. Material used to adhere a denture to the oral mucosa; should not be used long term to compensate for poorly designed, constructed, or ill-fitting dentures.
14. Fissuring at the corners of the mouth of a patient who wears dentures (two words)
15. This condition can cause a generalized redness on the tissues that support a denture; your patient may experience a burning sensation (two words).
16. Red, pebble-shaped, edematous lesions on the palate that are related to ill-fitting dentures, poor oral hygiene, and possible *Candida albicans* infection (two words).
17. Congenital absence of teeth that may require construction of dentures for a child patient.
18. Bony protuberance located on the buccal aspect of the alveolar ridge.
19. Mucosa that covers the dorsal surface of the tongue and contains filiform papillae.

CHAPTER 54

The Oral and Maxillofacial Surgery Patient

Learning Objectives

Upon successful completion of these exercises, you will be able to:

1. Identify and define key terms and concepts related to oral and maxillofacial surgery.
2. Identify causes, classifications, and treatment options for facial fractures.
3. Discuss dental hygiene interventions for patients before and after general surgery.
4. Plan and document dental hygiene care, oral health education, and dietary recommendations for patients before and after oral and maxillofacial surgery.

 KNOWLEDGE EXERCISES

Write your answers for each question in the space provided.

1. What is orthognathic surgery?

   _____

   _____

2. In your own words, define *intermaxillary fixation*.

   _____

   _____

3. Define exodontics.

   _____

   _____

4. List at least three reasons why it is important to provide dental hygiene care for a patient before oral and maxillofacial surgery, even when all of the patient's teeth will be removed during the surgical procedure.

   _____

   _____

   _____

   _____

5. List three personal factors that can affect communication with your patient when you are providing oral hygiene instructions to him or her before oral surgery.

   _____

   _____

   _____

6. List three types of printed instructions that you would provide as part of your presurgical patient education.

   _____

   _____

   _____

7. Identify specific components to include in instructions you provide your patient immediately after a surgical procedure.

_____

_____

_____

_____

_____

_____

_____

8. List postsurgical procedures you may be asked to participate in during follow-up care for your patient.

_____

_____

_____

9. Identify two possible causes of a fractured jaw.

_____

_____

10. List three clinical signs that can aid in recognition of a fractured jaw.

_____

_____

_____

11. Describe a comminuted fracture.

_____

_____

12. Which type of fractured jaw is more likely to occur in a small child?

_____

13. What is an arch bar, and how does it immobilize the mandibular jaw?

_____

_____

_____

14. Identify three advantages for using intermaxillary fixation (IMF) after surgical reduction of a fracture.

_____

_____

_____

15. List three contraindications for using an IMF.

_____

_____

_____

16. List three types of systems/materials used for immobilization after open surgical reduction of a skeletal fracture.

_____

_____

_____

17. List factors that make maxillary fractures more difficult to manage than mandibular fractures.

_____

_____

_____

_____

18. Describe a maxillary alveolar process fracture. (_Hint:_ Draw a diagram of what you are trying to describe.) List the components of treatment provided for the patient with this type of fracture.

_____

_____

_____

_____

19. Identify two reasons that a healthy liquid or soft diet is difficult to plan for a postsurgical patient.

_____

_____

20. List three vitamins that are essential in the diet of a patient who is healing after an oral/maxillofacial surgical procedure.

    _____

    _____

    _____

21. Provide three examples of feeding methods used for patients after a surgical fixation procedure.

    _____

    _____

    _____

22. List three foods that can supply needed nutrients as part of a soft diet prepared for a patient with only a single-jaw fixation appliance.

    _____

    _____

    _____

23. When is personal oral care and thorough biofilm removal by the patient resumed after an oral surgical procedure?

    _____

24. List three reasons why it is difficult for a postsurgical patient who has a fixation appliance or who is experiencing trismus to accomplish complete dental biofilm removal.

    _____

    _____

    _____

✔ COMPETENCY EXERCISES

Apply information from the chapter and use critical thinking skills to complete the competency exercises. Write responses on paper or create electronic documents to submit your answers.

1. Compare open and closed reduction procedures used for the treatment of a facial fracture.

2. Mr. Bright is scheduled in 2 weeks for oral surgery to remove all of his remaining maxillary teeth and receive an immediate denture. His patient record contains assessment data indicating that teeth 1, 3, 6–9, 13, and 16 are missing; tooth 2 is extremely sensitive owing to a carious lesion; teeth 4 and 5 are mobile; and his gingival tissue is sensitive and bleeds profusely. There is visible calculus and a high level of biofilm on all the remaining teeth. He has not had any regular dental care or oral hygiene instructions for many years. Create an infomap or table that will help you organize the following information.

    ■ Identify factors from this case scenario that can affect instrumentation techniques when you are providing presurgical scaling for Mr. Bright.

    ■ Identify why these factors are a problem.

    ■ Suggest procedures you might use to overcome each problem.

    ■ Use the format required in your school clinic to write a progress note for an imaginary patient visit that documents the use of one of the potential modifications you have described in the infomap table you created.

3. Your patient, Alicia Wentworth, is upset today when she comes to the office for her dental hygiene appointment. She tells you that her good friend, David, was recently injured in an automobile accident. She asks you to explain what a simple fracture of the mandible is and what a Le Fort II midfacial fracture is. Draw diagrams you can use to educate Alicia.

4. A week later, Alicia calls and leaves a message on the office voice mail. She says that David is coming home from the hospital and she has agreed to provide meals for him every day. His fracture has been treated using an IMF appliance and he must receive all his nutrition using a straw or a spoon-feeding technique. He is restricted to a full liquid diet. She asks you to call her back and recommend foods and preparation methods. She wants to know about how he can keep his mouth clean after he eats.

    Make notes that you can refer to when you call her back to give her the information she is asking for.

Everyday Ethics

Before completing the learning exercises below, reread and reflect on the Everyday Ethics scenario and Questions for Consideration in this chapter of the textbook. It may also be useful to review the Dental Hygiene Ethics discussion in Chapter 1, the Ethical Applications in the introduction pages for each section in the textbook, as well as the Codes of Ethics in Appendices I, II, and III.

Individual Learning Activity

- Imagine that you have observed what happened in the scenario, but are not one of the main characters involved in the situation. Write a reflective journal entry that
    - describes how you might have reacted (as an observer-not as a participant),

- expresses your personal feelings about what happened,

or

- identifies personal values that affect your reaction to the situation.

Discovery Activity

Ask a friend or relative who is not involved in healthcare to read the scenario and discuss it with you from the perspective of a "patient" who receives services within the healthcare system. Discuss what you learned from the concerns, insights, or difference in perspective that person expressed.

Factors To Teach The Patient

This scenario is related to the following factors listed in this chapter of the textbook:

- Why it is necessary to have dental and dental hygiene care completed before surgery

Mr. Brown is scheduled in about 2 weeks for some very serious surgery that is part of his treatment for pancreatic cancer. His physician has recommended that Mr. Brown visit his dental hygienist for a complete dental assessment before the surgery. As you go over his health history, you discover that he is very confused about why dental hygiene interventions are necessary as part of his treatment—after all, his illness has nothing to do with his mouth!

Use the information in Chapter 54 of the textbook and the examples of a patient conversations in Appendix D as a guide to write a statement explaining to Mr. Brown why this dental-hygiene appointment is such an important component of his total health and well-being.

CHAPTER 55

The Patient With Cancer

Learning Objectives

Upon successful completion of these exercises, you will be able to:

1. Identify and define key terms and concepts related to the patient with cancer.
2. Identify risk factors for oral cancer.
3. Identify standard cancer treatments and the oral effects of each.
4. Plan and document dental hygiene care for the cancer patient before, during, and after therapy.

 KNOWLEDGE EXERCISES

Write your answers for each question in the space provided.

1. Match the following terms related to the physical and oral effects of cancer treatment with the correct description.

TERM	DESCRIPTION OF EFFECT
_____ Mucositis	A. Diminishment or abatement of the symptoms of a disease
_____ Dysgeusia	B. Recurrence of a disease after its apparent cessation
_____ Neurotoxicity	C. Treatment that provides relief of symptoms but is not intended to cure
_____ Alopecia	D. A loss of hair
_____ Palliative	E. Virus that can cause oral infection during or after radiation therapy.
_____ Herpes simplex	F. Distortion of the sense of taste
_____ *Candida albicans*	G. Limited jaw opening because of spasm or fibro-sis of muscles or joint; may occur 3–6 mo after radiation treatment to the head and neck
_____ Trismus	H. Fungus that commonly causes oral infection related to treatment for cancer
_____ Immunosuppression	I. Inhibition of antibody responses resulting from leucopenia related to chemotherapy treatments
_____ Relapse	J. Inflammation of the oral mucosa
_____ Remission	K. Can cause a bilateral feeling of toothache related to chemotherapy treatments for cancer

2. What is cancer?

_____

_____

3. How are cancers classified and described?

_____

_____

_____

_____

4. What are the risk factors for developing cancer?

_____

_____

_____

_____

5. Why is it important to plan comprehensive and coordinated dental hygiene care for your patient before, during, and after treatment for cancer?

_____

_____

_____

_____

6. Identify the dental hygiene interventions you will most likely provide for your patient before the medical treatment for cancer begins.

_____

_____

7. Radiation therapy for cancer is most likely to have oral effects if the field of radiation is concentrated in your patient's head and neck area. Identify the long-term complications of radiation treatment on oral tissues.

_____

_____

_____

_____

8. Identify the signs and symptoms of radiation- and chemotherapy-induced stomatitis.

_____

_____

_____

_____

_____

_____

9. List recommendations you can make to help your patient reduce sensitivity and increase ability to maintain daily oral hygiene measures when mucositis is a problem during cancer treatment.

_____

_____

_____

_____

_____

_____

_____

10. Radiation to salivary glands can cause a serious reduction in secretion of saliva. Chemotherapy treatments can also induce a transient xerostomia. Identify the ways that xerostomia can affect the oral cavity.

_____

_____

_____

11. What suggestions can you make to help your patient manage xerostomia during and after cancer treatments?

_____

_____

_____

_____

_____

12. Identify measures that can prevent radiation caries.

_____

_____

_____

13. What are the systemic side effects of chemotherapy cancer treatment?

_____

_____

_____

_____

_____

14. List the types of oral infections that are common during and after radiation therapy and/or chemotherapy treatment for cancer.

_____

_____

_____

15. _____ is a destructive condition affecting blood vessels and bone that can occur after high-dose radiation treatment in the head and neck area. This condition results in a decreased ability to heal and increased susceptibility to infection.

16. What oral changes can influence/restrict nutritional intake and further compromise the health status of a patient who is undergoing cancer therapy?

_____

_____

_____

_____

17. In your own words, briefly describe a hematopoietic cell transplantation.

_____

_____

_____

_____

18. What is graft-versus-host disease?

_____

_____

_____

19. What patient factors can influence your patient's ability to attend to and comply with the counseling and oral hygiene instructions that you provide before, during, and after treatment for cancer?

_____

_____

_____

 COMPETENCY EXERCISES

Apply information from the chapter and use critical thinking skills to complete the competency exercises. Write responses on paper or create electronic documents to submit your answers.

Mrs. Marge Henley is scheduled today in the hospital dental clinic as an emergency patient. After he examines her, Dr. Singh calls you in to consult with him. Mrs. Henley is currently undergoing chemotherapy for cancer treatment and is experiencing severe oral symptoms related to the treatment. Dr. Singh has already written a prescription to treat the oral candidiasis. He asks you to counsel Mrs. Henley about daily oral care and to write a dental hygiene care plan for her continuing care during the cancer treatment.

When you carefully examine her, you discover that Mrs. Henley's oral tissues are heartbreakingly inflamed, blistered, and dry. She tells you that she has been feeling a bit guilty because her mouth has been so sore that she cannot brush and floss as often or as thoroughly as she used to do. Her sense of humor has remained intact, though, and she tells you with a twinkle in her eye that she eats vanilla pudding for breakfast, lunch, and dinner every day. She asks for any suggestions you have to help her get through this difficult time.

1. What areas of risk are associated with the assessment findings that have been recorded for Mrs. Henley?

2. Write at least two dental hygiene diagnosis statements to include in Mrs. Henley's written care plan.

3. Write a goal for each of the problems identified in the dental hygiene diagnosis statements you wrote for question 2. Include a time frame for meeting each goal. How will you measure whether your patient met the goal?

4. Using your institution's guidelines for writing in patient records, document Mrs. Henley's visit and write a statement regarding her next visit.

DISCOVERY EXERCISES

1. The National Oral Health Information Clearinghouse (NOHIC) is a resource center for oral health information geared to patients with special needs and the healthcare providers who serve them. Visit their Web site (http://www.nohic.nidcr.nih.gov) to discover a wonderful series of education pamphlets about oral cancer and the oral complications of cancer treatment.

2. Investigate the medical and dental literature using a PubMed search to discover which types of cancer may be treated with drugs, such as bisphosphonates, that can have a long-term effect on oral tissues. (*Idea:* This topic would make an excellent table clinic presentation;-)

QUESTIONS PATIENTS ASK

What sources of information can you identify that will help you answer your patient's questions in this scenario?

"How can I possibly keep my mouth clean when it is so sore and/or dry that it hurts to use the toothbrush? And why is that so important anyway?" "When is the best time to have my teeth worked on while I am undergoing treatment for my cancer?" "How soon after my radiation treatment can I get my new dentures and/or partial dentures?" "Will the kind of cancer treatment I am receiving now affect my ability to receive dental care, such as having implants placed, later on?"

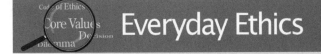

Everyday Ethics

Before completing the learning exercises below, reread and reflect on the Everyday Ethics scenario and Questions for Consideration in this chapter of the textbook. It may also be useful to review the Dental Hygiene Ethics discussion in Chapter 1, the Ethical Applications in the introduction pages for each section in the textbook, as well as the Codes of Ethics in Appendices I, II, and III.

Discovery Activities

■ Investigate the practice act in your state to determine the legal issues involved as the dental hygienist in this scenario contemplates what action to take.

■ Ask a dental hygienist who has been practicing for a year or more to read the scenario. Provide them with a copy of one of the Codes of Ethics as well. Share the responses you have made to answer each question and ask that person to discuss the situation with you. What insights did you have or what did you learn during this discussion?

 ## Factors To Teach The Patient

This scenario is related to the following factors listed in this chapter of the textbook:

■ Why the dental hygienist needs to conduct an oral soft-tissue screening and complete oral examination at regular, frequent intervals
■ How and when to use dental biofilm control methods, gel-tray application, use of saliva substitute, and all other details of personal care to reduce oral side effects caused by the disease and/or cancer treatment
■ Ideas for remembering to follow the instructions to keep the mouth healthier and more comfortable during cancer treatment
■ The reasons why a routine schedule of preventive periodontal scaling, fluoride application, and oral hygiene assessment done by a dental hygienist contributes to the success of cancer treatment

George Murphy, a 45-year-old construction worker, has recently been diagnosed with parotid gland cancer that has spread into his left neck. He will be having surgery to remove the left parotid gland with a left neck dissection followed by radiation therapy. He is scheduled today for a pretreatment dental examination. Mr. Murphy has not seen a dentist in more than 10 years and has dental caries lesions, moderately advanced periodontal disease, and very poor oral hygiene. You are asked to prepare a dental hygiene care plan to address Mr. Murphy's oral care needs during and after the radiation treatment.

Mr. Murphy tells you that he hates dentists because they always hurt him and that is why he never comes to see one. The only reason he is here today is because he was told that he could not proceed with his cancer treatment unless he gets his mouth into better shape.

Use the information in the "Personal Factors" section of Chapter 55 of the textbook and the examples of patient conversations in Appendix D as guides to prepare an outline for a conversation you will use to counsel Mr. Murphy regarding his oral condition.

WORD SEARCH

```
R  A  D  I  A  T  I  O  N  T  H  E  R  A  P  Y  A
U  U  R  J  O  K  G  O  N  T  R  I  S  M  U  S  U
Y  D  Z  N  W  V  R  A  V  Y  N  C  N  W  U  I  T
M  P  A  L  L  I  A  T  I  V  E  D  V  Z  O  M  O
I  N  S  I  T  U  D  X  B  W  O  P  Y  U  M  G  L
S  I  A  I  G  Y  C  W  J  L  P  M  Q  R  E  V  O
P  U  Y  Q  M  D  V  Y  J  T  L  U  O  E  T  T  G
H  Z  S  A  R  C  O  M  A  N  A  C  D  N  A  M  O
H  U  B  E  N  I  G  N  E  M  S  O  O  C  S  A  U
N  S  T  A  G  E  Y  G  S  T  M  S  W  A  T  L  S
I  O  N  C  O  L  O  G  Y  F  Z  I  S  R  A  I  T
I  H  Q  C  S  N  R  Z  C  H  P  T  D  C  S  G  O
P  A  I  O  I  B  H  R  U  Y  L  I  R  I  I  N  J
I  N  P  C  O  O  K  S  D  T  N  S  E  N  S  A  H
R  J  R  K  A  N  A  P  L  A  S  I  A  O  D  N  U
Z  A  H  N  A  G  D  U  M  X  T  A  U  M  E  T  M
C  H  E  M  O  T  H  E  R  A  P  Y  D  A  P  E  Z
```

WORD SEARCH CLUES

1. The study of tumors.
2. A chemical, physical, or biologic agent that may cause cancer.
3. Any new and abnormal growth; can be benign or malignant.
4. The irreversible alteration in adult cells toward embryonic cell types, characteristic of tumor cells.
5. Type of tumor that grows slowly by expansion and does not infiltrate surrounding tissue, does not spread by metastasis, and does not usually cause death unless its location interferes with vital functions.
6. Confined to the site of origin (two words).
7. The spread of cancer cells from one body tissue or organ to others through blood and lymph systems.
8. Type of tumor that grows at a rapid rate, gains access to blood and lymph channels to metastasize into other areas of the body, and usually causes death unless growth can be controlled.
9. Malignant tumor of epithelial origin.
10. Tumor composed of cells derived from connective tissue.
11. Treatment of an illness by using drugs.
12. Treatment of disease with ionizing radiation (two words).
13. Donor for this type of bone marrow transplant is the patient.
14. Inflammation of oral tissues.
15. Providing relief of symptoms.
16. This condition can limit the patient's ability to open mouth during dental hygiene treatment.
17. Clinical classification of a tumor; consists of three components.

The Patient With a Disability

Learning Objectives

Upon successful completion of these exercises, you will be able to:

1. Identify and define key terms and concepts relating to individuals with disabilities.
2. Identify oral conditions caused by or resulting from disabling conditions.

3. Describe procedures and factors that contribute to safe and successful dental hygiene treatment for individuals with disabilities.
4. Describe factors that enhance the prevention of oral disease for individuals with disabilities and their caregivers.

 KNOWLEDGE EXERCISES

Write your answers for each question in the space provided.

1. In your own words, summarize the precautions you can take and modifications you can make to ensure safety and comfort during dental hygiene treatment for your patient with a significant disability.

_____
_____
_____
_____
_____
_____
_____
_____

2. Briefly describe the components included in the two main sections of the World Health Organization International Classifications of Functioning, Disability and Health.

a. Part 1: Functioning and Disability

_____
_____
_____

b. Part 2: Contextual Factors

_____
_____
_____

3. Identify additional oral findings that can be caused by, or be a result of, your patient's disability.

_____
_____
_____
_____
_____

4. List oral manifestations related to drug therapies commonly used to treat patients with disabilities.

   _____

   _____

   _____

   _____

   _____

5. List at least three objectives for providing quality dental and dental hygiene care for individuals with disabilities.

   _____

   _____

   _____

   _____

   _____

6. For you to plan dental hygiene care that takes all of the needs of your patient with a disability into consideration, it is essential to gather as much information as possible before the first appointment. Identify three individuals (or groups) who can provide the needed information.

   _____

   _____

   _____

7. To avoid confusion, it is best to ask direct questions concerning the type and severity of your patient's disability. Identify four categories of information to obtain from the patient or caregiver.

   _____

   _____

   _____

   _____

8. List four factors to consider when scheduling appointments for an individual with a disability.

   _____

   _____

   _____

   _____

9. In your own words, define a barrier-free dental treatment facility.

   _____

   _____

10. What size parking space must be allowed for disabled individuals?

   _____

11. How wide must outdoor walkways and indoor passageways be to accommodate a wheelchair?

   _____

12. An appropriately constructed wheelchair ramp entrance has a handrail and a gentle slope that rises _____ inch for every _____ inches in length.

13. Lightweight doors with lever handles must open at least _____ inches wide for a wheelchair to pass through.

14. For providing oral hygiene instruction for a patient who is in a wheelchair, it is ideal to have a table or sink built at a height of _____ inches to _____ inches and that permits clearance underneath for knees and wheelchair arms.

15. A dental chair that is accessible for wheelchair transfers can be lowered to at least _____ inches from the floor.

16. Describe a way to position your wheelchair-bound patient for dental hygiene treatment if a portable headrest is not available to attach to the wheelchair.

   _____

   _____

17. List three basic types of wheelchair transfers.

   _____

   _____

   _____

18. What is the first thing you should do before starting a wheelchair transfer?

   _____

   _____

19. Who can give you advice in how best to help during a wheelchair transfer?

_____

_____

20. List three factors that take special consideration during a wheelchair transfer.

_____

_____

_____

21. Describe the position of the wheelchair with respect to the position of the dental chair when transferring your patient from the wheelchair to the dental chair.

    a. Mobile transfer

    _____

    _____

    _____

    b. Immobile transfer

    _____

    _____

    _____

    c. Sliding board transfer

    _____

    _____

    _____

22. It makes sense, when transferring your patient back to the wheelchair after treatment, to position the seat of the dental chair slightly _____ than the seat of the wheelchair.

23. If you are helping your patient with a mobile transfer from a wheelchair to the dental chair, where are your patient's arms and hands?

    _____

    _____

24. Describe the position of the first aide's hands/arms when two people are helping with an immobile patient transfer.

    _____

    _____

25. What is the responsibility of the second aide during an immobile patient transfer?

    _____

    _____

26. What is your role in assisting a patient with a walker, crutches, or a cane to seat themselves in the dental chair?

    _____

    _____

    _____

27. List factors that contribute to safety and comfortable positioning or stabilization of your patient with a disability while he or she is in the dental chair.

    _____

    _____

    _____

28. What precautions are required if body enclosure stabilization is considered.

    _____

    _____

    _____

29. Describe a techniques for safely stabilizing a patient's head during dental hygiene treatment.

    _____

30. List the types of aids that can be used to stabilize the patient's mouth while providing dental hygiene treatment or during daily oral care provided by caregivers.

    _____

    _____

    _____

31. List precautions to observe if you are using a mouth prop.

    _____

    _____

    _____

    _____

    _____

32. List the components of an oral disease prevention and control program for a patient with a disability.

_____

_____

_____

_____

_____

_____

_____

33. To plan oral hygiene instructions for your patient with a disability, it is important for you to understand the ability of your patient to perform daily living and self-care skills such as toothbrushing. Briefly describe the functioning ability for each ADL/IADL level.

  a. ADL/IADL level 0

  _____

  _____

  b. ADL/IADL levels 1 and 2

  _____

  _____

  c. ADL/IADL level 3

  _____

  _____

34. What is your role in providing oral hygiene instructions for an individual who is identified as having a moderate- or low-functioning ADL/IADL level?

  _____

  _____

35. When should you recommend that the use of a dentifrice should be limited or eliminated from the oral care regimen of a patient with a disability?

  _____

  _____

  _____

36. What recommendations can you make so that a patient who cannot use a dentifrice receives the benefits of fluoride?

  _____

  _____

  _____

  _____

37. Self-care aids can make a difference in the ability of a patient or caregiver to maximize effectiveness or oral care. List the general prerequisites of a good oral self-care aid.

  _____

  _____

  _____

  _____

38. Identify three general modifications that can be made to a toothbrush handle to enhance the ability of a patient with a disability to provide oral self-care.

  _____

  _____

  _____

39. What factors will you take into consideration when recommending the use of a power-assisted toothbrush for a patient with a disability?

  _____

  _____

40. Briefly describe modifications that can be made to help a patient with a disability care for a removable dental prosthesis.

  _____

  _____

41. In your own words, describe the position that a caregiver can use to be most effective when providing daily oral care for a person with disabilities.

  _____

  _____

  _____

  _____

42. Identify factors to take into consideration when planning dietary recommendations for your patient with a disability.

_____

_____

_____

_____

_____

_____

_____

43. Identify three factors that, if addressed during planning, can enhance/contribute to the success of a caregivers' education/in-service program you provide in a long-term care facility.

_____

_____

_____

44. Identify ways to evaluate the success of an in-service program.

_____

_____

45. Identify topics to include in an in-service presentation that teaches caregivers how to examine oral tissues.

_____

_____

_____

_____

_____

46. Identify four additional oral care/disease prevention techniques to teach during staff in-service training.

_____

_____

_____

_____

_____

_____

_____

COMPETENCY EXERCISES

Apply information from the chapter and use critical thinking skills to complete the competency exercises. Write responses on paper or create electronic documents to submit your answers.

1. In your own words, explain the relationship between the terms *impairment, disability,* and *handicap.*

2. Steve McKnight is your patient with cerebral palsy. He is charming and witty. He works for a company that develops voice technology for computers. He has significant physical impairments associated with his condition and moves about with difficulty, using crutches and special leg braces to walk. He is fiercely independent, preferring to manage as many tasks as possible on his own.

   Steve moves his hands with difficulty and cannot grasp small objects very well. He feeds himself using specially adapted utensils. When you talk to him about his daily oral care, he mentions that he used a power-driven toothbrush for a while but that it was heavy and, when it started to vibrate, he could barely hold it up to his mouth. He sighs and says that he really wishes he could find a regular toothbrush that he could hold on to without dropping it in the sink all the time.

   Find appropriate materials and make a device to adapt a toothbrush and floss handle that would help Steve continue to be independent in his daily oral care. Share your design with your classmates. Does your design meet the general prerequisites for a self-care aid as described in the textbook?

3. Your next patient tells you that her daughter, Sara (age 14), has a fractured right elbow and will spend the next several months handicapped by a cast that holds her arm stiff in a slightly bent position. She can maneuver her wrist about but cannot bend her arm. Describe how your patient can modify a toothbrush that will allow Sara to independently accomplish biofilm removal until her arm heals.

 ## DISCOVERY EXERCISE

Explore the Americans with Disabilities Act Website at http://www.ada.gov.

Everyday Ethics

Before completing the learning exercises below, reread and reflect on the Everyday Ethics scenario and Questions for Consideration in this chapter of the textbook. It may also be useful to review the Dental Hygiene Ethics discussion in Chapter 1, the Ethical Applications in the introduction pages for each section in the textbook, as well as the Codes of Ethics in Appendices I, II, and III.

Individual Learning Activity
Imagine that you are the dental hygienist in this scenario. Answer each of the questions for consideration at the end of the scenario.

Collaborative Activity
Answer each of the questions for consideration at the end of the scenario in the textbook. Compare what you wrote with answers developed by another classmate and discuss differences/similarities.

Factors To Teach The Patient

This scenario is related to the following factors listed in this chapter of the textbook:

■ Practice a healthy lifestyle, including a healthy diet

Use the information in Chapter 56 about diet instruction, the principles of anticipatory guidance in Chapter 49, and the examples of patient conversations in Appendix D as a guide to write a conversation educating the mother of a 4-year-old child who has a disability about the general concepts of maintaining a tooth-healthy diet.

WORD SEARCH

```
I  X  X  H  Q  H  M  S  U  P  P  O  R  T  I  V  E
D  M  C  R  A  F  I  N  A  N  C  I  A  L  P  R  S
I  Y  G  W  T  N  C  C  A  R  E  G  I  V  E  R  H
S  Q  R  L  J  H  D  A  D  A  D  N  L  D  P  D  C
A  E  A  S  N  X  S  I  M  P  N  G  R  I  E  E  N
B  P  J  W  F  R  B  J  C  F  U  A  E  N  V  V  H
I  C  B  T  R  O  I  J  B  A  O  C  R  S  D  E  A
L  P  I  A  R  B  U  G  G  B  P  V  F  E  G  L  I
I  H  F  A  R  A  M  R  G  K  B  H  I  R  T  O  K
T  Y  U  S  T  R  N  N  H  R  F  X  R  V  D  P  A
Y  S  U  M  R  T  I  S  N  A  R  K  M  I  X  M  X
D  I  M  Q  C  D  I  E  F  P  N  N  Q  C  Z  E  O
K  C  T  C  I  Z  R  T  R  E  D  D  E  E  T  N  E
Y  A  L  L  D  X  S  A  U  F  R  I  E  W  V  T  Q
E  L  S  F  T  T  V  X  K  D  R  K  S  D  R  A  Z
N  G  S  D  N  N  R  C  S  A  E  E  M  N  Z  L  L
T  G  U  A  R  D  I  A  N  K  N  I  E  H  I  G  H
```

WORD SEARCH CLUES

1. An aid that can be used to help transfer an individual from a wheelchair to the dental chair and back again (two words).
2. Refers to the disadvantage that can limit fulfillment of a normal role for a person with impairment.
3. A dental treatment room that is not wheelchair accessible is an example of this kind of barrier that can hinder access to oral care.
4. Person who performs or helps to perform daily life activities.
5. The need for longer appointment time—and the dental professional's need to be reimbursed for providing that time—can constitute this type of barrier that limits oral-care options for an individual with a disability.
6. Dental professionals who do not feel adequately trained to provide safe treatment is an example of this type of barrier to care for individuals with a disability.
7. Refers to a disability of indefinite duration with an onset before the age of 18.
8. The individual responsible for making decisions if a person is declared incapacitated in a legal process; requires written proof for decision making.
9. Refers to the restriction that results from impairment.
10. Accessible; obstacles to passage or communication have been removed.
11. A term that refers to several techniques for moving a person from a wheelchair to a dental chair and back.
12. Refers to dental hygiene care delivered with the help of a dental assistant. (two words)
13. Education program about some specific topic, such as oral care for individuals with disabilities, that is provided for parents, teachers, volunteers, nurses, or other health professionals (without the hyphen).
14. The Americans with Disabilities Act, *not* the American Dental Association!
15. Padding and other body stabilization methods used to facilitate patient comfort and safety.
16. Level of function identified by an ADL/IADL level of 0.

CHAPTER 57

The Patient Who Is Homebound

Learning Objectives

Upon successful completion of these exercises, you will be able to:

1. Identify and define key terms and concepts related to the homebound, bedridden, or terminally ill patient.

2. Prepare materials necessary for visiting a homebound patient.

3. Plan and document adaptations to dental hygiene care plans and oral hygiene instructions for the homebound patient.

 KNOWLEDGE EXERCISES

Write your answers for each question in the space provided.

1. What characteristics help define a person who may not be able to access dental hygiene care in a traditional private practice office setting?

   _____

   _____

   _____

   _____

2. What are the barriers that prevent a homebound individual from receiving oral health services?

   _____

   _____

   _____

   _____

   _____

   _____

   _____

3. List three objectives of providing dental hygiene care in a home or residential care facility setting.

   _____

   _____

   _____

   _____

   _____

4. Identify three unique objects or implements, not usually associated with providing care in a dental office, to include when planning to provide care for a homebound patient.

   _____

   _____

   _____

5. List three factors that can influence scheduling an appointment time to provide dental hygiene care for a homebound or nursing home patient.

_____

_____

_____

6. List five unhealthy mental characteristics associated with inactivity and the monotonous existence of a homebound patient.

_____

_____

_____

_____

_____

7. When is a firm pillow important for patient positioning during dental hygiene care?

_____

_____

8. Describe a patient who is comatose.

_____

_____

9. In your own words, define the concept of hospice care for the terminally ill.

_____

_____

_____

_____

_____

10. Define palliative care.

_____

_____

11. What common oral infection is often found in a patient with a terminal illness?

_____

_____

✔️ COMPETENCY EXERCISES

Apply information from the chapter and use critical thinking skills to complete the competency exercises. Write responses on paper or create electronic documents to submit your answers.

1. You are one of the dental hygienists on a dental care team that visits the Nightingale Long Term Care Center each month to provide oral care for residents. Your first patient of the day is Bruce Wilkerson, a handsome 29-year-old who has been in a coma since a diving accident 8 years ago. After looking at the information in Bruce's medical record, you enter his room and greet him. As you prepare your armamentarium, position him for oral care, and place towels under his chin, you keep up a cheerful one-sided conversation. Explain why it is important to talk with this patient even though he will definitely not respond to your remarks.

2. Miss Louise Piranian is a 96-year-old resident in the Nightingale Long Term Care Center. She is amazingly feisty and young acting for her age, and she delights the nursing staff with her antics. Her favorite trick is to slip her upper denture out and grin widely with no front teeth! She also wears a lower partial denture, but she won't take that one out because it is too hard to get back in.

   Miss Louise loves to entertain guests at her daily tea party and can talk and talk and talk about all sorts of interesting topics while keeping everyone's teacup full. Lately she is getting a bit forgetful, though, so the Nightingale Center nursing staff is putting together a plan to make sure all her daily personal care needs are met.

   Write your recommendations for a daily oral health plan for Miss Louise that takes into account daily oral care regimens, nutrition, and care of her denture.

3. Mrs. Malcolm has been a patient in your clinic for about 15 years. She has always had fairly good oral hygiene and a healthy mouth has been important to her. You haven't seen her in quite a while, though, because Mrs. Malcolm has spent a lot of time in the hospital over the last year. You recently heard that she has been receiving hospice care in her home.

   Dr. Gable, the dentist in your clinic, has agreed to provide some basic comfort care at home for Mrs. Malcolm, and she suggests that you accompany her. When you arrive, you find that Mrs. Malcolm, although very weak, is awake and able to speak with you. She complains of having a very dry mouth and you notice that her lips are coated with a dry looking, crusty material. She mentions that her lower partial denture does not fit very well anymore and often slips around whenever she tries to eat. It is rubbing on her left cheek. She says her mouth feels and tastes bad and that her gums were bleeding when her daughter tried to help her brush her teeth a couple of days ago.

Write at least three dental hygiene diagnosis statements for Mrs. Malcolm's care plan.

4. Write a goal and evaluation method for one of the diagnosis statements you identified in question 3. Include a time frame for meeting that goal.

5. Describe ways that you can arrange your dental hygiene instruments and materials for providing dental hygiene care to Mrs. Malcolm in her home bedroom.

6. Mrs. Malcolm's daughter, Amy, mentions that she bought some lemon and glycerin swabs at the drugstore to help with the dry mouth her mother has been experiencing. What information can you provide Amy that will help her relieve her mother's dry mouth?

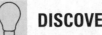 **DISCOVERY EXERCISE**

Use the information in Boxes 57-3 and 57-4 in the textbook as well as additional information from dental supply catalogs and web sites to put together a plan and a budget for everything you would need for a portable dental hygiene practice.

QUESTIONS PATIENTS ASK

What sources of information can you identify that will help you answer your patient's questions in this scenario?

"There are so many agencies now that offer health and personal care services to homebound individuals—why don't they have someone who can come to my house/nursing home so that I could get my teeth cleaned?" "Is there a dentist around here who will make house calls?" "Why doesn't the staff in my mother's nursing home help her brush her teeth every day?"

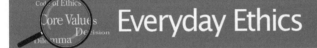 Everyday Ethics

Before completing the learning exercises below, reread and reflect on the Everyday Ethics scenario and Questions for Consideration in this chapter of the textbook. It may also be useful to review the Dental Hygiene Ethics discussion in Chapter 1, the Ethical Applications in the introduction pages for each section in the textbook, as well as the Codes of Ethics in Appendices I, II, and III.

Individual Learning Activities
- Imagine that you are the dental hygienist in this scenario. Answer each of the questions for consideration at the end of the scenario.

- Imagine that you have observed what happened in the scenario, but are not one of the main characters involved in the situation. Write a reflective journal entry that
  - describes how you might have reacted (as an observer- not as a participant),
  - expresses your personal feelings about what happened,
    or
  - identifies personal values that affect your reaction to the situation.

Factors To Teach The Patient

This scenario is related to the following factors listed in this chapter of the textbook:

- The contribution of good oral health to general health
- How a clean mouth can contribute to wellness and quality-of-life factors
- How to care for the patient's natural teeth: toothbrushing, flossing, rinsing, and other personal needs
- How to use a suction toothbrush, power brush, or other device to provide oral care for the patient

Today you are giving hands-on training in providing daily oral care for a group of nurse's aides at the Nightingale Long Term Care Center. You have set up a suction toothbrush at the bedside of Bruce Wilkerson (introduced in question 1 of the competency exercises). Besides showing and telling the nurse's aides how to brush someone else's teeth and care for the suction toothbrush afterward, you also want to explain the reasons for providing daily oral cleansing for all of the residents/patients in the center.

Use the examples of patient conversations in Appendix D as a guide to write an outline of information you need to present to the group of nurse's aides.

Use the conversation you create to role play this situation with several fellow students. If you are pretending to be a nurse's aide in the role-play, be sure to ask questions. If you are the dental hygienist, try to anticipate questions and answer them in your explanation.

CHAPTER 58

The Patient With a Physical Impairment

Learning Objectives

Upon successful completion of these exercises, you will be able to:

1. Identify and define key terms and concepts related to physical impairment.
2. Describe the characteristics, complications, occurrence, and medical treatment of a variety of physical impairments.

3. Identify oral factors and findings related to physical impairments.
4. Plan and document modifications for dental hygiene care based on assessment of needs that are specific to a patient's physical impairment.

 KNOWLEDGE EXERCISES

Write your answers for each question in the space provided.

1. Define the following terms and concepts related to movement.

   a. Akinesia

   _____

   _____

   b. Ankylosis

   _____

   _____

   c. Ataxia

   _____

   _____

   d. Athetosis

   _____

   _____

   e. Bradykinesia

   _____

   _____

   f. Diplegia

   _____

   _____

   g. Dysphagia

   _____

   _____

   h. Flaccidity

   _____

   _____

i. Hemiplegia

_____

_____

j. Kyphosis

_____

_____

k. Lordosis

_____

_____

l. Muscle atrophy

_____

_____

m. Myopathy

_____

_____

n. Orthosis

_____

_____

o. Palsy

_____

_____

p. Paralysis

_____

_____

q. Paraplegia

_____

_____

r. Paresis

_____

_____

s. Parkinsonism

_____

_____

t. Polyarthritis

_____

_____

u. Quadriplegia

_____

_____

v. Rigidity

_____

_____

w. Sclerosis

_____

_____

x. Scoliosis

_____

_____

y. Spasticity

_____

_____

z. Tetraplegia

_____

_____

aa. Tremor

_____

_____

bb. Triplegia

_____

_____

2. Describe the sensorimotor effects of the following lesions.

a. Complete spinal cord injury lesion

_____

_____

b. Incomplete spinal cord injury lesion

_____

_____

3. Identify the appropriate descriptive term and the number of vertebrae associated with each of the following letters.

- C

  Descriptive term: _____

  Number of vertebrae: _____

- T

  Descriptive term: _____

  Number of vertebrae: _____

- L

  Descriptive term: _____

  Number of vertebrae: _____

4. A patient's level of disability depends on the level of the spinal cord injury. Paralysis occurs in the limbs and muscle groups innervated by nerve fibers extending at and below the injured vertebrae. Individuals who are most likely to need adaptive measures for daily oral health care procedures are those with a spinal cord injury above _____.

5. Paralysis of limbs, the need for wheelchair use, and potential complications can require that you be prepared to modify standard patient care techniques, especially when your patient's spinal cord injury is located at T6 or above. Identify modifications you might make during dental hygiene treatment to accommodate this patient's comfort and safety.

  _____

  _____

  _____

  _____

  _____

  _____

  _____

  _____

  _____

  _____

6. What causes a decubitus ulcer and how can you help prevent this condition during dental hygiene treatment of a patient with paralysis?

  _____

  _____

  _____

  _____

7. Describe the correct response to hyperreflexia.

  _____

  _____

  _____

  _____

  _____

  _____

8. Mouth-held appliances can aid many patients who have upper body disabilities in performing a variety of basic procedures that contribute to independence. List the criteria for an adequate oral orthosis.

  _____

  _____

  _____

  _____

9. In your own words, define *CVA*.

  _____

  _____

  _____

  _____

10. What is a TIA?

  _____

  _____

11. List the causes of CVAs.

  _____

  _____

  _____

12. What conditions increase an individual's risk for CVA?

_____

_____

_____

_____

_____

_____

_____

13. What patient assessment technique, commonly used by dental hygienists, can provide information that may indicate your patient's increased risk for CVA.

_____

_____

14. Describe signs and symptoms commonly observed in a patient with a history of CVA.

_____

_____

_____

_____

_____

_____

15. What is aphasia?

_____

_____

16. If your patient has a history of CVA damage to the right side of the brain, that patient would exhibit _____-side hemiplegia, have difficulty with action requiring _____ _____ and would likely behave in an _____ and _____ manner.

17. If your patient has a history of CVA damage to the left side of the brain, that patient would exhibit _____-side hemiplegia, have difficulty with _____ communication, and would likely behave in a _____ and _____ manner.

18. Osteoarthritis is a chronic degenerative joint disease that is common in individuals who are over _____ years old.

19. Describe the location and progression of osteoarthritis symptoms.

_____

_____

_____

20. Describe osteoarthritis symptoms that can occur in the temporomandibular joint.

_____

_____

21. What is rheumatoid arthritis?

_____

_____

_____

22. In your own words, describe the symptoms of rheumatoid arthritis.

_____

_____

_____

_____

_____

23. What is juvenile rheumatoid arthritis?

_____

_____

_____

24. How does rheumatoid arthritis affect the temporomandibular joint?

_____

_____

25. What modifications to standard treatment techniques can you use to increase the comfort of your patient who has arthritic involvement of the temporomandibular joint while you are providing dental hygiene treatment?

_____

_____

_____

26. What is the relationship between rheumatoid arthritis and periodontal disease?

_____

_____

27. Drugs used for treatment of arthritis include pain medications such as NSAIDs. What additional drugs are used to control rheumatoid arthritis?

_____

_____

_____

_____

28. If your patient has severe degenerative joint disease, what additional important question will you be sure to incorporate when you are updating his or her health history?

_____

_____

_____

29. Complete Infomaps 58-1 and 58-2 with just enough basic information to help you identify and differentiate among the listed developmental and acquired disabling conditions.

INFOMAP 58-1	DEVELOPMENTAL CONDITIONS (ONSET BEFORE AGE 18)		
CONDITION	**CAUSE/OCCURRENCE**	**BASIC CHARACTERISTICS**	**CONSIDERATIONS FOR DENTAL HYGIENE CARE**
Cerebral Palsy			
Muscular Dystrophy, Duchenne			
Muscular Dystrophy, Facioscapulohumeral			
Myelomeningocele			

INFOMAP 58-2	ACQUIRED IMPAIRMENT (ONSET AFTER AGE 18)		
CONDITION	**CAUSE, OCCURRENCE, PATHOLOGY**	**BASIC CHARACTERISTICS**	**CONSIDERATIONS FOR DENTAL HYGIENE CARE**
Bell's Palsy			
Multiple Sclerosis			
Amyotrophic Lateral Sclerosis (ALS)			
Myasthenia Gravis			
Parkinson's Disease			
Scleroderma, Progressive Systemic Sclerosis			
Post-Polio Syndrome (PPS)			

30. What percent of patients with cerebral palsy also have brain damage that causes intellectual or cognitive impairment?

_____

_____

31. What additional disabling conditions can sometimes accompany a diagnosis of cerebral palsy?

_____

_____

_____

_____

32. What oral characteristics are associated with cerebral palsy?

_____

_____

_____

_____

_____

_____

_____

_____

33. What symptoms of muscular dystrophy can directly affect your patient's oral health status?

_____

_____

_____

34. Describe the categories that are used to identify types of multiple sclerosis.

_____

_____

_____

_____

_____

_____

35. ALS is also sometimes called what?

_____

36. Describe early/onset symptoms for each of the two types of ALS.

_____

_____

_____

_____

37. Myasthenia gravis and scleroderma are both disabling conditions that have special significance for dental professionals. Why?

_____

_____

_____

_____

_____

38. Care is taken when raising the dental chair after treatment of your patient with Parkinson's disease who is being treated with dopamine replenishment medications, because of the possibility of

_____.

COMPETENCY EXERCISES

Apply information from the chapter and use critical think-ing skills to complete the competency exercises. Write responses on paper or create electronic documents to submit your answers.

Read the Chapter 58 Patient Assessment Summary to help you answer questions 1 through 3.

1. Anitha Jones presents for an initial visit dental hygiene appointment. Laura, Anitha's new caregiver, introduces herself as she assists you in transferring Anitha to the dental chair. While you are helping transfer Anitha to the dental chair, you note that she cannot control the constant disorganized movements of her arms, legs, and head. When you mistakenly startle her by reaching quickly to move the dental light out of the way, this uncontrolled movement becomes intensified. Anitha's hand flings out and bumps into the instrument tray, scattering instruments all over the floor. Anitha's face muscles are in constant motion; she drools and breathes through her mouth. Describe steps you will take to determine modifications in your usual patient care procedures that will help to keep both you and Anitha safe and comfortable during dental hygiene treatment.

CHAPTER 58—PATIENT ASSESSMENT SUMMARY

Patient Name: Ms. Anitha Jones	Age: 30	Gender: M [F]	☑ Initial Therapy
			☐ Maintenance
Provider Name: D.H. Student	Date: Today		☐ Re-evaluation

Chief Complaint:

Patient has recently moved into the area. She presents for routine 3-month maintenance and new patient examination.

ASSESSMENT FINDINGS

Health History

- Medical diagnosis of cerebral palsy
- Spasticity, athetosis, facial movements
- No intellectual or cognitive disability.
- Takes anti-seizure medication once per day, but caregiver who accompanies her to the appointment is not sure what it is.
- ASA Classification—III
- ADL level—3

At Risk for:

Social and Dental History

- *Previous history of excellent professional dental care*
- *Personal dental literacy is high*
- *New caregiver with low dental knowledge*

At Risk for:

Dental Examination

- Difficulty controlling jaw and face movements during examination
- Bruxism; incisal attrition and history of anterior fractures
- Evidence of past lip and cheek-biting trauma
- Mouth breathing; slight anterior gingivitis
- Increased gag reflex
- Current posterior restorations in good repair
- Healthy periodontal tissues; probing depths <3 mm

At Risk For:

---

2. When she is trying to communicate, it takes Anitha a long time to say anything and you cannot under-stand her very well. What communication strategies will help you successfully determine answers to the questions you need to ask in order to complete your patient assessment?

3. As you complete assessment data, you realize that Anitha has enjoyed regular professional and per-sonal dental care throughout her life. A caregiver has always provided daily oral biofilm removal. Laura, the new caregiver, admits to having very little dental knowledge, but she very much wants to learn how to

keep Anitha's mouth as healthy as her previous care-giver has done. Use the assessment summary data for Anitha and a copy of the Dental Hygiene Care Plan template (Appendix B) to complete a dental hygiene care plan for Anitha that includes appropriate education for Laura.

4. Mr. O'Brien, who has been recovering for about 9 months since experiencing a CVA, has been receiving physical and occupational therapy to help him learn how use his left hand to do what he used to do with his, now partially paralyzed, right hand and arm. He is very proud of his growing independence

and slowly tells you about how he can now comb his own hair and brush his own teeth. While you are performing an oral examination, you note that his biofilm control is very poor and that there is a bolus of left-over food pocketed in his right cheek. The paralyzed muscles on that side of his face have affected his ability to self-clean and even to detect the food that is pouching there after he eats.

Explain how you can counsel Mr. O'Brien about his oral health needs and encourage him to let his wife help him clean his mouth, especially on the paralyzed side, while still respecting his desire to independently care for his own personal needs?

Everyday Ethics

Before completing the learning exercises below, reread and reflect on the Everyday Ethics scenario and Questions for Consideration in this chapter of the textbook. It may also be useful to review the Dental Hygiene Ethics discussion in Chapter 1, the Ethical Applications in the introduction pages for each section in the textbook, as well as the Codes of Ethics in Appendices I, II, and III.

Cooperative Learning Activity

Answer each of the questions for consideration at the end of the scenario in the textbook. Compare what you wrote with answers developed by another classmate and discuss differences/similarities.

Discovery Activity

Investigate the practice act in your state to determine the legal issues involved as the dental hygienist in this scenario contemplates what action to take.

Factors To Teach The Patient

This scenario is related to the following factors listed in this chapter of the textbook:

- That daily, thorough biofilm removal is particularly necessary to reduce the occurrence of oral disease
- That regular maintenance appointments are important to promote oral health
- Why maintaining periodontal health has added value for teeth used as abutments for a mouth-held implement
- How to clean and maintain the mouth-held implement
- The need to maintain teeth in order to tolerate a mouth-held aid

Once a month, your employer, Dr. Tom Buckner, and his entire dental team provide care in a little dental clinic inside a nearby assisted-living residence. Your next patient, Terry Biensfield, 25 years old, sustained a level C5 spinal-cord injury in a motorcycle accident several years ago. He has

worked hard in his physical-therapy sessions to maximize his level of function in activities of daily living by using adaptive aids. You have taught him how to brush his own teeth using a modified, long-handled toothbrush attached to one hand, but he still needs some caregiver support and reminders that he must complete his daily oral care routine.

Last month, Dr. Buckner and the physical therapist devised a mouthstick appliance that allows Terry to use a computer. Terry has been practicing with the computer every day, when he participates in an online discussion for people with spinal-cord injuries. He now has lots of new ideas for ways he can use his mouthstick to be more independent and creative in his daily life.

Use the example of patient conversations in Appendix D as a guide to write a statement explaining to Terry how important it is for him to maintain his present level of oral health so that his teeth can continue to support the use of a mouthstick.

The Patient With a Sensory Impairment

Upon successful completion of these exercises, you will be able to:

1. Identify and define key terms and concepts related to sensory impairment.
2. Describe the causes of sensory impairments.

3. Identify factors that affect interpersonal communication and patient education.
4. Plan and document adaptations that enhance dental hygiene care for a patient with a sensory impairment.

 KNOWLEDGE EXERCISES

1. A reference to a patient with a disability always begins with a statement about the person before defining the disability. Using the Americans with Disabilities Act (ADA) definition and terminology from this chapter, how would you describe an individual who is blind?

   _____

   _____

2. In what way does the ADA define the responsibility of the dental practitioner in meeting the needs of a patient with a hearing or vision impairment?

   _____

   _____

   _____

   _____

3. In your own words, define *visual impairment*.

   _____

   _____

4. Define *total blindness*.

   _____

   _____

5. Explain the term *legally blind*.

   _____

   _____

   _____

6. For each descriptive term below that describes types of visual impairment often corrected by prescription eyeglasses, provide the medical term and characteristics associated with it.

   a. Farsighted

   _____

   _____

   b. Nearsighted

   _____

   _____

7. An astigmatism, also often corrected with prescription glasses, is caused by what?

_____

_____

8. An _____ measures visual acuity and prescribes lenses for the correction of visual defects; an _____ is the technician who prepares the adaptive lenses prescribed by the specialist.

9. An _____ is a physician specializing in treatment of defects, injuries, and diseases of the eye.

10. _____ _____ during pregnancy is the cause of at least half of the blindness in children.

11. _____ is an inflammation of the retina.

12. What is retinopathy?

_____

_____

13. Identify and describe the condition that causes blindness in infants who must be treated at birth with very high concentrations of oxygen.

_____

_____

_____

14. In your own words, define *glaucoma*.

_____

_____

15. What action during dental hygiene treatment can cause pain for your patient with glaucoma?

_____

_____

16. What term refers to a visual impairment that can be caused by a vitamin deficiency?

_____

17. Through observation, how can you identify a potential visual impairment in an older patient who does not admit to failing sight?

_____

_____

18. Why do you always speak to patients who have a significant visual impairment each time before you enter or leave the room and each time before you touch them during dental hygiene treatment?

_____

_____

19. A person can hear when the _____ _____ vibrates and sound waves are transmitted to nerve endings by the ossicles of middle ear, to cochlea in the inner ear, and then to the brain.

20. What is tinnitus?

_____

_____

21. What is vertigo?

_____

_____

22. What is the abbreviation for decibel?

_____

23. Your patient is considered deaf when his or her hearing impairment is at what level?

_____

_____

24. What descriptive phrase is used for a patient who has a hearing impairment but uses an aid to facilitate communication?

_____

25. List factors that may contribute to hearing loss.

_____

_____

_____

_____

_____

26. What is an audiologist?

_____

_____

27. How does the audiologist determine an individual's hearing ability?

_____

_____

28. An otologist would most likely be the health care worker involved with treating otitis media. What is otitis media?

_____

29. Identify the four types of hearing loss and briefly identify the damaged body structure(s) associated with each type.

_____

_____

_____

_____

30. How does a hearing aid function?

_____

_____

31. Why should you remind your patient who uses a hearing aid to either turn it off or take it out during dental hygiene treatment?

_____

_____

_____

32. Describe a cochlear implant.

_____

_____

33. In your own words, what is American Sign Language (ASL)?

_____

_____

34. What is speech reading?

_____

_____

35. If your patient is speech reading, what can you do to enhance his or her understanding during oral hygiene instructions?

_____

_____

_____

_____

36. The best way to teach skills, such as biofilm removal, to your patient with a hearing loss is by _____ rather than by explanation.

 ## COMPETENCY EXERCISES

1. You have completed Mr. Corkman's dental hygiene treatment for today, and you direct him down to Jenny, the appointment manager, so he can schedule his next visit while you clean and disinfect the treatment room for your next patient. When he gets to the end of the hallway, you hear him say, "Delighted to meet you, Benny!" You observe him at the front desk for a bit and then walk up to him and remind him that he turned his hearing aid off when you were using the ultrasonic scaler during his treatment. What signs did you observe that indicated Mr. Corkman had forgotten to turn it on again?

2. Ask one of your student colleagues to role play the part of Anastasia Binghamton, 16 years old, your patient who is profoundly deaf. Her preferred method of communicating is using a combination of ASL and finger spelling. Use the pictures in Figures 59-2 and 59-3 in the textbook to help you practice asking her the following questions.

   ■ Are there any changes in your health history?

   ■ Is there any pain in the area where tooth 32 was extracted last month?

   ■ Can you please open wider so that I can polish the back teeth?

   ■ I will show you how to position your toothbrush in order to get all the bacteria off the gums.

   ■ The dentist will be right in to examine your mouth.

   ■ Please make your next appointment in 6 months.

3. Patty Ricalde, 25 years old, is one of your favorite patients. She usually arrives for her appointment clinging to the arm of her younger sister; both of them are out of breath, laughing uproariously, and looking as though they had just returned from some astonishing adventure. Sometimes they have, as you found out last year, when they came in with photographs of a desert hiking adventure in southern Utah!

Sometimes, when you listen to the two of them, you forget that Patty is designated as legally blind. She also wears a hearing device that allows her to communicate with anyone who will take the time to talk slowly and clearly.

You will be developing a new dental hygiene care plan for Patty, and you want to designate her ADL level to indicate her ability to manage daily oral care (*Hint:* Refer to Table 23-3 in the textbook).

Discuss and provide a rationale for the ADL level that you assign to Patty.

4. What ASA classification will you assign to Patty? (*Hint:* Refer to Table 23-1 in the textbook.)

5. Patty arrives without her sister, but with a huge golden retriever guide dog she calls Harrison. You are a bit flustered and you hold out your hand to greet Patty without first letting her know you have come into the room with her. She bumps into you as she turns to return your greeting. You aren't quite sure what to do next, as Patty's sister has always helped guide Patty to your treatment room and helped her get settled in the chair, and today you will obviously have to help her yourself. You cover your distress by complimenting her on the beauty of her dog and bending down to hug him.

You gently take Harrison by the collar and lead him down the hall to the door of your treatment room. Patty follows you and her dog into the room. You raise the chair up a bit higher, so the seat is just above the level of Patty's knees and you turn her around and gently ease her back until she is sitting against the edge of the dental chair. You tell her you will place the dog out in the hall where there is significantly more room. She seems uneasy about that, but you reassure her that no one will be going by to step on him there, as your treatment room is the last one down the hall.

As you return to the room, Patty pushes herself up and back into the chair, turns, and slides her feet up on the footrest. You wince as her head just misses the dental light, but she doesn't hit it and you breathe a sigh of relief. You notice the time, so you quickly update her health history (no significant findings), lower the chair, and tell Patty to grab hold of the armrests before you tilt her back. You complete your oral assessment and begin scaling.

Later, after polishing her teeth, you squirt lots of water so she can rinse her mouth. She raises herself from the chair, swallows twice, and then apologizes and asks for a cup to rinse. After you help her rinse with a cup, you are feeling that this appointment has been very stressful for you, and you would love to have a quiet minute to recover your calm. As Patty gets out of the dental chair, you walk out into the hallway to bring Harrison back in to her.

What could you have done differently to manage Patty's care to reduce both her stress and your own during this appointment?

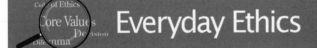

Everyday Ethics

Before completing the learning exercises below, reread and reflect on the Everyday Ethics scenario and Questions for Consideration in this chapter of the textbook. It may also be useful to review the Dental Hygiene Ethics discussion in Chapter 1, the Ethical Applications in the introduction pages for each section in the textbook, as well as the Codes of Ethics in Appendices I, II, and III.

Individual Learning Activity
Imagine the scenario from the patient's perspective. How might the patient's response to the questions following the scenario be different from those of the dental hygienist involved?

Collaborative Learning Activity
Work with another student colleague to role-play the scenario. The goal of this exercise is for you and your colleague to work though the alternative actions in order to come to consensus on a solution or response that is acceptable to both of you.

Factors To Teach The Patient

This scenario is related to the following factors listed in this chapter of the textbook:

■ The importance of oral care for the guide dog

When you have completed care for Patty Ricalde (introduced in the competency exercises) for the day, she tells you laughingly that her vet said she needs to clean Harrison's teeth regularly to keep him healthy. You reply that, of course, regular oral hygiene is as important for him as it is for Patty. You agree to teach her how. Because your next patient is due, you don't have time today, but you agree to meet her during your lunch hour tomorrow. She already has a toothbrush and some special chicken-flavored toothpaste. You decide that to be thorough, you had better plan this doggy oral hygiene instruction carefully before you meet with Patty tomorrow.

Keeping in mind that Patty is blind and wears a hearing aid, use the examples of patient conversations in Appendix D as a guide to prepare a conversation to teach Patty about maintaining her guide dog's oral health.

CHAPTER 60

The Patient With a Developmental or Behavioral Disorder

Learning Objectives

Upon successful completion of these exercises, you will be able to:

1. Identify and define key terms and concepts related to the patient with a developmental disorder.
2. Identify the dimensions, intellectual functioning levels, risk factors, and etiologies associated with developmental disorders.
3. Describe the specific characteristics of individuals with an intellectual disability, Down syndrome, and autistic spectrum disorders.
4. Plan and document modifications necessary for dental hygiene care and effective oral hygiene instruction for persons with developmental or behavioral disorders.

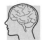 **KNOWLEDGE EXERCISES**

Write your answers for each question in the space provided.

1. Identify the major groups of disorders that are usually first diagnosed before or during adolescence.

   _____
   _____
   _____
   _____
   _____
   _____
   _____
   _____

2. List the five interrelated dimensions that contribute to testing the functioning level of an individual with an intellectual disorder.

   _____
   _____
   _____
   _____
   _____

3. In your own words, briefly summarize the characteristics for each classification of intellectual functioning that will impact the dental hygienist's approach to providing oral health education and oral hygiene instruction.

   a. Mild

   _____
   _____
   _____

b. Moderate

_____

_____

_____

c. Severe

_____

_____

_____

d. Profound

_____

_____

_____

4. Identify the four categories of risk factors for intellectual disorders.

_____

_____

_____

_____

5. What behavior-related factors during pregnancy may result in an infant with an intellectual disorder?

_____

_____

_____

6. What can happen during the infant's birth that can lead to an intellectual disorder?

_____

_____

_____

_____

_____

_____

7. When an infant is born normal, what two early childhood situations can lead to intellectual disorders?

_____

_____

8. Identify characteristic physical features or anomalies you might observe when performing an extraoral examination for your patient with an intellectual disorder.

_____

_____

_____

9. List five intraoral findings common in individuals with intellectual disorders.

_____

_____

_____

_____

_____

10. List five characteristics that can help you identify an individual with Down syndrome.

_____

_____

_____

_____

_____

11. What level of functioning do individuals with Down syndrome usually reach?

_____

_____

12. Most individuals with Down syndrome have pleasant personalities. Identify three personal characteristics that make these individuals likable and easy to be around.

_____

_____

_____

13. Why do patients with Down syndrome often present for dental treatment with very cracked and dried lips?

_____

_____

14. Identify physical/medical health problems commonly found in individuals with Down syndrome that require special consideration or modifications during dental hygiene treatment.

    _____

    _____

    _____

15. Briefly describe the characteristics that distinguish each of the five variations of pervasive development disorder.

    _____

    _____

    _____

    _____

    _____

    _____

    _____

    _____

    _____

16. Describe two types of treatment used to manage symptoms and increase the ability of the patient with autism to live a normal life.

    _____

    _____

17. Identify the 5 steps from the D-TERMINED program that you can use to help your patient with an autistic spectrum disorder or other intellectual disorder learn how to cooperate during dental hygiene interventions and self-care recommendations.

    _____

    _____

    _____

    _____

    _____

✓ COMPETENCY EXERCISES

Apply information from the chapter and use critical thinking skills to complete the competency exercises. Write responses on paper or create electronic documents to submit your answers.

1. Next week you will be starting a new part-time position as the dental hygienist for 50 resident patients in a small private residential facility. You will go once a week to work with Dr. Sally Roderick, the dentist who has been providing dental care at the residence for 25 years. The individuals living in the residence are classified as having severe or profound intellectual disorder. You are excited about the opportunity to work with Dr. Roderick and to learn about this population, which you have only read about in your textbook.

   To prepare for this new challenge, create a list of planning measures you can take and modifications you can make to your usual treatment procedures so you can increase your effectiveness when providing dental hygiene care for these patients.

2. On the first day at the residence center, you find that Dr. Roderick has done very well providing patients with restorative care, but not much attention has been paid to dental hygiene care and education. The patient in your clinic chair right now is Bonne. She is 22 years old and is classified as having a profound intellectual disability.

   One of the nurse's aides, who is her regular caregiver, helps you place Bonne in the papoose board and sits by the side of the dental chair to help when she can. You have some difficulty examining Bonne's mouth, but you can readily see that she has extensive biofilm buildup and significant amounts of calculus in all areas of her mouth.

   You know that it will take more than one appointment to assess Bonne's dental hygiene needs thoroughly and to make a full plan for care. However, Dr. Roderick asks you to write up a formal dental hygiene care plan for what you will accomplish in the next three or four appointments so that it can be recorded in Bonne's medical record. You know that you must plan enough time for the complete assessment that you need to accomplish before you can fully understand Bonne's oral condition. You must also plan for daily biofilm control.

   Use the Dental Hygiene Care Plan Template in Appendix B to develop a formal, written care plan for clinical procedures and educational interventions you will provide during the four appointments you will schedule in the next few weeks for Bonne and her caregiver.

4. Today when you saw Bonne in the clinic, you reviewed her medical history, provided a limited intraoral assessment examination, and developed a written care plan that will help you get through four initial assessment and educational visits with Bonne and her caregiver. Use your institution's guidelines for writing in patient records to document these procedures.

Everyday Ethics

Before completing the learning exercises below, reread and reflect on the Everyday Ethics scenario and Questions for Consideration in this chapter of the textbook. It may also be useful to review the Dental Hygiene Ethics discussion in Chapter 1, the Ethical Applications in the introduction pages for each section in the textbook, as well as the Codes of Ethics in Appendices I, II, and III.

Individual Learning Activity
Imagine that you have observed what happened in the scenario, but are not one of the main characters involved in the situation. Write a reflective journal entry that

- describes how you might have reacted (as an observer-not as a participant),
- expresses your personal feelings about what happened, or
- identifies personal values that affect your reaction to the situation.

Collaborative Learning Activity
Answer each of the questions for consideration at the end of the scenario in the textbook. Compare what you wrote with answers developed by another classmate and discuss differences/similarities.

Factors To Teach The Patient

This scenario is related to the following factors listed in this chapter of the textbook:

For the patient:
- How to perform oral self-care procedures
- Why assistance from others is an important supplement to the patient's own efforts
- How to use and show cooperation skills

For the caregiver:
- Why a total preventive program is important
- How to incorporate behavior modification into oral care procedures
- The importance of repeating "show-tell-do" instructions often

Use information in Chapter 60 in the textbook and the examples of patient conversations in Appendix D as guides to develop a conversation you will use to provide oral hygiene instructions for a patient who is classified with a moderate intellectual disability. Include the patient's caregiver as you discuss strategies for daily oral care.

Use the conversation you create to role-play this situation with a fellow student. If you are the patient or the caregiver in the role-play, be sure to ask questions. If you are the dental hygienist, try to anticipate questions and answer them in your explanation. Modify your conversation based on what you learned.

CROSSWORD PUZZLE

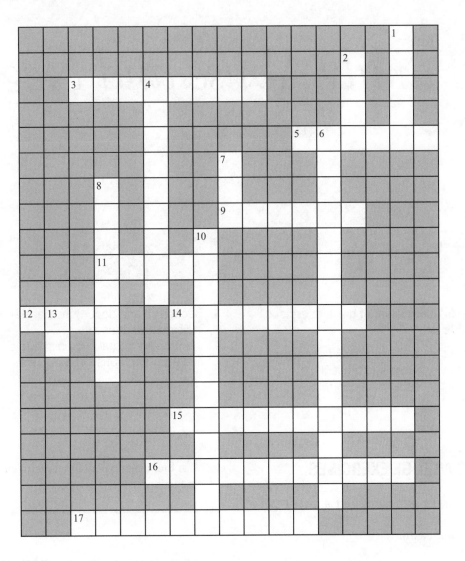

ACROSS

3. One of the autistic spectrum disorders that is characterized impairment in social interactions.
5. Inability or refusal to speak.
9. Refers to coexisting medical conditions
11. A vertical fold of skin on either side of the nose; a normal characteristic of persons of some races that is associated with Down syndrome.
12. Persistent craving/eating of nonnutritive substances or unnatural articles of food.
14. Classification of intellectual disability in which the individual would most likely need to have all daily oral hygiene measures provided by a caregiver.
15. Involuntary utterance of vulgar words.
16. Abnormality in morphologic development.
17. Repeated regurgitation of food.

DOWN

1. Trisomy 21 syndrome (two words).
2. An autism spectrum disorder that occurs only in girls; characterized by repetitive hand movements.
4. The involuntary repetition of a word or sentence just spoken by another person.
6. The reflection or transmission of ultrasonic waves in body tissues; can be used to examine a fetus to determine birth defects.
7. Sudden nonrhythmic motor movement or vocal sound
8. Category of intellectual disability in which the individual could most likely attend to personal oral care with some reminders from a caregiver.
10. Very large tongue.
13. Numeric rating of the relationship of mental age to chronologic age.

Family Abuse and Neglect

Upon successful completion of these exercises, you will be able to:

1. Identify and define key terms and concepts related to family abuse and neglect.
2. Describe various categories of family maltreatment.
3. Recognize and document signs and behavioral indicators of abuse.
4. Identify the dental hygienist's role in recognizing and reporting abuse and neglect.

 KNOWLEDGE EXERCISES

Write your answers for each question in the space provided.

1. Define *forensic dentistry*.

   _____

   _____

2. Identify three programs you can explore further to help you learn more about how to assess and respond to suspected abuse during a patient/provider interaction.

   _____

   _____

   _____

The factors involved in the recognition and management of suspected maltreatment of children, the elderly, people with disabilities, and women are similar. When answering the following questions, be sure to take all of these potential at-risk groups into consideration, unless the question specifics a particular group or groups.

3. List four major types of maltreatment that can occur in families.

   _____

   _____

   _____

   _____

4. Identify two types of maltreatment of elders that do not usually occur in cases involving children.

   _____

   _____

5. In your own words, define *dental neglect*.

   _____

   _____

6. When children state that there is no one at their house to help them brush their teeth, what additional appearance and behavioral indicators might lead you to suspect that your patient is neglected?

_____

_____

_____

_____

7. Identify the signs of lice infestation.

_____

_____

_____

8. Identify personal appearance factors that might lead you to suspect that an individual is being physically abused.

_____

_____

_____

_____

9. In your own words, describe the raccoon sign.

_____

10. What is an area of baldness that is caused by pulling out hair by the roots?

_____

11. What is the medical term used to document a bruise?

_____

12. Describe what you might notice about an accidental injury versus characteristics you might observe when the injuries are inflicted or deliberate.

_____

_____

_____

_____

13. Identify intraoral signs of physical abuse.

_____

_____

_____

_____

_____

_____

14. Identify general signs of physical abuse and neglect in a child patient.

_____

_____

_____

_____

_____

15. In what way do these general signs compare with what you might notice if an elderly patient is being mistreated?

_____

_____

_____

16. Extremely aggressive behavior by a child when you try to examine his or her mouth can be a behavioral indicator for _____ abuse as well as for physical abuse.

17. Identify intraoral signs of sexual abuse.

_____

_____

_____

_____

18. List nonabuse-related conditions that can mimic the physical signs of abuse.

_____

_____

_____

19. One important role for the dental hygienist in cases of suspected abuse is to document the observable facts in the patient's record. What information is necessary to have available when you are reporting abuse to state authorities?

_____

_____

_____

_____

COMPETENCY EXERCISES

Apply information from the chapter and use critical thinking skills to complete the competency exercises. Write responses on paper or create electronic documents to submit your answers.

1. Read the information in the Everyday Ethics case study for this workbook chapter. Using your institution's guidelines for writing in patient records, document your findings regarding Sarah. (_Important Note:_ Write your progress note entry so that it includes only factual, objective information about the dental hygienist's observations and no subjective statements or personal opinions.)

2. Outline the thought process you will use when making a decision to report suspected child abuse to state authorities. Discuss your outline with a small group of your student colleagues. Use the results of this discussion to write an office protocol for reporting suspected abuse.

DISCOVERY EXERCISES

1. Investigate the laws and the processes for reporting child, elder, or spouse abuse in your state.

2. Investigate the agencies in your area where abused elders or battered spouses can obtain help or emergency assistance.

3. Investigate the PANDA program, the AVDR Tutorial for Dentists, or Project RADAR to learn more about recognizing and reporting family abuse and neglect.

Everyday Ethics

Before completing the learning exercises below, reread and reflect on the Everyday Ethics scenario and Questions for Consideration in this chapter of the textbook. It may also be useful to review the Dental Hygiene Ethics discussion in Chapter 1, the Ethical Applications in the introduction pages for each section in the textbook, as well as the Codes of Ethics in Appendices I, II, and III.

Collaborative Learning Activities
■ Identify a situation in which you have resolved an ethical dilemma and share the story with a classmate. Discuss how that person might have acted differently to resolve the situation.

■ Work with a small group to develop a 2- to 5-minute role-play that introduces the Everyday Ethics scenario described in the chapter (a great idea is to video record your role-play activity). Then develop separate 2-minute role-play scenarios that provide at least two alternative approaches/solutions to resolving the situation. Ask classmates to view the solutions, ask questions, and discuss the ethical approach used in each. Ask for a vote on which solution classmates determine to be the "best."

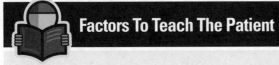

Factors To Teach The Patient

This scenario is related to the following factors listed in this chapter of the textbook:

■ The value of oral hygiene with age-appropriate materials
■ What the bacterial biofilm is on teeth, using a disclosing agent
■ How to use the new toothbrush the child just received
■ Why it is especially important to brush the teeth and tongue just before going to sleep

Johnny is 8 years old. This is his first dental hygiene visit with you, and his dental history indicates that he has not seen a dentist since a dental examination was required by the HeadStart program when he was 3 years old. His parents scheduled this dental appointment as a result of a directive from state authorities after a report by his teacher.

Johnny is very shy, but after he gets to know you a bit during his appointment, he seems interested in what you are doing and asks all kinds of questions. You note during your intraoral examination that his teeth are completely covered with dental biofilm. Johnny states he doesn't really have a very good toothbrush. He obviously is not performing daily self-care, and you suspect that his parents are not helping or encouraging him in any way. Fortunately, there are no carious lesions, but his gingival tissue is red and bleeds easily when you touch it.

Use the examples of patient conversations in Appendix D as a guide, and use language appropriate for a child to explain why Johnny needs to brush his teeth every day.

The Patient With a Seizure Disorder

 KNOWLEDGE EXERCISES

Write your answers for each question in the space provided.

1. What is the etiology of a seizure?

   _____

   _____

2. Although most seizure disorders tend to be stable, some individuals experience a random pattern of seizures that disrupt their lives. List some activities that may be compromised for an individual who experiences recurrent seizures.

   _____

   _____

   _____

3. Identify factors that can trigger a seizure in a susceptible patient during dental hygiene treatment.

   _____

   _____

   _____

   _____

4. If your patient has a history of seizure activity, when should you contact/consult with your patient's physician?

   _____

   _____

   _____

5. In what three ways are epileptic syndromes classified?

   _____

   _____

   _____

6. List the subcategories for the partial and generalized epileptic seizures.

   a. Partial seizures

   _____

   _____

   _____

   b. Generalized seizures

   _____

   _____

7. A partial seizure involves only part of the brain. In your own words, briefly describe the clinical manifestations of a partial seizure.

   _____

   _____

   _____

   _____

8. A generalized seizure affects both sides of the brain at the same time. In your own words, briefly describe the clinical manifestations of an absence seizure.

   _____

   _____

   _____

   _____

9. Describe a tonic–clonic seizure.

   _____

   _____

   _____

   _____

10. List other medical conditions you should consider if your patient is manifesting some clinical signs of a seizure, particularly if the patient's medical history does not indicate a seizure disorder. (*Hint:* Think "differential diagnosis.")

   _____

   _____

   _____

   _____

   _____

   _____

   _____

11. If your patient does have a seizure during dental hygiene treatment, what emergency measures will you take to protect your patient from injury?

   _____

   _____

   _____

   _____

12. What oral injuries are associated with generalized seizures?

   _____

   _____

   _____

13. What action should you take in the event that your patient's tonic–clonic seizure continues for longer than 5 minutes?

   _____

   _____

   _____

14. Describe status epilepticus.

   _____

   _____

15. Identify surgical interventions that are used to medically treat patients with seizure disorders.

   _____

   _____

   _____

16. Which treatment for seizure disorders will require you to modify the use of some dental devices during dental hygiene treatment?

   _____

   _____

   _____

17. Your patient with a seizure disorder is likely to be taking an antiepileptic medication. Of the medications listed in Table 62-1 in the textbook, phenytoin (Dilantin) is the most likely to induce gingival hyperplasia in your patient. In your own words, describe the mechanism, incidence, appearance, and effects of phenytoin-induced gingival hyperplasia.

_____

_____

_____

_____

_____

_____

_____

_____

18. What medications, in addition to phenytoin, are associated with gingival overgrowth?

_____

_____

_____

19. Identify dental hygiene treatment and education interventions that can prevent or inhibit the growth of gingival tissues in your patient who is taking phenytoin or another medication that causes gingival enlargement.

_____

_____

_____

_____

20. What surgical options are available for treating phenytoin-induced gingival hyperplasia?

_____

_____

✓ COMPETENCY EXERCISES

Apply information from the chapter and use critical thinking skills to complete the competency exercises. Write responses on paper or create electronic documents to submit your answers.

1. You can tell that your new patient has a very business-like approach to his health care. Mr. Arakawa is a 45-year-old chief executive officer in a major corporation in town. As you lead him back to your treatment room, he stops briefly at the front desk to make sure of the procedure for submitting today's charges to his dental insurance. He mentions that he is on a tight schedule and wants to be sure about what time his appointment will end.

   He fills out the health history form you hand him with short, efficient strokes of his pen and hands it back to you. The only positive answers on the form are for seizure activity and medication, but he does not indicate what drug he is taking. You know that to completely understand Mr. Arakawa's condition, you must ask him more questions. Create a list of questions you will ask Mr. Arakawa as you clarify his health history information.

2. When you begin to ask Mr. Arakawa the questions you formulated, he briskly states that his history of seizures is not relevant to his dental treatment. He states that his previous dental provider never asked such questions, and, besides, he has not had a seizure for a long time. He tells you about the medication he is taking but is clearly not happy about answering the other questions you are asking.

   You know that he needs to understand why it is important for you to learn about his history of seizures. What information will you include in your discussion with Mr. Arakawa as you convince him to comply with your request for information about his seizures?

3. Your education/counseling approach is successful and you find out that Mr. Arakawa has been experiencing seizures for almost 30 years. The severity of the tonic–clonic type seizures he experiences has decreased since his teenage years, and in fact, the seizures are now fairly well under control.

The medication he is currently taking is an etho-suximide (Zarontin), but his previous prescription was a phenytoin (Dilantin), which he took for almost 20 years. About 10 years ago, he had gingival surgery to control gingival overgrowth he experienced from taking the phenytoin and fears that his gums are growing again.

Mr. Arakawa experienced some fairly serious dental trauma when he lost consciousness and fell during a seizure, and his maxillary anterior teeth have been replaced with a porcelain bridge. He has often bitten his lips and tongue when he is convulsing. One time when he was young, he experienced a seizure during routine dental treatment and that is why he was at first reluctant and embarrassed to share much information about his seizures with you. He describes the aura that he experiences before a seizure, which appears as flashes of light just outside the direct view of his left eye. He also mentions that sometimes changing patterns of light have caused a seizure to happen and asks you to be careful when positioning the dental light during his treatment. His last seizure was about 2 years ago.

Using your institution's guidelines for writing in patient records, document what you have learned about Mr. Arakawa's medical condition.

4. You know that many medications prescribed to control seizures have numerous side effects, other than gingival hyperplasia, that are a concern for dental professionals. Refer to the list of potential side effects in the "Treatment" section of Chapter 62 in the textbook and indicate which side effects have implications for patient education or treatment modifications during Mr. Arakawa's dental hygiene appointments.

5. When you examine Mr. Arakawa's mouth, you observe areas of advanced gingival hyperplasia. Use the decision tree in Figure 62-3 in the textbook to indicate what the next step would be in deciding appropriate treatment for this condition.

Everyday Ethics

Before completing the learning exercises below, reread and reflect on the Everyday Ethics scenario and Questions for Consideration in this chapter of the textbook. It may also be useful to review the Dental Hygiene Ethics discussion in Chapter 1, the Ethical Applications in the introduction pages for each section in the textbook, as well as the Codes of Ethics in Appendices I, II, and III.

Collaborative Learning Activity
Answer each of the questions for consideration at the end of the scenario in the textbook. Compare what you wrote

with answers developed by another classmate and discuss differences/similarities.

Discovery Activity
Ask a dental hygienist who has been practicing for a year or more to read the scenario. Provide them with a copy of one of the Codes of Ethics as well. Share the responses you have made to answer each question and ask that person to discuss the situation with you. What insights did you have or what did you learn during this discussion?

Factors To Teach The Patient

This scenario is related to the following factors listed in this chapter of the textbook:

- Relationship of systemic health to oral health
- Importance of careful daily care of mouth
- Antiepileptic medication side effects, including gingival enlargement and how to minimize its growth
- Seek immediate care if any oral change or injury is suspected

Use the information provided in Chapter 62 in the textbook and the examples of patient conversations in Appendix D

as a guide to prepare a conversation that you could use to provide patient education for Mr. Arakawa (introduced in the competency exercises). As you prepare the conversation, remember that you have already observed Mr. Arakawa's businesslike approach to health care. Make sure your education approach suits his personality and level of readiness for behavior change.

Use the conversation you create to role-play this situation with a fellow student. If you are the patient in the role-play, be sure to ask questions. If you are the dental hygienist, try to anticipate questions and answer them in your explanation.

CROSSWORD PUZZLE

ACROSS

2. Former term for a type of tonic–clonic epileptic seizure (two words).
6. Impaired digestive function.
8. Double vision.
11. Refers to a state of continuous, unremitting muscular contractions.
12. Describes the degree of awareness or responsiveness.
13. A disorder for which the cause is hidden.
21. Refers to a group of functional disorders of the brain characterized by recurrent seizures.
23. Remedy for seizures.
25. Uncontrolled motor activity, such as repeated swallowing.
26. Refers to shocklike contractions of muscles or groups of muscles.
27. Drug that inhibits convulsions.
30. Refers to a symptom that indicates the onset of a disease or condition.
31. Nerve that is stimulated by a pacemaker-like device implanted to reduce seizures.
32. Refers to expression or appearance of the face.

DOWN

1. Type of seizure in which there is alternate contraction and relaxation of muscles (two words).
3. A type of seizure in which the person experiences a brief impairment of consciousness; manifests in a blank stare, fixed posture, and sometimes rhythmic face movements before a return to awareness with no recollection of the seizure.
4. Refers to a seizure that involves only part of the brain.
5. Refers to the phase following a seizure when rest, reassurance, and palliative care for any oral trauma are administered.
7. A life-threatening emergency related to seizure disorders (two words).
9. Describes a muscle that is without normal tone or tension.
10. Refers to a seizure that affects the entire brain at the same time.
14. Refers to a seizure condition with a primary (genetic or neurologic abnormality) etiology.
15. Abnormal burning, prickling, or tingling sensation.
16. The sudden recurrence or intensification of sharp spasms or convulsions.
17. Former term for absence seizure (two words).
18. Refers to irregular muscle action.
19. Term associated with symptoms such as pallor, flushing, sweating, pupillary dilation, cardiac arrhythmia, or incontinence.
20. Class of anticonvulsant drugs highly correlated with gingival hyperplasia.
22. Refers to a seizure disorder that does not resolve following treatment with a basic, single drug therapy.
24. Unprovoked, unpredictable, and involuntary symptoms of a motor, sensory, cognitive, or emotional nature.
25. A peculiar prodromal sensation experienced by some people immediately preceding a seizure.
28. Active, acute phase of an epileptic seizure.
29. Sudden, involuntary contraction.

The Patient With a Psychiatric Disorder

Learning Objectives

Upon successful completion of these exercises, you will be able to:

1. Identify and define key terms and concepts related to psychiatric disorders.
2. Describe the symptoms, treatment, and oral implications of a variety of psychiatric and mood disorders.
3. Plan and document dental hygiene care and oral health education for a patient with a psychiatric disorder.

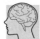 **KNOWLEDGE EXERCISES**

Write your answers for each question in the space provided.

1. Why is it more appropriate to refer to your patient as "an individual with bulimia" rather than as "a bulimic"?

   _____

   _____

2. In what way are agitation, bradykinesia, akinesia, and catatonia related? How are they different?

   _____

   _____

   _____

   _____

3. What is a psychotropic medication?

   _____

   _____

4. In your own words, define *schizophrenia*.

   _____

   _____

5. List three phases of schizophrenia.

   _____

   _____

   _____

6. Identify five behavioral characteristics that can both precede and follow the active phase of schizophrenia. (See Box 63-2 in the textbook.)

   _____

   _____

   _____

   _____

   _____

7. List five types of profoundly unusual behavior that are considered symptoms of the active phase of schizophrenia.

_____

_____

_____

_____

_____

8. Identify the concept or term defined by each of the following statements.

   a. A false sensory perception in the absence of an actual external stimulus

   _____

   b. A mental impression derived from misinterpretation of an actual sensory stimulus; a false perception

   _____

   c. A false belief firmly held though contradicted by social reality

   _____

   d. A psychiatric disorder characterized by delusions of persecution, illusions of grandeur, or a combination of both

   _____

9. Unfortunately, many people diagnosed with schizophrenia also qualify for a diagnosis of _____. This condition can aggravate psychiatric symptoms and complicate treatment.

10. Schizophrenia is associated with an excess of dopamine at specific synapses in the brain. List the brand names of three antipsychotic medications that block dopamine receptors.

   _____

   _____

   _____

11. In your own words, define _dysarthria_.

   _____

   _____

12. What is tardive dyskinesia?

   _____

   _____

13. During a scaling and root planing procedure, how can you facilitate safety and comfort of your patient with tardive dyskinesia?

   _____

14. Major depressive disorder and bipolar disorder are the primary _____ disorders discussed in the textbook chapter.

15. List reasons why the elderly are more susceptible to major depressive episodes.

   _____

   _____

   _____

16. List five characteristics that, if demonstrated by your patient, can help you identify a major depressive episode.

   _____

   _____

   _____

   _____

   _____

17. Identify five types of medications that are prescribed to stabilize the mood for individuals with depression.

   _____

   _____

   _____

   _____

   _____

18. What oral condition is a frequent side effect of medications used to treat depression?

   _____

19. What preventive measures can you recommend for your patient to help combat the effects of the medications used to treat depression?

   _____

   _____

   _____

20. Why might you offer tinted protective eyewear for a patient who is taking medications to treat depression?

_____

_____

21. If your patient's depression is not well controlled by medication, what personal/emotional factors can influence the way in which you need to approach oral hygiene instructions.

_____

_____

_____

22. List two specific behaviors you should avoid in your approach to oral health education for a patient with depression.

_____

_____

23. Identify three situations in which electroconvulsive therapy is used to treat an individual with depression.

_____

_____

_____

24. Define _euphoria_.

_____

_____

25. In what way is bipolar disorder different from major depressive disorder?

_____

_____

26. How is bipolar depression treated?

_____

_____

27. What drug used to treat bipolar disorder can impart a metallic taste in your patient's mouth?

_____

28. Provide five characteristics common to the manic phase of bipolar disorder.

_____

_____

_____

_____

_____

29. Define _postpartum depression_.

_____

_____

30. Compare postpartum blues and postpartum psychosis.

_____

_____

_____

_____

31. List the four types of anxiety disorders described in the textbook.

_____

_____

_____

32. Briefly describe each of the three types of treatment provided for a patient with anxiety disorder.

_____

_____

_____

_____

_____

33. What oral problems are associated with anxiety disorders?

_____

_____

_____

_____

34. List three risk factors for the occurrence of a dental psychiatric emergency during a dental hygiene appointment.

_____

_____

_____

35. In your own words, describe measures you can take to prevent or prepare for a psychiatric emergency.

_____

_____

_____

_____

_____

_____

_____

_____

36. If your patient has a panic attack while you are providing dental hygiene care, what will you do?

_____

_____

_____

37. Identify and briefly describe the three types of serious eating disorders.

_____

_____

_____

_____

_____

38. Discuss the effects of perimylolysis as it relates to bulimia.

_____

_____

_____

_____

COMPETENCY EXERCISES

Apply information from the chapter and use critical thinking skills to complete the competency exercises. Write responses on paper or create electronic documents to submit your answers.

1. Study the list of potential effects of antipsychotic medications in Table 63-1 in the textbook. Identify at least three modifications you would make beyond your usual clinical routines to ensure the comfort and safety of your patient who is taking an antipsychotic medication.

2. When you check his health history before calling Jack into your treatment room at the VA hospital, you note that he has been diagnosed with schizophrenia. You greet him cheerfully, talk to him brightly all the way down the hall to your room about how beautifully the sun is shining today. You ask him, with a smile, if there have been any changes in his medications since he was last seen in the dental clinic.

   You suspect that he is displaying the negative symptoms of the active phase of his disorder. Describe the type of responses that Jack displays in this situation. Make sure you don't just list the symptoms mentioned in Box 63-2 in the textbook, but rather, describe what you might observe about Jack's demeanor or behavior based on the symptoms.

3. Shaun Kennedy, a newspaper reporter, has been your patient for several years. You always enjoy the stories he tells about working for the newspaper. His oral hygiene has never been particularly good, and you have been really working with him each time he comes in to make sure he understands how his risk for oral disease increases when he doesn't thoroughly remove the dental biofilm from his teeth every day. You know that he is receiving treatment for bipolar disorder but, so far, you have not noticed that he ever displays any symptoms of either the manic phase or the depressive phase of his disease.

   Today Shaun is talking a mile a minute about a new novel he has started writing. As he gets more excited about telling you the plot of the novel, he actually pushes your hands aside, leaps up from the chair, and walks back and forth in your small treatment space! You would really like to convince him to get back in the dental chair so you can complete your oral hygiene instructions in a timely manner. What can happen if you pressure him to comply? Given Shaun's behavior today, how can you sensitively and realistically approach this situation?

4. Compare and contrast the four types of anxiety disorders. (*Hint:* Create an Infomap with identifying symptoms, severity, and predisposing factors, for each type.)

5. Isabella Stamos, 13 years old, is a beautiful girl with long curly blond hair, huge green eyes, and an already successful modeling career. You still have not started your intraoral examination, but after talking with her and observing her for several minutes, you suspect that she has an eating disorder. What clinical clues or signs can you look for to help confirm your impressions? What questions will you ask Isabella to help you determine if your suspicions are correct?

6. After you have questioned Isabella and completed an intraoral examination, it becomes clear that she is battling with bulimia nervosa. What ethical factors will you take into consideration when you discuss your assessment findings and Isabella's oral health needs with her mother at the end of the appointment?

Everyday Ethics

Before completing the learning exercises below, reread and reflect on the Everyday Ethics scenario and Questions for Consideration in this chapter of the textbook. It may also be useful to review the Dental Hygiene Ethics discussion in Chapter 1, the Ethical Applications in the introduction pages for each section in the textbook, as well as the Codes of Ethics in Appendices I, II, and III.

Individual Learning Activity
Imagine that you are the dental hygienist in this scenario. Answer each of the questions for consideration at the end of the scenario.

Discovery Activity
Ask a dental hygienist who has been practicing for a year or more to read the scenario. Provide them with a copy of one of the Codes of Ethics as well. Share the responses you have made to answer each question and ask that person to discuss the situation with you. What insights did you have or what did you learn during this discussion?

Factors To Teach The Patient

This scenario is related to the following factors listed in this chapter of the textbook:

- The causes and effects of enamel erosion; the high acidity of the vomitus from the stomach
- How to rinse after vomiting but not brush immediately; demineralization begins promptly after the acid from the stomach reaches the teeth, and brushing can cause abrasion of the demineralizing enamel
- The need for multiple fluoride applications through use of home dentifrice, rinse, and brush-on gel, as well as professional application of varnish or gel tray at regular dental hygiene appointments

You have talked with Isabella (introduced in the competency exercises in this chapter) about some ways she can receive help with her eating disorder, but as a dental hygienist, you know that the most important thing you can do is educate her about the risks to her oral health.

Use the examples of patient conversations in Appendix D as a guide, taking into account the personal factors that often accompany this disorder, educate Isabella about the negative oral findings common in a patient with bulimia. Discuss strategies for protecting her teeth and gums until she gets her eating behaviors under control.

CHAPTER 64

The Patient With a Substance-Related Disorder

Learning Objectives

Upon successful completion of these exercises, you will be able to:

1. Identify and define key terms and concepts related to alcohol and drug use.
2. Identify physical and behavioral factors associated with alcohol and drug use.

3. Describe health-related effects of alcohol and drug use, abuse, and withdrawal.
4. Plan and document dental hygiene care and oral hygiene instructions for the patient with a substance-related disorder.

 KNOWLEDGE EXERCISES

Write your answers for each question in the space provided.

1. Define the following terms and concepts in your own words to help you differentiate them and understand what they mean.

    a. Abuse

    _____

    _____

    b. Dependence

    _____

    _____

    c. Addiction

    _____

    _____

    d. Tolerance

    _____

    _____

    e. Alcoholism

    _____

    _____

    f. Polysubstance dependence

    _____

    _____

2. What is the difference between chemical, physical, and psychological dependence?

    _____

    _____

    _____

    _____

    _____

    _____

3. Identify the levels in the spectrum of alcohol use.

_____

_____

_____

_____

_____

_____

4. Identify the signs of alcoholism.

_____

_____

_____

_____

5. What is *acne rosacea?*

_____

_____

6. What factors contribute to the etiology of alcoholism?

_____

_____

_____

7. How is the concentration of alcohol in the blood measured?

_____

_____

8. What behavioral characteristics, if you observe them in an otherwise healthy patient, might indicate that your patient is intoxicated?

_____

_____

_____

_____

9. Define *nystagmus.*

_____

_____

10. The liver is the organ most severely affected by chronic alcohol abuse. Briefly describe the adverse effects of excessive or prolonged alcohol use on each of the following body systems.

a. Immune system

_____

_____

b. Digestive system

_____

_____

c. Cardiovascular system

_____

_____

d. Nervous system

_____

_____

e. Reproductive system

_____

_____

11. In what ways does excessive alcohol consumption affect nutritional intake?

_____

_____

12. Describe the two types of complications that can occur if an individual abruptly withdraws from alcohol use.

a. Alcohol hallucinosis

_____

_____

b. Alcohol withdrawal delirium (DTs)

_____

_____

13. Identify factors that can increase the severity of the symptoms that a person with alcoholism may experience if he or she abruptly ceases drinking.

_____

_____

_____

_____

14. What is the overall objective of treatment provided to support an individual who is recovering from alcoholism?

_____

_____

15. List the four components of an alcohol treatment program.

_____

_____

_____

_____

16. Your patient who is participating in an alcohol recovery program may be taking an alcohol-sensitizing agent such as Antabuse because these drugs act as a deterrent to consuming alcohol. If alcohol is taken, this drug interferes with the conversion of _____ to _____ in the liver and makes the patient very ill.

17. Identify the drug that is prescribed for the recovering alcoholic to help inhibit or decrease the desire to consume alcohol.

_____

18. Why can use of alcohol during pregnancy seriously threaten the health of the baby?

_____

19. What three additional factors linked with the mother's alcohol intake, in addition to the mother's general health status, are additional factors that may influence the baby's health?

_____

20. Describe the facial features that are observed in an infant with FAS.

a. Eyes

_____

b. Ears

_____

c. Nose

_____

d. Lips

_____

21. Identify behavioral, cognitive, and psychomotor factors associated with FAS.

_____

_____

_____

_____

22. What is FAE?

_____

_____

23. What is ARBD?

_____

_____

24. List the categories of drugs that are most commonly abused.

_____

_____

_____

_____

_____

25. Identify oral manifestations associated with the use of each of the following drugs.

a. Methamphetamine

_____

_____

_____

_____

_____

b. Speed, Ecstasy and other amphetamine-based drugs

_____

_____

_____

_____

c. Cocaine

_____

_____

_____

_____

_____

_____

d. Cannabis

_____

_____

_____

_____

26. Which body systems can be adversely affected by excessive use of drugs?

_____

_____

_____

_____

_____

_____

_____

_____

27. Identify medications commonly used to assist in lessening withdrawal symptoms during treatment for drug abuse.

_____

_____

_____

28. Why is it important to include a medical alert for possible substance abuse in the patient's chart?

_____

_____

_____

29. List actions that health care providers can take to avoid prescription pad theft

_____

_____

_____

_____

_____

_____

_____

_____

_____

_____

COMPETENCY EXERCISES

Apply information from the chapter and use critical thinking skills to complete the competency exercises. Write responses on paper or create electronic documents to submit your answers.

1. Explain why it is especially important to inspect intra-oral tissues each time you assess a patient who has a past or current history of excessive alcohol consumption or drug use.

2. The CAGE questionnaire (Box 64-6) provides a reliable score for determining potential alcohol dependence and is beneficial for use as a screening tool in clinical settings. Discuss the kind of communication approach that would be most successful in eliciting honest answers from patients.

3. Your afternoon patient is 20 minutes late for her appointment; she is a well-dressed woman in a business suit and is the new patient in the office. As you review her medical history, you notice her breath smells of alcohol and she answered "yes" to the question concerning having 1 or more drinks a day. You explain the office policy that a "yes" answer to that question requires you to give her an additional questionnaire; you ask if she is willing to answer additional questions and she complies. The patient answers "yes" for all four questions in the CAGE questionnaire; she immediately engages you in a discussion concerning her answers. The patient admits that

she has been trying to stop drinking because she has noticed red areas in her mouth, she states that no matter how much she brushes her gums bleed and they are red and swollen all the time. The patient lives alone and feels very guilty about her habit; lately she needs a drink in the morning before going to work and at night before going to sleep. She has no family; however, her colleagues make annoying comments about her breath and criticize her for drinking. The patient has also answered "yes" to increasing pains in her stomach.

- According to the CAGE questionnaire; explain what degree of suspicion of alcohol consumption you would assign to this patient and why.

- What medical referral would this patient require and why?

- Is this patient at a high risk for drug abuse and why?

4. Your next patient is Justin Townsley, age 21. He has just returned home from his first year away at college. His mother has made a dental hygiene appointment for him because he has not had his teeth examined in at least 3 years. She also wants him to have his wisdom teeth extracted before he is no longer covered under her dental insurance plan. When you go to greet Justin in the reception area, you overhear the end of a cell phone conversation in which he is planning to meet his buddies later on this evening to go out partying. "And, we'll stay out all night so we can have even more fun *this* time than we did *last* time," he says just before he hangs up the telephone to greet you. He stumbles just a bit as he rises from the chair but recovers quickly to follow you to the treatment room. As he walks past you into the chair, you distinctly catch the odor of alcohol on his breath.

Justin's health history is unremarkable except for having an arm broken in an automobile accident last year. He states that he does not take any regular medications. When you take his pulse and blood pressure today, both are slightly elevated.

Your intraoral findings include generalized poor oral hygiene, significant calculus deposits, coated tongue, dry oral mucosa, red and swollen gingiva,

generalized 4- to 6-mm probing depths, and generalized bleeding on probing. Justin states that "the left side of my jaw has been aching a lot lately, probably from grinding my teeth." A front tooth and the cusp of an upper premolar are both slightly chipped, findings that were not previously noted in his dental record. As you are working to complete your oral assessment, Justin keeps up a constant conversation about how much fun he has had this year while he was away at college. He sheepishly admits that his daily oral care has suffered, saying, "I stay up all night sometimes—to study for all those mid-term and final exams, you know. Sometimes I just forget to brush." You decide that you need to ask Justin about his drinking and the possible use of stimulant drugs. Identify the assessment findings that lead you to this decision.

- What oral signs and symptoms will you look for as you continue your assessment?

- What additional follow-up questions will you ask Justin to help you determine his patterns of alcohol and/or drug use?

5. Your careful and sensitive questioning leads you to believe that Justin's level of alcohol consumption and possible use of street drugs is probably having some detrimental impact on his health status. You are concerned enough that you discuss the matter with him and you give him a brochure about the oral effects of alcohol. You plan to bring your concerns for his health up again at his subsequent appointments. When you write a dental hygiene care plan for Justin, you will plan two additional visits for scaling and root planing his entire mouth. What education/counseling and oral hygiene instructions/home care interventions will you plan to help Justin maximize healing and tissue response during and after oral debridement? (*Hint:* If you write dental hygiene diagnosis statements for Justin it may help you decide on your planned interventions.)

6. Using your institution's guidelines for writing in patient records, document progress notes for your first appointment with Justin.

Everyday Ethics

Before completing the learning exercises below, reread and reflect on the Everyday Ethics scenario and Questions for Consideration in this chapter of the textbook. It may also be useful to review the Dental Hygiene Ethics discussion in Chapter 1, the Ethical Applications in the introduction pages for each section in the textbook, as well as the Codes of Ethics in Appendices I, II, and III.

Individual Learning Activity

Imagine that you have observed what happened in the scenario, but are not one of the main characters involved in the situation. Write a reflective journal entry that

- describes how you might have reacted (as an observer, not as a participant),
- expresses your personal feelings about what happened, or
- identifies personal values that affect your reaction to the situation.

Discovery Activity

Summarize this scenario for faculty member at your school and ask them to consider the questions that are included. Is their perspective different from yours or similar? Explain.

Factors To Teach The Patient

This scenario is related to the following factors listed in this chapter of the textbook:

- Drug abuse is a great risk to overall health.
- The risk of oral cancer is increased by the use of alcohol.
- Routine oral screening is needed at least twice a year to check for signs of early cancer.
- Drinking alcohol and using other drugs (prescription or over-the-counter) can lead to medical emergencies. Always check each drug and its action before using it in combination with alcohol or in combination with another drug.

Discussing your concerns about potential substance abuse with a patient like Justin Townsley (introduced in competency exercises Question 4) requires building trust.

You will be more successful in educating Justin and changing his health behaviors if you approach him without disapproval or judgment, but instead give him important information that motivates him to make changes in his own behaviors.

Use information in Chapter 64 of the textbook and the example of patient conversations in Appendix D as guides to develop a conversation you will use to discuss the negative effects that alcohol and other drugs can have on Justin's health status.

Use the conversation you create to role-play this situation with a friend or fellow student. If you are the patient in the role-play, be sure to ask questions. If you are the dental hygienist, try to anticipate questions and answer them in your explanation. Modify your conversation on the basis of what you learned.

CHAPTER 65

The Patient With a Respiratory Disease

Upon successful completion of these exercises, you will be able to:

1. Identify and define key terms and concepts related to respiratory diseases.
2. Differentiate between upper and lower respiratory tract diseases.

3. Describe a variety of respiratory diseases.
4. Plan and document dental hygiene care and oral hygiene instructions for patients with compromised respiratory function.

 KNOWLEDGE EXERCISES

Write your answers for each question in the space provided.

1. Identify the components of an additional Standard Precaution that can be implemented to help prevent transmission of respiratory infections.

_____

_____

_____

2. What vital signs, related to respiratory function, are assessed at each patient visit?

_____

_____

_____

_____

3. Define *dyspnea*.

_____

_____

4. What medical test measures various aspects of breathing and lung function?

_____

5. When performing a pulse oximetry test, what level of blood oxygen saturation signifies poor oxygen exchange?

_____

6. What should you do if you recognize that your patient is experiencing symptoms of respiratory distress during dental hygiene treatment?

_____

_____

7. A patient in respiratory distress may experience hypoxia. What patient signs and symptoms characterize hypoxia?

_____

_____

_____

_____

8. _____ is defined as a breathing rate of greater than 20 breaths per minute. A patient who is breathing very rapidly can experience _____, which may lead to dizziness and possible syncope.

9. What body structures are considered to be in the upper respiratory system?

_____

_____

_____

_____

10. What body structures comprise the lower respiratory system?

_____

_____

_____

_____

11. What are the pleura?

_____

_____

12. Identify two functions of the mucus secreted from goblet cells in respiratory mucosa?

_____

_____

13. What happens when an inflammatory disease causes an overproduction of mucus?

_____

_____

_____

14. _____ is the profuse mucous membrane discharge that often accompanies upper respiratory infections.

15. Identify three upper respiratory diseases that are more likely to be viral rather than bacterial infections.

_____

_____

_____

16. What medication is used primarily to treat bacterial respiratory infections but is not prescribed for infections caused by a virus or fungus?

_____

17. How are upper respiratory infections transmitted?

_____

_____

18. How can you best prevent transmission of pathogens while you are providing dental hygiene treatment?

_____

_____

19. What type of upper respiratory infection can cause tooth pain?

_____

20. Identify two oral side effects of medications commonly used to treat upper respiratory infections.

_____

_____

21. What oral lesions can accompany the infectious stage of an upper respiratory infection?

_____

_____

_____

_____

22. List the lower respiratory tract diseases described in this chapter.

_____

_____

_____

_____

_____

23. Identify three types of organisms that can cause pneumonia.

_____

_____

_____

24. What medical treatment is provided for each of the three types of pneumonia?

_____

_____

_____

25. What pathogen causes a type of pneumonia most often associated with immune-impaired individuals?

_____

26. Pneumonia infection that occurs from person-to-person transmission (not in a healthcare facility) is called:

_____

27. What is a potential oral health related cause for HCAP or NCAP pneumonia?

_____

_____

28. What signs and symptoms are associated with tuberculosis?

_____

_____

_____

_____

29. How is tuberculosis transmitted?

_____

_____

30. How is clinically active tuberculosis diagnosed?

_____

_____

_____

_____

31. What two diagnostic tests are used to determine a latent tuberculosis infection?

_____

_____

32. What medication regimen is used to treat the clinically active stage of tuberculosis?

_____

_____

_____

33. What oral condition is associated with the causative agent of tuberculosis?

_____

34. List five types of asthma based on pathophysiology.

_____

_____

_____

_____

_____

35. List the four NAEPP classifications of asthma.

_____

_____

_____

_____

36. What are the signs and symptoms of an asthma attack?

_____

_____

_____

_____

_____

37. True or False. Corticosteriods and mast call stabilizers are examples of short-term control medications for asthma.

_____

_____

38. List the drugs an individual with asthma should avoid.

    _____

    _____

    _____

39. What ingredient in local anesthetic solutions can cause an asthma attack?

    _____

    _____

40. What oral condition(s) may occur in patients being treated for asthma?

    _____

    _____

    _____

41. What is the primary cause of COPD?

    _____

    _____

42. Patients with COPD who are chronic smokers have an increased risk for which oral conditions?

    _____

    _____

    _____

_____

_____

43. The term *blue bloater* is related to _____ _____.

44. Describe the cough of an individual with chronic bronchitis?

    _____

    _____

45. What are the symptoms of emphysema?

    _____

    _____

    _____

    _____

46. Cystic fibrosis is an autosomal recessive gene disorder that affects the _____ tract, the _____ tract, and the _____.

47. What oral changes are likely to occur as cystic fibrosis progresses?

    _____

48. Complete **Infomap 65-1** below to compare three types of hypersensitivity reactions.

INFOMAP 65-1		
CONDITION	**PATHOGENESIS**	**SIGNS/SYMPTOMS**
Allergic Rhinitis (Hay Fever)		
Atopic Asthma		
Anaphylaxis		

COMPETENCY EXERCISES

Apply information from the chapter and use critical thinking skills to complete the competency exercises. Write responses on paper or create electronic documents to submit your answers.

1. Charles Marcin, a handsome blond 67-year-old man, has been a patient in your practice for many years; but this is the first time you have met him.

His health history confirms your first impression of Mr. Marcin as a patient with COPD, and you remember the term *pink puffer* from your textbook. You observe Mr. Marcin carefully as he walks the short distance from the reception room to your treatment room. He rests with his head bent and his hands on the back of the dental chair to catch his breath before he sits down.

Describe what you observe as you watch Mr. Marcin's breathing pattern and explain how it is different from the breathing pattern of an individual with other respiratory diseases.

2. When he can talk again, Mr. Marcin reminds you to call him Charlie. He says he has recently had a bit of a cold but is feeling somewhat better now. He tells you that his cough has pretty much gone away, and he isn't blowing his nose every 5 minutes any more. He complains that this is already his second cold this year, and once he was treated for a sinus infection. He mentions his teeth are stained because he has been drinking so much hot tea lately, and he is excited about being in your office today so that he can have an especially bright smile for his daughter's wedding this coming weekend. You think back to everything you learned about respiratory diseases as you plan Mr. Marcin's appointment for today. What safety and comfort factors will you need to assess and consider as you provide care during Mr. Marcin's dental hygiene appointment today?

3. Mr. Mitch Angelo is currently taking several medications to treat his asthma. When you are examining his mouth, you notice enamel erosion on the lingual areas of the anterior teeth. Explain what is happening that may be contributing to this oral condition.

4. When you have completed the first quadrant of scaling and root planing, you mention to Mr. Angelo that the gingival tissue in that area might be a bit sensitive later on today. He asks you what he should do if he feels pain. Which analgesics does a patient with asthma need to avoid?

5. When you update his medical history, Mr. Ben Samuelson, a 45-year-old businessman, tells you that he has been taking a new medication called isoniazid. When you question him further, he states that he does not know why he is taking it. What follow-up questions will you ask Mr. Samuelson?

6. What additional steps will you take before beginning your assessment of Mr. Samuelson's oral condition?

7. Explain the role of oral bacteria as a potential pathogenic agent in pneumonia, particularly if the patient is debilitated or chronically ill.

Everyday Ethics

Before completing the learning exercises below, reread and reflect on the Everyday Ethics scenario and Questions for Consideration in this chapter of the textbook. It may also be useful to review the Dental Hygiene Ethics discussion in Chapter 1, the Ethical Applications in the introduction pages for each section in the textbook, as well as the Codes of Ethics in Appendices I, II, and III.

Collaborative Learning Activity
Answer each of the questions for consideration at the end of the scenario in the textbook. Compare what you wrote

with answers developed by another classmate and discuss differences/similarities.

Discovery Activity
Summarize this scenario for faculty member at your school and ask them to consider the questions that are included. Is their perspective different from yours or similar? Explain.

Factors To Teach The Patient

This scenario is related to the following factors listed in this chapter of the textbook:

■ The need for frequent handwashing to help prevent transmission of respiratory disease.
■ The need for thorough daily cleaning of toothbrushes to help prevent spread of infections.
■ How using a new toothbrush and cleaning dentures/orthodontic appliances after bacterial infections can decrease the possibility of reinfection.
■ Why elderly patients and those with chronic cardiovascular disease, diabetes, and other immunosuppressed

conditions should receive a pneumonia vaccine and annual influenza immunizations.

Because of Mr. Marcin's chronic emphysema (patient introduced in competency exercises for this chapter), you are concerned about his recurring upper respiratory infections. Use the information in Chapter 65 in the textbook and the examples of patient conversations in Appendix D as guides to write a statement explaining ways that Mr. Marcin can reduce his risk for more serious acute respiratory diseases.

The Patient With a Cardiovascular Disease

Learning Objectives

Upon successful completion of these exercises, you will be able to:

1. Identify and define key terms and concepts related to cardiovascular disease.
2. Describe the cause, symptoms, prevention, and treatment of major cardiovascular diseases.
3. Identify clinical considerations and oral health factors related to cardiovascular conditions.
4. Plan and document dental hygiene care for a patient with cardiovascular disease.

 KNOWLEDGE EXERCISES

Write your answers for each question in the space provided.

1. Identify two ways to classify heart diseases.

   _____

   _____

2. Identify the various tissues in the heart that can be affected by cardiovascular disease.

   _____

   _____

   _____

   _____

3. Refer to Figure 66-1 in the textbook to help you visualize the veins, arteries, and chambers of a healthy heart. Describe the sequence of the normal flow of blood through the heart.

   _____

   _____

   _____

   _____

   _____

   _____

   _____

   _____

   _____

4. Congenital heart disease is the result of anatomic anomalies that occur during the first _____ weeks of fetal development. The exact cause is often unknown but is either _____, _____, or a combination of the two.

5. Refer to Figures 66-2 and 66-3 from the textbook to help you describe how the normal path of blood flow is compromised in each of the two types of congenital heart disease.

   a. Ventricular septal defect

   _____

   _____

   _____

b. Patent ductus arteriosus

_____

_____

_____

6. What is the etiology of rheumatic heart disease?

_____

_____

_____

7. Describe the flow of blood through the heart when there is a mitral valve prolapse.

_____

_____

_____

8. In your own words, describe the progression and diagnosis of infective endocarditis.

_____

_____

_____

_____

_____

9. List steps you can take to prevent infection during oral assessment and dental hygiene treatment if you suspect your patient is at risk for infective endocarditis.

_____

_____

_____

_____

_____

10. Recording your patients' blood pressure is an essential step in patient assessment before dental hygiene care. Blood pressure is recorded as a fraction; systolic/diastolic pressure in millimeters of mercury. In your own words, define systolic and diastolic blood pressure.

a. Systolic

_____

_____

b. Diastolic

_____

_____

11. Patient screening and early detection of hypertension are important components of dental hygiene care because, in the early stages, this condition is often unrecognized owing to lack of clinical symptoms. Identify the symptoms and sequelae of long-standing hypertension.

a. Symptoms

_____

_____

b. Sequelae

_____

_____

12. List the systolic and diastolic values that determine normal adult blood pressure, prehypertension, and stages 1 and stage 2 hypertension.

_____

_____

_____

_____

13. What is malignant hypertension?

_____

_____

14. What blood pressure level triggers concern for your child patient?

_____

_____

15. List anatomical or physical factors that influence an individual's blood pressure.

_____

_____

_____

_____

16. Treatment of primary hypertension includes patient education and counseling regarding reduction of risk factors. Identify the modifiable patient risk factors associated with essential hypertension.

_____

_____

_____

_____

_____

17. List the causes of secondary hypertension.

_____

_____

_____

18. Your patient who is taking an antihypertensive medication is susceptible to what condition after dental hygiene treatment?

_____

_____

19. Ischemic heart disease arises from _____ _____ to the heart muscle.

20. What is the principal cause of ischemic heart disease?

_____

_____

21. What are the modifiable (lifestyle) risk factors for ischemic heart disease?

_____

_____

_____

_____

_____

_____

22. If your patient's medical history indicates ischemic heart disease, angina pectoris is one manifestation you should be prepared for during dental hygiene treatment. What are the signs and symptoms of angina pectoris?

_____

_____

_____

_____

23. What is the difference between stable and unstable angina?

_____

_____

_____

_____

24. If your patient's medical history indicates medication for angina pectoris, where should the container with nitroglycerin be kept during a dental hygiene appointment?

_____

_____

25. The vasodilator (nitroglycerin) tablet is placed under the patient's tongue. What can you do to help the tablet to dissolve more quickly?

_____

_____

26. If your patient experiences an angina attack during dental hygiene treatment, what will you do? The steps are listed below. Number the list in the correct order (1 = first step; 9 = last step).

_____ Administer vasodilator (nitroglycerin)

_____ Administer oxygen

_____ Re-administer vasodilator (if indicated)

_____ Call for staff/colleague assistance

_____ Call for medical assistance

_____ Position patient in upright position

_____ Check patient response

_____ Check purchase date/potency of nitroglycerin

_____ Terminate dental hygiene treatment

27. When do you record vital signs after an angina attack that has been resolved by administering the patient's nitroglycerin?

_____

_____

28. Myocardial infarction is the most extreme manifestation of ischemic heart disease. What is the cause of myocardial infarction?

_____

_____

_____

29. What is the most common artery associated with myocardial infarction?

_____

_____

30. The symptoms of myocardial infarction are similar to those of angina pectoris. When should you summon immediate medical assistance for your patient who is experiencing these symptoms and be ready to administer basic life support?

_____

_____

_____

31. If your patient, who is experiencing symptoms of angina, suddenly becomes unconscious, what should you do?

_____

_____

_____

32. After a myocardial infarction, your patient's elective dental and dental hygiene treatment is postponed until:

_____

33. What is congestive heart failure?

_____

_____

34. Identify the underlying causes and precipitating factors associated with congestive heart failure.

_____

_____

_____

_____

35. If your patient's medical history indicates chronic congestive heart failure, what symptoms can you observe that will indicate whether the right or the left side of the heart is affected?

a. Left side of heart

_____

_____

_____

b. Right side of heart

_____

_____

36. Most sudden deaths in individuals with cardiovascular disease are attributed to what cause?

_____

37. What is the purpose of an artificial pacemaker?

_____

_____

38. Describe the two general types of artificial pacemakers.

_____

_____

39. What types of dental equipment are most likely to interfere with the functioning of your patient's pacemaker?

_____

_____

40. List the symptoms experienced by the patient during a pacemaker malfunction.

_____

_____

_____

_____

_____

_____

41. If your patient indicates that he or she has a pace-maker, what additional information will you document during the health history review?

_____

_____

_____

_____

_____

42. What surgical interventions can be used to treat ischemic heart disease?

_____

_____

_____

43. Identify the clinical procedures that will protect your patient who is receiving anticoagulant therapy for a cardiovascular condition.

_____

_____

_____

_____

_____

COMPETENCY EXERCISES

Apply information from the chapter and use critical thinking skills to complete the competency exercises. Write responses on paper or create electronic documents to submit your answers.

1. Review your school's dental clinic policy and guidelines for screening and treating patients with hypertension and answer the following questions.

   ■ At what intervals are patients' blood pressure readings recorded in the patient record? At what level are patients referred for a physician consult?

   ■ At what level is administration of local anesthetic compromised?

   ■ At what blood pressure classification or level will you suspend planned dental hygiene treatment and reschedule your patient after medical intervention?

2. What is the goal of providing dental hygiene treatment before and after cardiac surgery?

3. When you update her health history at her 3-month dental hygiene visit, Mrs. LaShawn Peal tells you that her physician has recently prescribed anticoagulant therapy to treat a cardiac condition. She states that she doesn't really understand what the medication is for, exactly, and that the Prothrombin Time test you ask her about was not recommended by her physician. She minimizes the issue and tells you that if her doctor isn't worried about this kind of thing, then neither is she. She protests vehemently when you mention that you need to contact her physician for a consultation before you begin her dental hygiene maintenance treatment. Using patient appropriate language, explain why you will require a physician consult before you begin dental hygiene treatment for Mrs. Peal.

4. When you contact Mrs. Peal's physician, he tells you that he will order the test. Mrs. Peal can stop by any time to have it done. You return to the treatment room to explain the situation to Mrs. Peal. Using your institution's guidelines for writing in patient records, document why Mrs. Peal was dismissed today and her dental hygiene appointment rescheduled.

DISCOVERY EXERCISE

Visit the American Heart Association Web site at http://www.heart.org and use the Web site search box to learn more about conditions that put your patient at risk for infective endocarditis and access the latest guidelines for premedication.

Everyday Ethics

Before completing the learning exercises below, reread and reflect on the Everyday Ethics scenario and Questions for Consideration in this chapter of the textbook. It may also be useful to review the Dental Hygiene Ethics discussion in Chapter 1, the Ethical Applications in the introduction pages for each section in the textbook, as well as the Codes of Ethics in Appendices I, II, and III.

Individual Learning Activity
Imagine that you have observed what happened in the scenario, but are not one of the main characters involved in the situation. Write a reflective journal entry that
- describes how you might have reacted (as an observer, not as a participant),

- expresses your personal feelings about what happened, or
- identifies personal values that affect your reaction to the situation.

Collaborative Learning Activity
Work with a small group to develop a 2- to 5-minute role-play that introduces the Everyday Ethics scenario described in the chapter (a great idea is to video record your role-play activity). Then develop separate 2-minute role-play scenarios that provide at least two alternative approaches/solutions to resolving the situation. Ask classmates to view the solutions, ask questions, and discuss the ethical approach used in each. Ask for a vote on which solution classmates determine to be the "best."

Factors To Teach The Patient

This scenario is related to the "Stress Reduction Procedures" listed in the Factors to Teach the Patient section of this chapter in the textbook:

When you read the patient record before seating Mr. Pedro Valdez (age 58) for his dental hygiene maintenance appointment, you note that he has a very complex history of cardiovascular disease, including myocardial infarction 6 years ago. When you call his name in the reception area, he looks up at you while coughing into a tissue. He comments that you are not the dental hygienist he usually sees for his appointment. He rises wearily from the chair, complains briefly he has been waiting quite a long time, and walks with you to your treatment room.

As you stroll slowly beside him, you notice he is pale, and the back of his neck is sweating. When he reaches the

dental chair, he collapses into it breathing heavily. While you take his blood pressure, you note that his skin feels quite cold, his fingernail beds look bluish, and his wrists and ankles appear quite swollen. You record a blood pressure of 135/95 mmHg on his right arm and a resting pulse of 83 bpm. When you begin to lower the dental chair for your intraoral examination, he becomes agitated, leans forward in the chair, and tells you that he has to sit up straight to be comfortable.

Use the information in Chapter 66 in the textbook and the examples of patient conversations in Appendix D as guides to prepare an outline for a conversation that you might use to discuss the ways you will help Mr. Valdez to be comfortable and safe during his dental hygiene treatment.

CROSSWORD PUZZLE

ACROSS

1. Mechanism that maintains a reliable heart rhythm.
4. Refers to the lipid plaque that deposits on the lining of an artery.
7. The record that is produced when a beam of ultrasonic waves is directed to record the position and motion of structures in the heart.
10. Temporary cessation of breathing.
12. A term meaning passageway (as in patent ductus arteriosus).
13. Deficiency of blood to supply oxygen (to the heart); result of constriction or obstruction of a blood vessel.
15. Refers to narrowing or constriction (of an artery).
17. Variation (of the heart) from its normal rhythm.
18. Characterized by hardening, thickening, and loss of elasticity.
20. Labored or difficult breathing that may be a symptom of cardiovascular disease.
22. Localized area of ischemic necrosis in the heart.
25. The record that is produced by recording electric currents generated by the heart; EKG.
26. The middle layer of the heart wall.
27. A term that refers to the surgical procedure that redirects blood flow around a narrowed heart artery.
28. Refers to a localized dilation of the wall of a blood vessel.

DOWN

1. Refers to the downward displacement of the mitral valve between the left atrium and the left ventricle of the heart.
2. Refers to a blood clot attached to the interior of a blood vessel.
3. Refers to the channel inside a blood vessel.
5. Deficiency of oxygen and increase of carbon dioxide in the blood.
6. Dividing wall between left and right ventricles in the heart.
8. Bluish coloration caused by reduced hemoglobin in the blood.
9. Refers to the blockage or closing (of a blood vessel).
10. A substance that interferes with coagulation of the blood.
11. Narrowing of the lining of a blood vessel by fatty deposits containing cholesterol.
14. Oxygenated blood that flows from the heart to nourish body tissues.
16. Abnormally rapid heart rate; usually more than 100 bpm.
19. Caused by an object (blood clot, air bubble, or clump of bacteria) that suddenly blocks an artery.
21. Irregularity of heartbeat caused by turbulent flow of blood flowing through a valve that has failed to close.
23. A disease that causes acute, spasmodic pain attack.
24. Related to absence of oxygen in tissues; symptoms include deep respirations, cyanosis, increased pulse rate, and reduced coordination.
25. Abnormal accumulation of fluid in body tissues.

CHAPTER 67

The Patient With a Blood Disorder

Learning Objectives

Upon successful completion of these exercises, you will be able to:

1. Identify and define key terms and concepts related to hematologic conditions.
2. Recognize blood components and normal reference values.

3. Describe the causes, symptoms, and oral effects of red and white blood cell disorders, bleeding disorders, and clotting deficiencies.
4. Plan and document dental hygiene education and treatment for patients with a blood disorder.

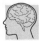

KNOWLEDGE EXERCISES

Write your answers for each question in the space provided.

1. Early signs of systemic conditions are often recognized first by a dental hygienist. Identify five oral signs associated with blood disorders.

   _____

   _____

   _____

   _____

   _____

2. List seven formed elements that make up blood.

   _____

   _____

   _____

   _____

   _____

   _____

   _____

3. What is the composition of plasma?

   _____

   _____

4. Identify the functions of three of the plasma proteins.

   _____

   _____

   _____

5. Why are red blood cells termed *corpuscles*?

   _____

   _____

6. What is the purpose of red blood cells?

_____

_____

7. Identify two main types of disorders in which red blood cells are destroyed.

_____

_____

8. Identify two causes of diminished production of red blood cells.

_____

_____

9. What genetic disorders are characterized by absent or decreased production of normal hemoglobin?

_____

_____

10. What is a normal hemoglobin value?

_____

_____

11. When the diagnosis is anemia, what has happened to the hemoglobin value?

_____

_____

12. Identify five basic causes of anemia.

_____

_____

_____

_____

_____

13. Iron-deficiency anemia is more often seen in younger people than in older people; and more often in _____ than in _____.

14. What can cause iron-deficiency anemia?

_____

_____

15. Which megaloblastic anemia is caused by a vitamin B_{12} deficiency?

_____

16. What oral findings are related to both iron-deficiency anemia and anemia related to vitamin B_{12} deficiency?

_____

_____

17. Which foods can you suggest to your patients as good sources of vitamin B_{12}?

_____

_____

_____

_____

_____

18. Dietary factors are important in the treatment of folate-deficiency anemia, but this type of megaloblastic anemia may be more frequently related to _____ than to inadequate intake.

19. What severe condition affecting newborns is also a result of folic acid deficiency?

_____

20. Sickle cell disease is a form of _____ anemia.

21. Individuals from which two ethnic populations are most at risk for sickle cell disease?

_____

_____

22. In your own words, briefly describe the clinical course of the chronic and acute phases of sickle cell disease.

a. Chronic

_____

_____

_____

b. Acute

_____

_____

_____

23. Briefly describe preventive and disease state treatments for sickle cell disease.

    a. Preventive

    _____

    _____

    _____

    b. Disease state

    _____

    _____

    _____

24. List radiographic bone changes and oral manifestations associated with sickle cell disease that can be identified by the dental hygienist.

    _____

    _____

    _____

    _____

25. A red blood cell count that is _____ normal levels is characteristic of polycythemia

26. What causes the relative form of polycythemia?

    _____

27. What causes the primary form polycythemia?

    _____

28. Identify health related factors that can contribute to the secondary form polycythemia.

    _____

    _____

    _____

29. Which of the three types of polycythemia can result in purplish red tongue, mucous membrane, and gingiva?

    _____

30. Identify two main types of white blood cells.

    _____

    _____

31. What is the main function of leukocytes?

    _____

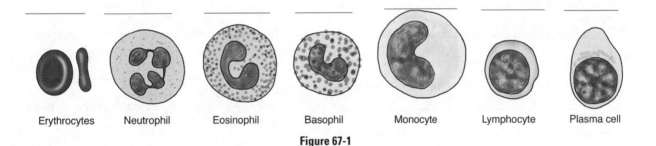

Erythrocytes   Neutrophil   Eosinophil   Basophil   Monocyte   Lymphocyte   Plasma cell

Figure 67-1

32. On the lines provided above the drawings in Figure 67-1, place the letter that matches the correct description of each white blood cell from the list below. NOTE: Not every cell pictured is a white blood cell, so some of the cells pictured will not be matched by a description in the list below.

    A. Functions to increase vascular permeability so that phagocytic cells can pass into inflamed areas

    B. Stains bright pink under the microscope; increases markedly during allergic conditions

    C. Multiplies when needed and moves back and forth between vessels and extravascular tissue

    D. Actively phagocytic; changes into macrophage in connective tissue

    E. Also called PMN; first in line to phagocytosis when the body is invaded by bacteria

33. What is the normal reference value of leukocytes in the blood?

    _____

34. White blood cell counts that differentiate by type can be used to detect and monitor disease because each cell type either _____ or _____ in association with certain conditions.

35. Identify the specific type of white blood cell associated with these approximate percentages of the total WBC count.

    a. 60–70%

    _____

    b. 20–35%

    _____

    c. 2–6%

    _____

    d. 1–3%

    _____

    e. 1%

    _____

36. Describe how leukopenia, a decrease in the total number of white blood cells, occurs.

    _____
    _____

37. Identify two specific causes of leukopenia.

    _____
    _____

38. In your own words, describe agranulocytosis.

    _____
    _____
    _____
    _____

39. What condition is characterized by the most extreme increase in white blood cells circulating in the blood?

    _____

40. What is lymphocytopenia?

    _____
    _____

41. Identify three general types of bleeding disorders.

    _____
    _____

42. Acquired coagulation disorders are related either to liver disease or to a deficiency in _____.

43. Identify the clotting factor associated with each of the following coagulation disorders.

    a. Hemophilia A

    _____

    b. Hemophilia B

    _____

    c. Von Willebrand disease

    _____

    d. "Christmas disease"

    _____

    e. "Classic hemophilia"

    _____

44. Which is more common: hemophilia A or hemophilia B?

    _____

45. What is the most common hereditary platelet dysfunction?

    _____

46. Which hemophilia occurs in both males and females?

    _____

47. In your own words, describe the effects of hemophilia.

    _____
    _____
    _____

48. List risk factors for increased bleeding.

    _____
    _____
    _____
    _____
    _____
    _____
    _____

49. What actions are taken if uncontrolled bleeding happens during a dental hygiene appointment?

_____

_____

_____

 COMPETENCY EXERCISES

Apply information from the chapter and use critical thinking skills to complete the competency exercises. Write responses on paper or create electronic documents to submit your answers.

1. When you update his health history, Jeremiah Bell tells you that that his gums, which have always been healthy, have been bleeding profusely when he flosses. Once he woke up in the morning with blood in his mouth and on his pillow. What questions will you ask him?

2. Mr. Bell replies that he has seen his physician to be tested for a blood disorder and hands you a sheet of paper reporting the results of four tests. Which tests would you expect to see included in the report that evaluate bleeding time? (*Hint:* Table 67-1 will help you to answer this question).

3. If the report handed to you by Mr. Bell indicates a diagnosis of leukemia, what results would you expect to see for the blood tests?

4. You and the attending dentist decide together to postpone clinical dental hygiene treatment for Mr. Bell until you can arrange a telephone consultation with his physician. You provide oral hygiene instruction for Mr. Bell with an emphasis on what he can do on a daily basis to minimize oral effects of his blood disorder. Using your institution's guidelines for writing in patient records, document this appointment.

5. Mr. Weber presents for his continuing care appointment. He states that since his myocardial infarction eight months ago, he is taking Warfarin daily. He is sure of neither the amount nor his last anticoagulation test. What laboratory test(s) would you need to know before proceeding? What levels would be recommended for you to proceed today with treatment? State an example dialogue with his physician.

DISCOVERY EXERCISE

Explore the American Dental Association Web site or do a PubMed literature search to find information about the latest guidelines for management of dental patients who are taking anticoagulant or antiplatelet medications.

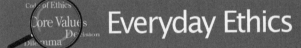

Everyday Ethics

Before completing the learning exercises below, reread and reflect on the Everyday Ethics scenario and Questions for Consideration in this chapter of the textbook. It may also be useful to review the Dental Hygiene Ethics discussion in Chapter 1, the Ethical Applications in the introduction pages for each section in the textbook, as well as the Codes of Ethics in Appendices I, II, and III.

Individual Learning Activity
Imagine that you are the dental hygienist in this scenario. Answer each of the questions for consideration at the end of the scenario.

Collaborative Learning Activity
Work with another student colleague to role-play the scenario. The goal of this exercise is for you and your colleague to work though the alternative actions in order to come to consensus on a solution or response that is acceptable to both of you.

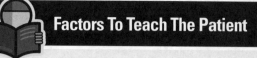

Factors To Teach The Patient

This scenario is related to the following factors listed in this chapter of the textbook:

- Meticulous hygiene techniques to practice daily: toothbrushing, flossing, and other interdental cleaning devices
- How to self-evaluate the oral cavity for deviations from normal; any changes should be reported to the dentist and dental hygienist

When Mr. Bell (introduced in competency exercises in this chapter) returns in a few weeks for his follow-up appointment, he tells you that he has just started treatment for leukemia. He has been advised that it is very difficult to control all of the symptoms of his condition. He is very concerned about his oral health.

Use the information in Chapter 67 in the textbook the examples of patient conversations in Appendix D to outline your education plan for Mr. Bell.

Use the outline you created to role-play this situation with a fellow student. If you are the patient in the role-play, be sure to ask questions. If you are the dental hygienist, try to anticipate questions and answer them in your explanation.

CROSSWORD PUZZLE

ACROSS

5. Formation/development of blood cells, usually in the bone marrow.
8. Increase in total number of leukocytes.
12. Occurs if 100% oxygen is not administered at the conclusion of a nitrous-oxide sedation procedure (two words).
13. Type of bleeding time test; normal range less than 5 minutes.
16. Condition characterized by an increase in number and concentration of red blood cells; hemoglobin and hematocrit values are raised.
18. Loss of structural differentiation with revision to a more primitive type of cell.
19. Darker color blood containing only 20–70% oxygen.
20. Temporary treatment that can limit the spread of a hematoma
22. Test used for blood evaluation; normal range 11–15 seconds (two words).
23. Reduction in leukocytes in blood to less than 500/mL.
24. Nose bleed.
25. Pinpoint-size hemorrhage.
26. Blood fluid composed of 90% water and 10% proteins, inorganic salts, gases, and other substances.
27. Large agranulocyte with indented nucleus that is actively phagocytic.

DOWN

1. Diminished number of neutrophils.
2. Pain in the tongue.
3. Condition that can be caused by a variety of factors; characterized by an increase in the number of circulating white blood cells.
4. Test used for blood evaluation; normal range 4–8 minutes (two words).
6. Inflammation of the tongue.
7. Granulocyte that increases markedly during allergic conditions.
9. A lowered number of platelets caused by decreased production in the bone marrow.
10. Destruction of decomposition of a cell wall.
11. Formation of red blood cells.
14. Bright red blood; 97% saturated with oxygen.
15. Type of purpura; circulating platelets are decreased.
17. Some general signs and symptoms of this condition are paleness, weakness, headache, vertigo, and brittle nails.
21. Defective development or congenital absence of an organ or tissue.
22. Hemorrhage into tissues.

The Patient With Diabetes Mellitus

Learning Objectives

Upon successful completion of these exercises, you will be able to:

1. Identify and define key terms and concepts related to diabetes.
2. Explain the function and effects of insulin.
3. Identify risk factors for diabetes.
4. Describe etiologic classifications, signs and symptoms, diagnostic procedures, complications, and common medical treatment for diabetes.

5. React appropriately in a diabetic emergency.
6. Explain the relationship between diabetes and oral health.
7. Plan and document dental hygiene care and oral hygiene instructions for patients with diabetes.

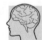 **KNOWLEDGE EXERCISES**

Write your answers for each question in the space provided.

1. What type of diabetes is related to genetics, obesity, and hormones during pregnancy?

_____

2. Identify the health-related factors besides pregnancy that can result in diabetes.

_____

_____

_____

_____

_____

_____

3. What genetic syndromes are sometimes associated with diabetes?

_____

_____

_____

4. Complete Infomap 65-1 by listing characteristics type 1 and type 2 that will help you learn to differentiate between the two types.

INFOMAP 68-1 · COMPARISON OF TYPE 1 AND TYPE 2 DIABETES

TYPE 1 CHARACTERISTICS	TYPE 2 CHARACTERISTICS

5. Diabetes is characterized by hyperglycemia. In your own words, define the *normal glucose blood level* and *hyperglycemia* using milligrams per deciliter and millimole per liter measurements.

_____

_____

_____

6. Define the following symptoms of hyperglycemia.

  a. Polyuria

  _____

  b. Polydipsia

  _____

  c. Polyphagia

  _____

7. List the common physical compilations associated with uncontrolled diabetes.

_____

_____

_____

_____

_____

_____

_____

8. What criteria are used to diagnose diabetes?

_____

_____

9. What self-administered tests are used for monitoring blood glucose levels during treatment of diabetes.

_____

_____

_____

10. If your patient tells you that the result of his fasting plasma glucose test this morning was less than _____ mg/dL, you know that his diabetes is well controlled and it is safe to provide dental hygiene treatment today.

11. If your patient tells you that her postprandial glucose level this morning was >200 mg/dL, you know that her diabetes is what?

    _____
    _____

12. What is the role of insulin in the human body?

    _____
    _____

13. Where is insulin produced in the human body?

    _____

14. What is exogenous insulin?

    _____

15. How is exogenous insulin administered?

    _____
    _____

16. What factors determine the dose of insulin administered for each patient?

    _____
    _____
    _____
    _____
    _____

17. Identify the duration of peak action for each of the classes of insulin.

    _____
    _____
    _____
    _____

18. If too much insulin is circulating in the blood because of inadequate nutritional intake, _____, sometimes referred to as _____ _____, can occur.

19. If too little insulin is administered to control hyperglycemia, _____ _____ or _____ can occur.

20. Oral hypoglycemic agents act differently from insulin to control blood glucose levels. What is the mechanism of action of biguanides and thiazolidinediones?

    _____
    _____

21. If your patient is taking sulfonylureas or meglitinides to control type 2 diabetes, what side effect is important for you to watch for during dental hygiene treatment?

    _____

22. Your patient with uncontrolled diabetes is at risk for many long-term health complications. Identify the body systems or organs (other than the mouth) that can be affected.

    _____
    _____
    _____
    _____

23. Diabetes can be controlled, but to date, there is no known cure. List five factors important for maintaining the overall good health and well-being of an individual with diabetes or at risk for diabetes.

    _____
    _____
    _____
    _____
    _____

24. In one sentence, describe the relationship between poorly controlled diabetes and periodontal disease.

    _____
    _____
    _____

25. Uncontrolled glucose levels place your patient at risk for _____, an opportunistic oral infection.

26. What is the role of the dental hygienist in planning care for patients who are at risk for diabetes or who are exhibiting signs and symptoms of diabetes?

_____

_____

_____

27. Why is stress prevention an important component of a dental hygiene care plan for a patient with diabetes?

_____

_____

28. Identify ways that the dental hygienist can reduce stress and prevent an emergency situation during an appointment with the patient with diabetes.

_____

_____

_____

29. Why should you be very careful to avoid undue tissue trauma when providing dental hygiene care for your patient with diabetes?

_____

_____

 COMPETENCY EXERCISES

Apply information from the chapter and use critical thinking skills to complete the competency exercises. Write responses on paper or create electronic documents to submit your answers.

1. In your own words, explain what can happen at the cellular level when glucose needed to supply energy cannot be accessed owing to either decreased supply or action of insulin.

   Read the Chapter 68 Patient Assessment Summary to help you answer the following questions.

CHAPTER 68 — PATIENT ASSESSMENT SUMMARY

Patient Name: Nicolas James Diamond	Age: 57	Gender: M̅ F	☑ Initial Therapy
			☐ Maintenance
Provider Name: D.H. Student	Date: Today		☐ Re-evaluation

Chief Complaint:
Patient presents for new patient examination. "I just want my teeth cleaned."

ASSESSMENT FINDINGS

Health History

- Diagnosed several years ago with type 2 Diabetes—Only monitors blood sugar levels when he isn't feeling well, tries to control the condition through diet and exercise.
- No medical visits for 2 y—no current medications
- Blood Pressure 145/95, Pulse 86 bpm.
- Tobacco use: 1–2 packs per day for 35 y
- Alcohol use: 1–2 drinks daily (usually beer)
- ASA Classification—III
- ADL level—0

At Risk for:

Social and Dental History

- 35 y in previous dental practice—dentist was a college roommate of his who recently retired.
- No previous periodontal therapy—only received "dental cleanings" every 6 mo.
- Limited dental knowledge

At Risk for:

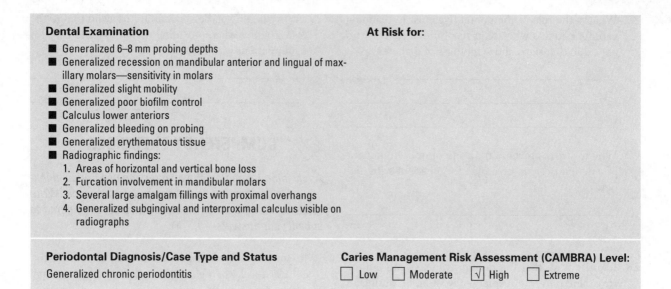

Dental Examination

At Risk for:

- Generalized 6–8 mm probing depths
- Generalized recession on mandibular anterior and lingual of maxillary molars—sensitivity in molars
- Generalized slight mobility
- Generalized poor biofilm control
- Calculus lower anteriors
- Generalized bleeding on probing
- Generalized erythematous tissue
- Radiographic findings:
  1. Areas of horizontal and vertical bone loss
  2. Furcation involvement in mandibular molars
  3. Several large amalgam fillings with proximal overhangs
  4. Generalized subgingival and interproximal calculus visible on radiographs

Periodontal Diagnosis/Case Type and Status

Generalized chronic periodontitis

Caries Management Risk Assessment (CAMBRA) Level:

☐ Low   ☐ Moderate   ☑ High   ☐ Extreme

2. While you are waiting for Mr. Diamond, your first patient of the day, you look over the health history form he sent to the office a week earlier and note that he has been diagnosed with type 2 diabetes. Mr. Diamond finally arrives 15 minutes late for the appointment. He is extremely anxious, and states he is late because of the traffic. His morning, it seems, has not gone well, and everything is off schedule. As you bring him back to your treatment room, you notice that he is pale and trembling. He is perspiring profusely and seems agitated as he sits in the chair.

   What questions will you ask Mr. Diamond to add to the information you already know about his medical history?

3. Mr. Diamond responds irritably to your questions and gives vague answers. He says. "I have been having my teeth cleaned regularly for years and no one has ever asked these kinds of questions." When you take his vital signs, you note that his pulse is rapid and his blood pressure is a bit high. You are really conscious of your appointment time slipping away, so you tilt the dental chair back to do an intraoral examination and begin your oral assessment. After 10 minutes, Mr.

Diamond stops you and says, "Please sit me upright." You note that his breath is coming in rapid gasps.

   What is most likely to be happening and what will your response be?

4. By mutual agreement, the dental hygiene care planned for today's appointment is postponed. Using your institution's guidelines for writing in patient records, document Mr. Diamond's appointment.

5. During a follow-up appointment several weeks later, when Mr. Diamond's medical situation has been stabilized, you are able to collect the rest of the assessment data. Use the information in Mr. Diamond's Patient Assessment Summary and a copy of the Patient Specific Care Plan template in Appendix B to develop dental hygiene diagnosis statements and complete a dental hygiene care plan for providing initial therapy dental hygiene interventions for Mr. Diamond.

6. Discuss options for continuing care if Mr. Diamond's initial therapy outcomes are not optimal?

Everyday Ethics

Before completing the learning exercises below, reread and reflect on the Everyday Ethics scenario and Questions for Consideration in this chapter of the textbook. It may also be useful to review the Dental Hygiene Ethics discussion in Chapter 1, the Ethical Applications in the introduction pages for each section in the textbook, as well as the Codes of Ethics in Appendices I, II, and III.

Collaborative Learning Activity

Work with another student colleague to role-play the scenario. The goal of this exercise is for you and your colleague to work though the alternative actions in order to come to consensus on a solution or response that is acceptable to both of you.

Discovery Activity

Ask a friend or relative who is not involved in healthcare to read the scenario and discuss it with you from the perspective of a "patient" who receives services within the healthcare system. Discuss what you learned from the concerns, insights, or difference in perspective that person expressed.

Factors To Teach The Patient

This scenario is related to the following factors listed in this chapter of the textbook:

- Recognizing early warning signs of diabetes and seeking medical treatment
- Reviewing practice of meticulous oral hygiene to prevent dental and periodontal disease

Use the information from Chapter 68 in the textbook and the examples of patient conversations in Appendix D as guides to prepare a conversation that you might use to educate Ed (introduced in Everyday Ethics) about the need to consult his physician related to signs and symptoms of diabetes, how diabetes can affect his oral health, and what he can do to prevent further health complications.

Use the conversation you create to role-play this situation with a fellow student. If you are the patient in the role-play, be sure to ask questions. If you are the dental hygienist, try to anticipate questions and answer them in your explanation.

Emergency Care

Learning Objectives

Upon successful completion of these exercises, you will be able to:

1. Identify and define key terms, abbreviations, and concepts related to emergency care.
2. List factors and procedures essential for preventing and preparing for a medical emergency in a dental setting.
3. Describe basic life support: external chest compression and rescue breathing.
4. Describe oxygen administration and AED defibrillation, and identify contraindications for use.
5. Recognize signs and symptoms of a medical emergency, and identify an appropriate response.

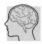

KNOWLEDGE EXERCISES

Write your answers for each question in the space provided.

1. Identify the patient assessment components that will help you know enough about your patient to help prevent an emergency during dental hygiene treatment.

   _____

   _____

   _____

   _____

   _____

   _____

2. Identify five *patient* factors that contribute to increased risk for medical emergency in a dental setting. (*Hint:* These are identified in several places throughout Chapter 69 in the textbook; some are psychosocial and some are specific to patient health status.)

   _____

   _____

   _____

   _____

   _____

3. Identify at least two dental treatment–related factors that contribute to greater risk for emergencies.

   _____

   _____

   _____

4. Recognizing the signs of patient stress is one important way to prevent medical emergencies. Identify ways you can reduce your patient's stress during dental hygiene treatment.

_____

_____

_____

_____

5. Where in the patient's dental record is medical information indicating that the patient is predisposed to medical emergencies listed?

_____

_____

6. What additional information should you document in the patient record about your patient's risk for medical emergency?

_____

_____

_____

_____

_____

7. What information must be clearly posted by the telephone in a dental clinic?

_____

8. What does EMS stand for?

_____

9. When a medical emergency happens in the dental setting, it is important to document all pertinent information as well as everything that happens during the event and as well as in the patient's record after the event. Why?

_____

_____

_____

10. In a medical emergency, your patient is "compensating" if the vital signs are what?

_____

11. In your own words, describe what happens if your patient goes into shock.

_____

_____

_____

12. When a patient is in shock, he or she is often placed in the Trendelenburg position. What does this mean?

_____

_____

13. In your own words, describe the purpose of basic life support (BLS) in the dental setting.

_____

_____

_____

14. If an emergency situation occurs, you will first quickly _____ the situation and then _____ promptly but not hastily to provide basic life support as indicated

15. What determines the need for external chest compressions?

_____

16. Where do you check for the pulse?

_____

_____

17. What is the purpose of providing chest compressions during basic life support?

_____

_____

18. Describe the patient's position when you perform chest compressions.

_____

19. In your own words, describe the landmarks used to determine hand placement during chest compressions.

_____

20. Chest compressions are intended to move the sternum downward with a firm, steady vertical pressure. How far down do the compressions move the thorax before releasing to allow the chest to return to normal?

_____

_____

21. How long do you continue to provide chest compressions?

_____

_____

22. Identify and define five key words from Box 69-1 in the textbook that are related to use of the automatic external defibrillator (AED).

_____

_____

_____

_____

_____

23. In your own words, describe what the AED does.

_____

_____

24. List three contraindications for using the AED.

_____

_____

_____

25. When providing rescue breathing during basic life support, what is the ratio of breaths to chest compressions.

_____

_____

26. Describe two ways to open your patient's airway.

_____

_____

_____

27. How do you identify whether each breath in rescue breathing is effective?

_____

28. Describe what to do if the breath is not effective.

_____

_____

_____

29. List the steps for performing rescue breathing.

_____

_____

_____

_____

30. What does FBAO stand for?

_____

31. Identify three measures you can take to prevent aspiration of objects during dental treatment.

_____

_____

_____

32. What is happening if your patient suddenly looks distressed, tries to sit up in the dental chair, and touches his or her neck?

_____

_____

33. Define *dyspnea*.

_____

_____

34. Describe the actions of a patient with a "mild" airway obstruction.

_____

_____

35. What are the signs of a "severe" airway obstruction?

_____

_____

_____

36. If your patient is in distress and coughing but he or she appears to have good air exchange, what should you do?

_____

_____

37. Your patient begins gasping and making sounds when he or she breathes in, but the cough is not strong enough to expel the object and the patient is starting to panic. What should you do?

_____

_____

38. In your own words, briefly describe the chest thrust used to manage airway obstruction situations.

_____

_____

_____

39. When is a "finger sweep" performed?

_____

_____

40. What series of steps will you follow if you are responding to a foreign body airway obstruction (FBAO) emergency and the patient becomes unconscious just as you arrive at her side?

_____

_____

_____

_____

41. What is the term for insufficient oxygenation of the blood?

_____

42. What is the term for diminished oxygen in body tissues?

_____

43. Direct delivery of oxygen is useful in most emergencies, but it is contraindicated in which two situations?

_____

_____

44. If your patient is not breathing, _____ _____ oxygen delivery is indicated, and a bag mask or _____ _____ _____ is used to deliver _____ % to _____ % oxygen.

45. If a regular face mask oxygen delivery system is used, _____ to _____ L/min and _____ % oxygen is delivered to the patient.

46. If the patient is breathing and needs only low levels of oxygen, the use of a _____ _____ device is indicated. Supplemental oxygen is started at _____ to _____ L/min.

47. If a bag mask device is used, the bag is compressed at _____ to _____ second intervals for an adult and _____ second intervals for a child.

48. What should you do if your patient's chest does not rise and fall after applying an oxygen delivery system?

_____

_____

49. What are the steps for turning on an oxygen tank and using an oxygen delivery system?

_____

_____

_____

_____

✓ COMPETENCY EXERCISES

Apply information from the chapter and use critical thinking skills to complete the competency exercises. Write responses on paper or create electronic documents to submit your answers.

1. The only real way to become competent in responding to emergencies in the dental setting is to practice, practice, practice, and then practice some more. This exercise should be ongoing and include everyone in your dental clinic.

    First, all students, faculty, and support personnel should *study Tables 69-4 and 69-5 in the textbook and be able to list the procedure to follow in each emergency.* Next, refer to Figure 69-2 in the textbook and write the list of duties assigned to each emergency team member on three small cards. (Or use your school's already established emergency protocols and procedures instead.) Finally, write the signs and symptoms of each emergency health situation listed in Tables 69-4 and 69-5 on a 3 × 5 inch card. If you'd like, write the list of procedures to follow for each emergency on the back side of its signs and symptoms card so that you will have a handy reference for evaluating everyone's response to that situation.

    When everything is ready, randomly give three people one of the three emergency team member cards and one person one of the emergency situation cards. The person who receives the emergency situation card is the patient and acts out the signs and symptoms listed. The emergency team must respond appropriately to the situation.

It is a great idea to practice this in your clinic setting, if possible. Try to initiate a mock emergency drill when it is not expected, to add to the reality of the situation. When you and your colleagues become proficient at responding, try doing this role-play when patients are in the clinic receiving treatment. If you do this, talk quietly to each patient and make sure he or she knows what is going on; you will find that the patients are delighted to see you are practicing your emergency response. Some of them might even be willing to participate by pretending to be the patient who is experiencing the emergency!

DISCOVERY EXERCISES

1. Locate the emergency cart or kit in your school clinic. Use the emergency equipment list in Table 69-1 in the textbook to identify what items are included in the kit.

2. Does your school have a written plan for medical emergencies in the dental clinic? Is the procedure outlined similar to or different from the flowchart in Figure 69-3 in the textbook? In what ways is your school's emergency report form similar to or different from Figure 69-1 in the textbook?

3. Determine how emergency medical services are activated in your school and/or in your community.

Everyday Ethics

Before completing the learning exercises below, reread and reflect on the Everyday Ethics scenario and Questions for Consideration in this chapter of the textbook. It may also be useful to review the Dental Hygiene Ethics discussion in Chapter 1, the Ethical Applications in the introduction pages for each section in the textbook, as well as the Codes of Ethics in Appendices I, II, and III.

Individual Learning Activities
■ Imagine that you are the dental hygienist in this scenario. Answer each of the questions for consideration at the end of the scenario.

■ Identify a situation you have experienced that presents a similar ethical dilemma. Write about you would do differently now than you did at the time the incident happened—support your discussion with concepts from the dental hygiene codes of ethics.

Factors To Teach The Patient

This scenario is related to the following factors listed in this chapter of the textbook:

■ Stress minimization to prevent emergencies

It is clear that Mr. Montgomery is an extremely anxious dental patient. He is scheduled with you today for presentation of the dental hygiene care plan you have developed. His health history indicates that he has type 2 diabetes, hypertension, and angina. He has a past history of alcohol abuse, and he still uses tobacco.

Mr. Montgomery is extremely overweight and has trouble catching his breath after walking from the reception area

to your treatment room. His periodontal status is poor, and he will require multiple appointments for scaling and root planing. In your dental hygiene care plan, there are several dental hygiene diagnosis statements that address his risk for medical emergencies during treatment.

To minimize the risk of a medical emergency, you plan to educate Mr. Montgomery carefully about how his treatment will proceed. Use the examples of a patient conversations in Appendix D as a guide to prepare a conversation that you can use when you are talking to Mr. Montgomery about ways to reduce his stress during his dental hygiene treatment.

Patients With Special Needs

■ Chapters 48–69

COMPETENCY EXERCISES

Apply information from the chapter and use critical thinking skills to complete the Competency exercises. Write responses on paper or create electronic documents to submit your answers.

SECTION VIII—PATIENT ASSESSMENT SUMMARY

Patient Name: Nicolas James Diamond   Age: 57   Gender: ☑ M   F

☑ Initial Therapy

☐ Maintenance

Provider Name: D.H. Student   Date: Today

☐ Re-evaluation

Chief Complaint:
Patient presents for new patient examination. "I just want my teeth cleaned."

ASSESSMENT FINDINGS

Health History

- Diagnosed several years ago with Type 2 Diabetes—Only monitors blood sugar levels when he isn't feeling well, tries to control the condition through diet and exercise.
- No medical visits for 2 y—no current medications
- Blood Pressure 145/95, Pulse 86 beats per minute.
- Tobacco use: 1–2 packs per day for 35 y
- Alcohol use: 1–2 drinks daily (usually beer)
- ASA Classification – III
- ADL level – 0

At Risk for:

Social and Dental History

- 35 y in previous dental practice—dentist was a college roommate of his who recently retired.
- No previous periodontal therapy—only received "dental cleanings" every 6 mo.
- Limited dental knowledge

At Risk for:

Dental Examination   **At Risk For:**

- Generalized 6–8 mm probing depths
- Generalized recession on mandibular anterior and lingual of maxillary molars—sensitivity in molars
- Generalized slight mobility
- Generalized poor biofilm control
- Calculus lower anteriors
- Generalized bleeding on probing
- Generalized erythematous tissue
- *Radiographic findings:*
    1. Areas of horizontal and vertical bone loss
    2. Furcation involvement in mandibular molars
    3. Several large amalgam fillings with proximal overhangs
    4. Generalized subgingival and interproximal calculus visible on radiographs

1. Use the information in the Section VIII Patient Assessment Summary for Mr. Nicholas Diamond and a copy of the Patient Specific Care Plan template in Appendix B to develop a care plan for a series of dental hygiene therapy appointments.

2. The best way to become competent in planning and providing dental hygiene care for patients with special needs is, of course, to practice planning and providing care. The learning that comes from practicing your skills is always enhanced by taking time to record the process in some sort of written format so that you can later reflect on what you have done, how you did it, and why things did or did not work out as you had planned.

    Select one or more patients for whom you provide care in your school clinic who have one (or more) of the special needs identified in the textbook. To complete this exercise, gather the assessment data from each patient's record, a copy of the patient-specific dental hygiene care plan template in Appendix B, the information from the appropriate chapters in the textbook, and any other source of information you think might be important (such as a drug reference book).

    Use the patient-specific care plan template to develop a comprehensive written dental hygiene care plan for each patient you select.

DISCOVERY EXERCISES

1. Gather as much information as you can about a specific special-need condition that interests you. Use PubMed to help you search the professional literature and/or look for online sources of information about the condition. The information in the scientific literature will probably be the most valid and reliable about the condition you select. Online sources can be variable, and it is important to determine that the host of the Web site is a reliable source of data and provides information about the condition that is supported by scientific principles.

2. You and your student colleagues can share information and learn from each other if you each present a different type of case and discuss the cases in a sort of case-presentation seminar. Each patient case you present should contain the following information:

- Patient background and demographics

- A general description of your patient, including name, age, race, sex, height, weight, blood pressure, pulse, and respiration

- Other information about your patient that is important for understanding the special condition

- A statement describing the significance of these data for planning and providing dental hygiene care

- Medical history

- A definition of each medical problem with an explanation of its significance to the delivery of dental care

- A description of your patient's ASA level

- A statement of the physical and oral manifestations of your patient's conditions

- A note about the anticipated complications associated with patient management during dental hygiene care

- A statement of the anticipated complications or potential emergency situations that are related to your patient's medical history

- A description of the actions needed to prevent complications and emergencies during dental hygiene care

- Pharmacological and therapeutic considerations (Hint: Refer to a Physician's Desk Reference or other accepted drug information reference as a guide)

- Identification of specific medications your patient is taking currently and how they relate to the medical history

- A list containing the commercial and generic name of each drug, class or mechanism of action, usual dosage, indications for use, and anticipated adverse side effects for dentistry

- An evaluation of your patient's local anesthesia considerations

- Dental hygiene care delivery considerations

- A description of the general physical and oral manifestations of your patient's condition that affect dental hygiene care

- A description of your patient's ADL and IADL levels

- A description of your patient's OSCAR considerations

- Identification of and rationale for modifications to standard dental hygiene treatment procedures needed to meet your patient's special needs during dental hygiene care

- Identification of and rationale for modifications in providing oral hygiene instructions

- Identification of and rationale for modifications of oral hygiene aids

- A description of behavioral and psychosocial considerations for planning and providing care for your patient
- Identification of communication issues and needed actions to ensure that your patient is fully informed before he or she consents to the planned dental hygiene treatment

3. Use information you gathered from a literature and/or developed for your patient case presentation to prepare a table clinic summarizing the dental hygiene

care considerations for patients with the condition you have studied. (*Hint:* Check out the American Dental Hygienists' Association Web site [http://www.adha.org] for information and guidelines for constructing and presenting a table clinic.)

 FOR YOUR PORTFOLIO

- Include your written responses to the Everyday Ethics questions from any of the chapters in this section.

- It is likely that while you are a student, you will develop many dental hygiene care plans for a variety of patients with a wide range of special needs. Include all of these written care plans in your portfolio. Also, include the care plans you developed using the patient-assessment data summaries when completing the competency exercises in this workbook; be sure to indicate which care plans were developed for practice patient cases and which were developed for individuals for whom you provided dental hygiene care in your school clinic.

- An effective way to document your growing knowledge about planning patient care is to include a written reflection that describes, in detail, how the care plans you developed later in your student career are different from the care plans you developed when you were first providing patient care.

    Cite specific examples from your earlier and later care plans that document your increased competency in planning individualized, patient-specific dental hygiene care. The examples should show how your later plans are more complete, more comprehensive, and more professional than your earlier plans.

- If you develop and present a table clinic, include your presentation outline, along with any powerpoint presentation or handouts you created to accompany the table clinic. Or, include a photograph that shows you and your coauthor colleagues presenting your table clinic in a professional setting. A brief written reflection of what you learned from the experience of preparing and presenting the table clinic will add depth to your documentation.

CROSSWORD PUZZLE

ACROSS

4. Abnormal fluid accumulation.
6. Bony projection extending beyond the normal contour of a bony surface.
7. Type of tumor that has the properties of anaplasia, invasiveness, and metastasis.
9. Pertaining to the eye.
10. Developing slowly and persisting for a long period.
16. Pertaining to the jaws and face.
17. Refers to coexisting or simultaneously existing disease processes.
18. Difficulty in swallowing.
19. Pertaining to, or arising through the action of, many factors.
21. Healthcare team comprised of specialists from many disciplines.
23. Persistent patterns of heavy intake of substances that cause health consequences.
24. Loss of ability to communicate.
27. To discontinue bottle or breast-feeding.
28. Fold of skin near the eye; characteristic of a person with Down's syndrome.
30. Hemorrhage into the tissues, produces petechiae and ecchymoses.
32. Involuntary muscular contraction; in the heart muscle can be a cause of cardiac arrest.
35. Within the womb (two words).
36. Sudden, involuntary conctaction of a muscle or group of muscles.
37. Loss or abnormality of structure or function.
39. Temporary loss of consciousness caused by sudden fall in blood pressure.
40. Another name for a bruise.
41. Disturbance of trigeminal nerve causing spasms of masticatory muscles and limiting the opening of the mouth.
42. Restriction in performing an activity; the result of an impairment.
43. Nodular inflammatory lesion containing macrophages and surrounded by lymphocytes.
44. Symptom that indicates the onset of a disease or condition.

DOWN

1. The study of the aging process.
2. Abnormally low blood glucose.
3. Inflammation of the tongue.
5. Minute reddish spot on the skin or mucous membrane caused by hemorrhage.
8. The concurrent use of a large number of medications or drugs.
11. Habitual psychologic and physiologic dependence on a substance.
12. Tendency of biologic systems to maintain internal stability while continually adjusting to external changes.
13. Slow heartbeat.
14. Failure to carry out prescribed healthcare recommendations.
15. Pain in the tongue.
20. Artificial replacement of a body part.
22. The period immediately following birth.
24. Absence of oxygen.
25. Diminished availability of oxygen to body tissues.
26. Beginning abruptly with marked intensity.
29. Affording relief, but not cure.
31. Refers to hearing a constant noise such as ringing or buzzing.
33. Refers to baldness or hair loss.
34. Loss of cognitive function that is sufficient to interfere with daily functioning.
36. A combination of symptoms that are related to a single cause or occur commonly together.
38. Screening and classification; sorting and allocating relative priority for patient treatment.

ADEA Competencies for Entry into the Profession of Dental Hygiene

CORE COMPETENCIES (C)

C.1 Apply a professional code of ethics in all endeavors.

C.2 Adhere to state and federal laws, recommendations, and regulations in the provision of dental hygiene care.

C.3 Use critical thinking skills and comprehensive problem-solving to identify oral health care strategies that promote patient health and wellness.

C.4 Use evidence-based decision making to evaluate emerging technology and treatment modalities to integrate into patient dental hygiene care plans to achieve high-quality, cost-effective care.

C.5 Assume responsibility for professional actions and care based on accepted scientific theories, research, and the accepted standard of care.

C.6 Continuously perform self-assessment for lifelong learning and professional growth.

C.7 Integrate accepted scientific theories and research into educational, preventive, and therapeutic oral health services.

C.8 Promote the values of the dental hygiene profession through service-based activities, positive community affiliations, and active involvement in local organizations.

C.9 Apply quality-assurance mechanisms to insure contiuous commitment to accepted standards of care.

C.10 Communicate effectively with diverse individuals and groups, serving all persons without discrimination by acknowledging and appreciating diversity.

C.11 Record accurate, consistent, and complete documentation of oral health services provided.

C.12 Initiate a collaborative approach with all patients when developing individualized care plans that are specialized, comprehensive, culturally sensitive, and acceptable to all parties involved in care planning.

C.13 Initiate consultations and collaborations with all relevant health care providers to facilitate optimal treatments.

C.14 Manage medical emergencies by using professional judgement, providing life support, and utilizing required CPR and any specialized training or knowledge.

HEALTH PROMOTION AND DISEASE PREVENTION (HP)

HP.1 Promote positive values of overall health and wellness to the public and organizations within and outside the profession.

HP.2 Respect the goals, values, beliefs, and preferences of all patients.

Reprinted with permission from American Dental Education Association (ADEA). Competencies for entry into the allied dental professions (As approved by the 2010 House of Delegates). *J Dent Educ.* 2010 Jul;74(7):769–75.

HP.3 Refer patients who may have a physiological, psychological, and/or social problem for comprehensive evaluation.

HP.4 Identify individual and population risk factors and develop strategies that promote health-related quality of life.

HP.5 Evaluate factors that can be used to promote patient adherence to disease-prevention or health maintenance strategies.

HP.6 Utilize methods that ensure the health and safety of the patient and the oral health professional in the delivery of care.

COMMUNITY INVOLVEMENT (CM)

CM.1 Assess the oral health needs amd services of the community to determine action plans and availability of resources to meet health care needs.

CM.2 Provide screening, referral, and educational services that allow patients to access the resources of the healthcare system.

CM.3 Provide community oral health services in a variety of settings.

CM.4 Facilitate patient access to oral health services by influencing individuals or organizations for the provision of oral healthcare.

CM.5 Evaluate reimbursement mechanisms and their impact on the patient's access to oral health care.

CM.6 Evaluate the outcomes of community-based programs, and plan for future activities.

CM.7 Advocate for effective oral health care for underserved populations.

PATIENT/CLIENT CARE (PC)

ASSESSMENT

PC.1 Systematically collect, analyze, and record diagnostic data on the general, oral, and psychosocial health status of a variety of patients using methods consistent with medicolegal principles.

PC.2 Recognize predisposing and etiologic risk factors that require intervention to prevent disease.

PC.3 Recognize the relationshops among systemic disease, medications, and oral health that impact overall patient care and treatment outcomes.

PC.4 Identify patients at risk for a medical emergency, and manage the patient care in a manner that prevents an emergency.

DETNAL HYGIENE DIAGNOSIS

PC.5 Use patient assessment data, diagnostic technologies, and critical decision making skills to determine a dental hygiene diagnosis, a component of the dental diagnosis, to reach conclusions about the patient's dental hygiene care needs.

PLANNING

PC.6 Use reflective judgement in developing a comprehensive patient dental hygiene care plan.

PC.7 Collaborate with the patient and other health professionals as indicated to formulate a comprehensive dental hygiene care plan that is patient-centered and based on the best scientific evidence and professional judgement.

PC.8 Make referrals to professional colleagues and other health care professionals as indicated in the patient care plan.

PC.9 Obtain the patient's informed consent based on a thorough case presentation.

IMPLEMENTATION

PC.10 Provide specialized treatment that includes educational, preventive, and therapeutic services designed to achieve and maintain oral health. Partner with the patient in achieving oral health goals.

EVALUATION

PC.11 Evaluate the effectiveness of the provided services and modify care plans as needed.

PC.12 Determine the outcomes of dental hygiene interventions using indices, instruments, examination techniques, and patient self-reports as specified in patient goals.

PC.13 Compare actual outcomes to expected outcomes, reevaluating goals, diagnoses, and services when expected outcomes are not achieved.

PROFESSIONAL GROWTH AND DEVELOPMENT (PGD)

PGD.1 Persue career opportunities within health care, industry, education, research, and other roles as they evolve for the dental hygienist.

PGD.2 Develop practice management and marketing strategies to be used in the delivery of oral health care.

PGD.3 Access professional and social networks to pursue professional goals.

Patient-Specific Dental Hygiene Care Plan Template

Patient Specific Dental Hygiene Care Plan

Patient name_____ Age _____ Gender: M ☐ F ☐   Initial therapy ☐

                                                                        Maintenance ☐

Provider name _____ Date _____   Re-evaluation ☐

Chief complaint:

Assessment Findings

Medical history	At Risk For
Social and dental history	
Dental examination	

Periodontal Diagnosis/Case Type and Status:	Caries Management Risk Assessment (CAMBRA) level: Low ☐ Moderate ☐ High ☐ Extreme ☐

Dental Hygiene Diagnosis

Problem	Related to (Risk Factors and Etiology)

Planned Interventions
(to arrest or control disease and regenerate, restore or maintain health)

Clinical	Education/Counseling	Oral Hygiene Instruction/Home Care

Expected Outcomes

Goals	Evaluation Methods	Time Frame
1		
2		
3		
4		

Appointment Plan
(sequence of planned interventions)

Appt #	Plan for Treatment and Services		Plan for Education, Counseling and Oral Hygiene Instruction
		Quadrant	
1			
2			
3			
4			

Re-evaluation Findings

Re-treat ☐   Refer ☐   Continuing care interval _____

Description of post-treatment outcomes:

Example Dental Hygiene Care Plan

Patient Specific Dental Hygiene Care Plan

Patient name _Mrs. Lorna Patel_ Age _49_ Gender: M ☐ F ☒   Initial therapy ☒

Provider name _D.H. Student_   Date _Today_   Maintenance ☐   Re-evaluation ☐

Chief complaint: _Gum tissues bleed when brushing and flossing. Mouth is dry all the time_

Assessment Findings

Medical history	At Risk For
History of high blood pressure managed by medication	Heart disease and stroke
Cholesterol managed by medication	Xerostomia
Mitral valve prolapse	Postural hypotension
Allergy to penicillin	Inappropriate antibiotic prescription
Zocor 20 mg 1 per day	
Caltrate 1 per day	
Enapril 10 mg/hydrochlorothiazide 25 mg 1 per day	
Multiple vitamin 1 per day	
Clindamycin 2.0 g taken 1 hour before appointment	
ASA II	
ADL level 0	

Social and dental history	
1.5 years since last recall	Increased incidence of dental caries and periodontal conditions
Localized 4-5 mm probing depths	
Flosses daily	
Rinses with Listerine	
Mouth dry all the time	
Uses mints and candy for dry mouth	
Uses bottled water with no fluoride content	

Dental examination	
Moderate dental biofilm along cervical margins and proximal surfaces	Increased incidence of dental caries and periodontal conditions
Generalized supra- and subgingival calculus	Increased risk for TMJ problems
Light yellow stain	
Posterior gingiva red and bleeding on probing	
Generalized moderate attrition (evidence of bruxism)	
Numerous faulty MOD amalgam restorations	
Localized 4-5 mm maxillary and mandibular probing depths	

Periodontal Diagnosis/Case Type and Status:	Caries Management Risk Assessment (CAMBRA) level:
Generalized biofilm-induced gingivitis with localized chronic slight periodontitis	Low ☐ Moderate ☐ High ☐ Extreme ☒

Dental Hygiene Diagnosis

Problem	Related to (Risk Factors and Etiology)
Unnecssary pretreatment antibiotic prophylaxis	Lack of knowledge about current prophylactic premedication protocols
Current gingivitis and periodontitis	Inadequate dental biofilm Faulty restorations that provide trap for biofilm
Increased caries risk	Xerostomia and use of mints and candies Inadequate biofilm removal and fluoride intake Faulty restorations
Risk for TMJ problems	Attrition (evidence of bruxism)
Management of positioning during dental hygiene procedures	Medications (potential for postural hypotension)
Increased risk for heart disease and stroke	Periodontal infection History of hypertension and high cholesterol

Planned Interventions
(to arrest or control disease and regenerate, restore or maintain health)

Clinical	Education/Counseling	Oral Hygiene Instruction/Home Care
Scaling and root planing Selective polishing Fluoride application	Importance of current prophylactic premedication protocols Importance of management of xerostomia Increased risk of dental caries because of faulty restorations Increased risk of dental caries because of lack of fluoride and use of sugar-based candies Correlation of risk for heart disease and periodontal disease	Reinforce sulcular brushing technique Review flossing technique Discuss the use of Listerine vs nonalcoholic mouthwash (because of xerostomia) Frequent use of water and/or saliva substitutes Use of Xylitol gum/candies Reinforce the need for further dental intervention to manage faulty restorations and attrition

Expected Outcomes

Goals	Evaluation Methods	Time Frame
1 Eliminate gingivitis/ control periodontitis	1 Reduction of dental biofilm, gingival redness, gingival bleeding, and periodontal probing depths	1 4 week re-evaluation 1a Reassessment at maintenance appointment (3 months)
2 Increase use and frequency of sugarless mints and gum	2 Patient discussion	2 4 week re-evaluation
3 Increase fluoride exposure; use of daily fluoride rinse and fluoridated water	3 Patient discussion	3 4 week re-evaluation
4 Reduce attrition	4 Refer for night guard fabrication	4 4 week re-evaluation 4a Reassessment at maintenance appointment (3 months)
5 Eliminate faulty restorations	5 Refer for restorative dental care	5 4 week re-evaluation 5a Reassessment at maintenance appointment (3 months)
6 Maintain patient comfort and safety during dental treatment throughout treatment	6 Patient discussion	6 At all appointments

Appointment Plan
(sequence of planned interventions)

Appt #	Plan for Treatment and Services	Quadrant	Plan for Education, Counseling and Oral Hygiene Instruction
1	Assessment, scaling/root planing	X ▢ X ▢	Importance of managing xerostomia Systemic impact of periodontal disease Importance of biofilm removal Reinforce sulcular brushing technique
2	Complete scaling/root planing, selective polishing, fluoride treatment	▢ X ▢ X	Importance of fluoride Importance of managing xerostomia Importance of biofilm removal Demonstrate flossing technique Importance of follow-up for management of attrition and faulty restorations
3	Re-evaluation assessment – in 4 weeks		

Re-evaluation Findings

Re-treat ▢   Refer ▢   Continuing care interval __3 months__

Description of post-treatment outcomes:

Motivational Interviewing: Guidelines for Conversation During Patient-Education Instructions

Between 30% and 70% of dental patients may not comply with personal oral care and diet recommendations because the communication approach used by the clinician during oral health education does not motivate the necessary change in health behavior. Motivational interviewing (MI) is a patient-oriented method of counseling based on recognizing a patients' readiness to change health-related behaviors and then helping them to successfully move through each stage, as described in Chapter 3 in the textbook.

The MI approach during chair-side patient counseling includes the following components:

- RESPECT that is indicated by conversing with the patient in an upright, eye-level, face-to-face position, the use of everyday words rather than professional terms, and through not interrupting when the patient is speaking.
- OPEN-ENDED QUESTIONS that help the clinician assess readiness to change and help the patient explore reasons for behavior change. (Example: "So what brings you here today?" Or "Tell me what happened since your last appointment?"
- AFFIRMATIVE STATEMENTS and elimination of emotional words or confrontational words in order to indicate a positive, concerned, and pleasant approach. Example: "You didn't want to come today, but you did it anyway"

- REFLECTIVE LISTENING to check for understanding, create empathy and build a positive rapport. Example: "You are not sure you what to make a change, but you are aware smoking can cause oral cancer and that your family is worried about your smoking"
- SUMMARY of the patients' comments and concerns as well as written information supporting behavior change goals patients have set for themselves.

EXAMPLE PATIENT CONVERSATIONS

Provided below are examples of MI conversations for each of the Stages of Change listed in Table 3-5 in the textbook. Not every patient progresses through the stages in the same timeframe indicated by the conversation examples below. Some patients may remain in a particular stage for a longer period of time, or may go back to a previous stage before again progressing to successful behavior change. An example is the patient who tries to quit using tobacco, but regresses one or two times before quitting completely.

Ask permission to discuss health-related aspects of dental biofilm accumulation before you begin. Begin by applying disclosing agent to your patient's teeth. Calculate and record the "plaque score." Seat your patient in an upright position, position yourself at eye level, and then use the mirror to help your patient identify areas of biofilm colored by the disclosing agent on his or her teeth.

PRECONTEMPLATION STAGE: (*No intention of behavior change*)

Clinician: Mr. Santi, may I discuss your "plaque score" with you?

Patient: Go ahead, but I've been brushing and I am not going to floss if that is what you are going to suggest.

Clinician: Your "plaque score" implies you have an above-average accumulation of a bacterial biofilm, which can cause your gums to be inflamed. I understand you are not planning to floss. Can you tell me more about that?

Patient: I am an air-traffic controller, am very busy, and am pressed for time. When I've tried flossing in the past it hurt my gums and made them bleed.

Clinician: The job of an air-traffic controller must be very stressful. Do you think the stress of your job may cause you to compromise your health?

Patient: I have never thought about it.

Clinician: Bleeding gums is a sign of inflammation related to the accumulation of dental biofilm that may put you at an increase risk for health diseases. Would it be OK if I give you a brochure that explains how poor oral health is related to systemic diseases?

Patient: Yes, I think that will be OK.

Clinician: May we continue to discuss this at your next visit?

CONTEMPLATION STAGE: (*Considering change; aware of problem. Weighing pros and cons.*)

Patient: I've had a chance to read the brochure; perhaps I am comprising my health by not flossing.

Clinician: So what do you think would happen if you were to change your oral hygiene habits to include flossing?

Patient: It may stop my gums from bleeding, but I am still to busy to take the time to floss in the mornings.

Clinician: If you don't change by making the time and leave everything the same, what do you think will happen?

Patient: Well, I guess my gums will continue to look swollen and bleed; however, if I start flossing and my gums stop bleeding, I suppose that my mouth would be healthier, and if my mouth is healthier, I guess that means overall a healthier body. I understand that you are saying oral health is related to overall health.

Clinician: Yes, it is. I am sure you read that not flossing could lead to heart problems due to periodontal disease. What about other family members, how are their oral hygiene habits?

Patient: Oh, I see my children brushing and flossing all the time; they have recently voiced a concerned about my brushing habits.

Clinician: I will continue to follow up on your progress.

PREPRATION STAGE: (*Ready and actively planning to make a change*)

Clinician: So, Mr. Santi, I see your gums don't look as red and swollen around your front teeth today—tell me why the change.

Patient: I tried flossing only the front teeth before I went to bed one or two nights last week.

Clinician: Seems like you are making a first step toward changing your oral hygiene habits. How has this change made you feel?

Patient: Well … my wife kissed me goodbye this morning and my children let me know my breath smells better.

Clinician: Sounds like you have a built-in support group at home. Would you like to discuss other ways you can continue to improve your oral hygiene care?

Patient: Time is still my problem, especially in the mornings. If I brush, I don't have time to floss; if I floss, I don't have time to brush.

Clinician: Your job must require you to process a lot of information at one time. I believe in you and I believe you have the skills to make the change that will allow time to improve your oral hygiene while protecting your overall health. What do you think?

Patient: First, I need to know how to get my fingers in the back of my mouth, then I will work on making more time and let you know how I am doing.

Clinician: I would like to have you trying using a floss holder to reach your back teeth, if that would be ok with you?

Clinician: Let me show you how to use the floss holder. (Floss holder instructions are shown in Chapter 56 of the textbook.)

ACTION STAGE: (*Commitment is clear; the behavior change has been adopted.*)

Clinician: Mr. Santi, I want to follow up on your question on how to floss your back teeth. (*Hand Mr. Santi a Typodont and a piece of floss: ask the patient to demonstrate how he flosses his back teeth.*)

Clinician: Seems like you have the right idea. May I offer to improve on your technique by showing you how better to reach you back teeth? [Correct flossing technique is shown in textbook in Chapter 28] *After putting on gloves and mask, correct Mr. Santi's flossing technique by demonstrating in the patient's mouth.*

Clinician: Now, Mr. Santi, will you try flossing your teeth while I hold the mirror for you. (*After flossing, ask permission to demonstrate correct toothbushing methods for Mr. Santi.*)

Clinician: I can see you have been brushing; however, your "plaque index score" still shows that you are leaving biofilm mostly on your back teeth. May I demonstrate how you might brush to improve removing the biofilm in these areas?

Demonstrate correction toothbrush method [as shown in textbook Chapter 27] on a Typodont, then instruct the patient to begin brushing from the back of mouth and then demonstrate brushing in the front of the mouth as you observe.

Example: Bass method. With gloves on, hold the toothbrush in your hand and demonstrate in your patient's mouth before having the patient demonstrate in his or her mouth. (You can use the Typodont and a toothbrush to demonstrate; however, demonstrating in the patient's own mouth is more effective.)

As the patient looks in the mirror, encourage, guide, and correct technique as he or she is brushing.

Clinician: Now take the brush and try brushing in your mouth using the same brushing strokes I demonstrated. Great job, Mr. Santi, I see you have caught on to this method very well!

With gloves on, hold the toothbrush in your hand, and demonstrate in the patient's mouth how to brush the occlusal surfaces and the tongue while the patient looks in the mirror.

Clinician: Now that you have brushed the inside (lingual) and outside (facial) of all your teeth, let me demonstrate how to brush the tops (occlusal surfaces) of your teeth. Mr. Santi, look into the mirror and watch as I place the toothbrush with the bristles pointed down into the pits and grooves of your chewing surfaces. Vibrate the brush head in a circular movement, keeping the bristles in contact with the teeth while counting to 10; move the brush to the next few teeth and begin again. The dental biofilm also forms on the tongue; bring your tongue outward and **hold** the toothbrush in a vertical position with the bristles pointed downward toward tongue; using light pressure pull the brush forward gently over the tip of the tongue. Now show me in your mouth the way I demonstrated brushing your tongue and chewing surfaces.

Clinician: Again, you have caught on very well. Do you have any questions, Mr. Santi?

Let me review with you the order in which you will brush all your teeth surfaces; the goal is to brush twice daily, especially before you go to sleep; however, you will have to set a realistic goal for yourself. You may start by brushing the teeth in the back of your mouth on the tongue side then go to the facial side; repeat on the opposite side of the mouth. You may start with your upper teeth or your lower teeth. You may want to start with the areas you find most difficult to brush. Continue by brushing the teeth in the front of your mouth—both the tongue side and the facial side. Finish by brushing your chewing surfaces and tongue. Remember, Mr. Santi, it is best to floss your teeth before you begin your brushing routine.

Patient: This is a lot to remember. I can see I will have to rearrange my daily routine to make time for this process.

Clinician: I am not sure, but it seems that if you decide something is important enough, you are willing to make the time? It will have to be your decision to make this change; however, I will be here to encourage you to reach your goal.

MAINTENANCE STAGE: (*Engages in new behavior; the change has been continuous for at least 6 months.*)

Clinician: So, Mr. Santi this is your 3-month recall appointment. Are you feeling like you've accomplished your goals to improve your oral hygiene care?

Patient: I have given it my best. I am sure you will let me know how I am doing.

Clinician: Your exam shows much improvement. There are no signs of inflammation or bleeding points today; however, we may need to review flossing especially areas in between your back teeth.

End the patient's appointment with a positive, encouraging comment.

Clinician: Mr. Santi, by my observations today, you have really worked to reach your goals toward a healthier mouth. I am sure with the few changes we made today, we will see even more improvements in your oral hygiene by your next 3-month recall appointment.

Evaluation Rubric for Competency Exercises

Competence is the ability to apply knowledge and skills in a relevant way to solve problems, answer questions, or make decisions.

Objectively evaluating a learner's ability to recall factual information is relatively easy. Evaluation of student responses to exercises/learning activities that are intended to assess competence is often significantly more difficult. Competence is a complex interaction of skills that begins with an understanding of basic facts (**KNOWLEDGE**) and incorporates the **ANALYSIS** of all relevant factors in a specific situation and **SYNTHESIS** of information in order to answer questions or solve problems. Competence also includes being able to **SUPPORT** or clearly explain the rationale for decisions and as well as effectively **COMMUNICATE** the plan for action.

An academic grading rubric provides objective criteria useful for evaluating student work that has been submitted to demonstrate competence. The assignment of points for each of the criteria stated in the rubric will aid the faculty member in providing an objective grade or score. When the evaluation rubric is provided along with instructions for the assignment, students receive a guide to faculty expectations. When the finished assignment is graded, focused feedback will help the student understand errors or omissions that result in a lower score or grade for the assignment.

The example evaluation rubric on the next page can be used as a template for evaluating student responses to all of the competency exercises, including those related to FACTORS TO TEACH THE PATIENT and EVERYDAY ETHICS, in each chapter of the Student Workbook.

EVALUATION RUBRIC FOR COMPETENCY EXERCISES

CATEGORIES	EXCELLENT 3 points	ACCEPTABLE 2 points	UNSATISFACTORY 0–1 points
KNOWLEDGE Familiarity with and understanding of concepts and information. Points _____	Student includes relevant and accurate information from the main chapter. **AND** Student includes relevant information from related chapters in the textbook	Student includes relevant and accurate information from the main chapter.	Significant relevant information from the main chapter is missing **OR** Misunderstanding of one or more basic concepts is evident.
ANALYSIS Breaking down a complex topic into its component parts. Points _____	All components of the question, case scenario, or patient assessment data is considered in the student's answer.	Only minor details or components of the question, case scenario, or patient assessment data have not been addressed in the student's answer.	At least one major component has not been addressed.
SYNTHESIS Combining ideas to form a complex, cohesive whole using logical reasoning and deduction. Points _____	Connection or comparisons made between factors, concepts and facts/knowledge from the textbook chapter is very clear.	Connection or comparisons between factors, concepts and facts/knowledge from the chapter textbook is apparent, but not completely explained.	Important or obvious connections are missing from the students answer.
SUPPORT Providing rationale for statements Points _____	Student provides clear explanations that support conclusions, statements or connections made. Examples: • Linking basic information and intended actions or conclusions drawn • Explaining personal perspective • Defining controversy that requires further investigation	Explanations are provided that support conclusions, statements, or connections, but could be more completely or clearly explained.	Little evidence is provided to support conclusions, statements or connections
COMMUNICATION Conveying information Points _____	Meets professional writing standards for: • Grammar • Spelling • Appropriate use of either a formal or "patient friendly" writing style (based on the focus of the exercise).	Meets professional writing standards for: • Grammar • Spelling • Appropriate use of either a formal or "patient friendly" writing style (based on the focus of the exercise).	Errors in spelling or grammar. **OR** Writing style is too casual/conversational for professional writing. **OR** Inappropriate professional jargon is used for a patient discussion.

Total points _____ / 15 possible points

FACULTY FEEDBACK: